500

LOW GLYCEMIC INDEX
RECIPES

500
LOW GLYCEMIC INDEX RECIPES

Fight Diabetes and Heart Disease, Lose Weight,
and Have Optimum Energy with Recipes
That Let You Eat the Foods You Enjoy

DICK LOGUE

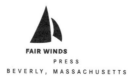

FAIR WINDS
PRESS
BEVERLY, MASSACHUSETTS

First published in the USA in 2010 by
Fair Winds Press, a member of
Quayside Publishing Group
100 Cummings Center
Suite 406-L
Beverly, MA 01915-6101
www.fairwindspress.com

16 15 14 13 12   5 6 7 8

ISBN-13: 978-1-59233-417-9
ISBN-10: 1-59233-417-2

Library of Congress Cataloging-in-Publication Data available

Cover and Book design by Fair Winds Press

Printed in the U.S.A.

*The information in this book is for educational purposes only. It is not intended to
replace the advice of a physician or medical practitioner. Please see your health care
provider before beginning any new health program.*

"To my family, who have dealt not only with the initial illness that caused me to change my diet (and theirs), but also have been my guinea pigs for any number of recipe tests. Some of them are in this book, some weren't nearly good enough."

Contents

What Is a Low-Glycemic-Index (GI) Diet?

Perhaps you've picked up this book because you've been hearing a lot lately about the glycemic index and how it can help you eat a more healthy diet. Perhaps you or someone you care about has diabetes, so things like carbohydrates, insulin production, and blood sugar levels are a special concern. Perhaps you are trying to lose weight and are confused about all the conflicting information about carbohydrates. Or perhaps you have one of my other books and are interested in what this new one had to offer. Maybe it's none of those reasons. Whatever the reason is, I can almost guarantee that there is information (and recipes!) here that will be useful to you.

I probably wouldn't have made that statement a year ago. I didn't know much about the glycemic index, other than that I thought it related to the amount of carbohydrates in food, and to be honest I wasn't very interested in it. I knew it was something that many doctors were talking about in relation to diabetic diets. But my mother had had diabetes for a number of years, and I thought from watching her and how she ate that I understood what was required to control your blood sugar level through diet. Basically she ate little or no sugar. She also was careful about not eating too many other carbohydrates, but not to an extreme. She still ate white bread with many meals as well as potatoes and other starches. This was common advice for people with diabetes when she was first diagnosed, and it worked pretty well for her. So I didn't give newer ideas much thought.

But my own doctor had been keeping a wary eye on my blood sugar levels, concerned that their slow rise from year to year and the family history of diabetes were signs that I would become diabetic myself. He suggested that I think about modifying my diet to be aware of the glycemic index values of the food I was eating as a way to help my body stabilize blood sugar levels. I wasn't really very happy with that suggestion. I already was on a low-sodium diet for congestive heart failure and about a year earlier had modified that diet to be aware of foods that could help me lower my cholesterol. It seemed like every time I had things pretty well worked out and was happy with what I could eat, it had to change because of some other factor.

But I dutifully began examining the facts about the glycemic index (often abbreviated GI) and how it related to the food we eat. I discovered that I hadn't really understood it, which didn't surprise me. However, I also discovered a lot of the foods that had been good things for fighting cholesterol were also low-GI foods. And I discovered that researchers were finding many benefits to low-GI foods beyond helping to stabilize blood sugar. And those things did surprise me. It was starting to sound like this might not be that difficult after all.

What Exactly Is the Glycemic Index?

The glycemic index does indeed relate to the carbohydrates in food. But it isn't so much a measure of the quantity of carbohydrates as their quality. Specifically it is a measure of how much the carbohydrates in foods affect your blood glucose level. Glucose is really what we are talking about when we use the term *blood sugar* as I did a few paragraphs ago. It is the most simple form of sugar, and its concentration in the blood is what we are measuring when we talk about "blood sugar levels." The digestive process converts other more complex sugars and starches, in other words carbohydrates, into glucose for use in the body. What the glycemic index measures is how quickly that process happens for different foods. High-GI foods break down quickly, causing a spike in the blood glucose level. Lower-GI foods break down more slowly but over a longer period of time, affecting blood glucose less.

The initial research on the glycemic index was done by Dr. David Jenkins and Dr. Thomas Wolever at the University of Toronto in the early 1980s. Prior to that time it was generally accepted that the diet my mother followed was the best for controlling blood sugar. It was believed that simple carbohydrates like granulated sugar broke down quickly and caused a sudden increase in blood glucose, while more complex carbohydrates like potatoes did not. Dr. Jenkins and his colleagues in Toronto tested a number of different foods, measuring the size and speed of their effect on blood glucose levels in the people eating them. He discovered that the common assumptions were not correct. In fact, some starches like potatoes, bread, and rice broke down much more quickly than the sugars in fruit and other foods.

The glycemic index for various foods was determined by testing people's blood glucose levels after they had eaten the foods. Pure glucose was assigned a value of 100, and other foods were given values based on how they raised the blood glucose level compared to glucose. Over the years a number of different studies have been done in Britain, France, Italy, Sweden, Australia, and Canada to determine the glycemic index of foods. Tables are available for over 700 different foods. While this isn't nearly every food, it does give us a good reference point for a lot of the more common foods containing carbohydrates. Foods such as meats, dairy products, and salad vegetables were not tested because they don't contain enough carbohydrates to raise the blood glucose level measurably. As expected, most foods have a GI value less than the 100 of pure glucose, although it was discovered that a few foods like jasmine rice actually affect the blood glucose level more than pure glucose. In general terms we call a food with a GI value of 55 or less low GI, 56 to 69 medium GI, and 70 or above high GI.

Why Is the Glycemic Index Important?

For most people, eating more low-GI foods is a good idea. If a person has diabetes or some other form of glucose intolerance, it means that they will not see the same kinds of spikes in blood glucose level. These spikes cause the body to produce more insulin than is really needed. That insulin level remains high after the high-GI food is no longer affecting the blood glucose level. Eating lower-GI foods causes the glucose and insulin levels to vary less over the course of the day, which stresses the body less. This is also good from a heart health standpoint. Studies have shown that high insulin levels are linked with higher blood pressure and cholesterol levels. High glucose levels also stress the cells, producing inflammatory responses that can contribute to blood clots and blockages in the arteries.

In addition, the slower digestive process for low-GI foods means that you'll feel less hungry between meals, making it easier to maintain a healthy body weight. The common belief about being hungry a few hours after eating Chinese food can actually be explained by the GI value of the rice and noodles that are often the main part of a Chinese meal. It also explains why people tend to feel so lethargic after a fast-food lunch. The glucose level goes up quickly, fueled by the high-GI foods, then falls just as quickly, leaving us suddenly tired in the middle of the afternoon.

What Is the Difference between Glycemic Index and Glycemic Load?

You may also have heard the term *glycemic load*, or GL. This measure is related to, but different from, the glycemic index. The glycemic index is measured when a person eats a standard amount of a food, usually the amount containing 100 grams of carbohydrates, and the blood glucose response is measured. This gives us a good number to use in comparing foods.

However, some researchers realized that this can be misleading because a serving of a particular food does not usually contain exactly 100 grams of carbohydrates. Researchers at Harvard University came up with a new measure called glycemic load, which took this into consideration. The glycemic load is based on the glycemic index, adjusted for the normal serving size of the food.

An example of how this works might be an apple. An apple has a GI of 38, meaning that a serving of apples containing 100 grams of carbohydrates affects blood glucose 38 percent as much as 100 grams of glucose. But an apple only contains about 15 grams of carbohydrates. So eating one apple does not really affect blood glucose as much as the GI might indicate. The GL takes this into consideration by multiplying the GI of a food times the carbohydrates per serving, then dividing by 100. So the GL of an apple is 38 × 15 / 100 or about 6.

There is still some debate about whether GI or GL is a better measure of the quality of a food. On the one hand, GL takes the actual serving size into consideration, so it gives us a better picture of the actual affect on blood glucose of a particular food. However, people on the other side of the debate point out that the GL does not accurately tell you whether a food is one of the slow-acting ones that we are trying to eat more of. A food with a GI of 80 with a small serving size would have the same GL as a food with a GI of 40, but twice as large a portion. However, the food with the 80 GI would be the kind that is quickly digested, causing more of a spike in insulin levels and leaving us feeling hungry again sooner.

What Are the Benefits of a Low-GI Diet?

To summarize, let's look at some of the major health benefits of choosing lower-GI foods.

Help Control Diabetes

This is one of the first benefits we think about with a low-GI diet. Choosing foods that are digested more slowly prevents spikes in blood glucose levels and the resulting spikes in insulin levels. Eliminating this roller-coaster effect means the body is stressed less and that you feel better because your glucose and insulin levels are more consistent. In addition, low-GI foods tend to be lower in carbohydrates overall, which is also good for a person with any form of glucose intolerance.

Lose Weight

This area has gotten a lot of interest lately. A number of diets have focused on reducing the amount of carbohydrates you eat. That is not what we are recommending when we talk about low-GI diets. We want to concentrate on the *type* of carbs you eat. A low-GI diet may indeed provide fewer overall carbs, but the big benefit comes again from the slower digestion of low-GI foods. This means that you are not as likely to be hungry again soon after eating, craving another high-GI fix to make you feel full and satisfied.

Heart Health

A low-GI diet has a number of benefits for heart health as well, some of them direct and some indirect. First of all, many of the foods we are going to be talking about on a low-GI diet are the same ones that I talked about in my *500 Low-Cholesterol Recipes* book. Whole grains, legumes, and fruits and vegetables all are low-GI foods and all can contribute to lower cholesterol levels. On a less direct basis, as mentioned before, high insulin levels such as the ones caused by a high-GI diet can also contribute to increased cholesterol levels as well as encourage the deposit of fatty acids in the arteries, contributing to increased risk of stroke and heart attack. A number of the risk factors for heart disease are the very things a low-GI diet can help with, including cholesterol level, diabetes or prediabetes, and being overweight.

How This Book Came About

Perhaps the best way to start telling you who I am is by telling you who I'm not. I'm not a doctor. I'm not a dietitian. I'm not a professional chef. What I *am* is an ordinary person just like you who has some special dietary needs. What I am going to do is give you 500 recipes I have made for myself and my family that I think will help you focus on controlling the amount and type of carbohydrates in your diet and your family's. Many of them are the kind of things people cook in their own kitchens all the time, but modified to make them healthier without losing the flavor.

I've enjoyed cooking most of my life. I guess I started in seriously about the time my mother went back to work, when I was 12 or so. In those days it was simple stuff like burgers and hot dogs and spaghetti. But the interest stayed. After I married my wife, we got pretty involved in some food-related stuff—growing vegetables in our garden, making bread and other baked goods, canning and jelly making—that kind of thing. She always said that my "mad chemist" cooking was an outgrowth of the time I spent in college as a chemistry major, and she might be right.

Some of you may already know me from my low-sodium cooking website and newsletter or from my other books focused on low-sodium, low-cholesterol, and high-fiber recipes. I started thinking about low-sodium cooking after being diagnosed with congestive heart failure in 1999. One of the first and biggest things I had to deal with was the doctor's insistence that I follow a low-sodium diet—1,200 mg a day or less. At first, like many people, I found it easiest to just avoid things that had a lot of sodium. But I was bored. And I was convinced that there had to be a way to create low-sodium versions of the food I missed. So I learned all kinds of *new* cooking ideas. I researched where to get low-sodium substitutes for the foods that I couldn't have anymore, bought cookbooks, and basically redid my whole diet.

Along the way I learned some things. And I decided to try to share this information with others who may in the same position I had been in. I started a website, www.lowsodiumcooking. com, to share recipes and information. I sent out an e-mail newsletter with recipes that now has over 17,000 subscribers. And I wrote my first book, *500 Low-Sodium Recipes.*

Along the way, I also discovered that other areas of the diet besides sodium were important. When I was told that my blood sugar levels indicated I was borderline diabetic, I became interested in the role of carbohydrates in the diet. I became more aware of the work that had been done on glycemic index and glycemic load and began incorporating these concepts into the food we prepared and ate. And I decided that another book focused on these kinds of recipes would be helpful to a lot of people.

How Is the Nutritional Information Calculated?

The nutritional information included with these recipes was calculated using the AccuChef program. It calculates the values using the latest U.S. Department of Agriculture Standard reference nutritional database. I've been using this program since I first started trying to figure out how much sodium was in the recipes I've created. It's inexpensive, easy to use, and has a number of really handy features. For instance, if I go in and change the nutrition figures for an ingredient, it remembers those figures whenever I use that ingredient. AccuChef is available online from www.accuchef.com. They offer a free-trial version if you want to try it out, and the full version costs less than $20 US.

The glycemic index values are calculated using the Glycemic Index Meal Planner software. This software is available from Glycemic Diet Software at www.glycemicdietsw.com. It is specifically designed to calculate the glycemic index and glycemic load for meals and costs $14.95 US. The software calculates both GI and GL, but it's sometimes difficult to get a definitive figure for a particular recipe or meal. As explained earlier, not all foods have been tested. The software appears to use the figures that were developed by Jennie Brand-Miller of the University of Sydney. It includes a lot of items, but for many the distinctions may be ones that we can't accurately assign to a recipe, such as where a potato was grown. It also includes a number of international foods not available to me in the United States. The tables are available on a number of websites. A particularly complete one is published by David Mendosa at www.mendosa.com/gilists.htm. Another issue in trying to come up with figures for individual recipes is that the software only allows you to choose a quantity that is ¼, ½, or some even multiple of the standard portion size. For these reasons I've decided only to publish the GI ranking low, medium, or high for these recipes. Other than a few items in the breakfast and bread section, all of the recipes fall into the low-GI range of 55 or less.

Of course that implies that these figures are estimates. Every brand of tomatoes or any other product, is a little different in nutritional content. These figures were calculated using products that I buy here in southern Maryland. If you use a different brand, your nutrition figures may be different. Use the nutritional analysis as a guideline in determining whether a recipe is right for your diet.

1

What Should I Be Eating on a Low-GI Diet?

Changing to a Lower-GI Diet

So now that we've talked about the "why?" of a low-GI diet, the next obvious question is "how?". It's really not as difficult as you may be thinking. The short answer is that you need to become more aware of the GI range of the foods you are eating. I'm not going to tell you that you should never eat another high-GI item. I know that's not realistic. What I am going to tell you is that you need to be careful about how often you eat high-GI foods and in what quantity. I'm going to give you 500 recipes to help you think about low-GI foods that you can easily incorporate in to your diet and your family's. These are generally everyday things, the kind of food that you've been eating and liking all your life. But even if you use these recipes, you also need to think about the overall GI rating of everything you eat. If you eat three or four low- to medium-GI foods in a meal, the total amount of carbohydrates and the GI rating for the entire meal will be pretty high. So you need to balance those things that have a moderate amount of carbohydrates and GI rating with some things that are at the low end of the scale.

One of the questions many people may have is the relationship of a low-GI diet to the popular low-carb diets. Plans like the Atkins diet have been popular in recent years, and some people have experienced success losing weight on them. However, there is also a high incidence of gaining weight back once you begin to ease up on the dietary restrictions. And a number of medical authorities question whether severe restriction of carbohydrates and the amount of fat many people eat to help replace the carbs is healthy over a long period of time. What we are looking for here is a diet for the rest of your life. A diet that leaves you feeling satisfied with both the quantity, and perhaps even more importantly, the taste of the foods you eat. I can tell you from personal experience that one of the things that has pleased me the most about eating a lower-GI diet was finding that the flavor of things like whole grain breads and pasta and brown rice was actually better than the bland taste of their more refined, less healthy alternatives. The changes we are talking about are not going to make you aware of the restrictions; they are going to make you aware of how good healthy food can be.

What Foods Are Low GI?

Let's get down to the real nitty-gritty of what foods you should be eating and what you should be avoiding in order to maintain a lower overall glycemic index. First let's look at some specific examples of the glycemic index of some foods, and then we'll talk about some general characteristics that tend to make a food lower or higher in GI. The values are taken from the studies done by Jennie Brand-Miller at the University of Sydney.

Some Low-GI Foods (GI less than 55) and Their Glycemic Index

Yogurt, low fat (sweetened)	14
Artichoke	15
Asparagus	15
Broccoli	15
Cauliflower	15
Celery	15
Cucumber	15
Eggplant	15
Green beans	15
Lettuce, all varieties	15
Peppers, all varieties	15
Snow peas	15
Spinach	15
Tomatoes	15

Zucchini	15
Cherries	22
Pearl barley	25
Grapefruit	25
Milk, whole	27
Kidney beans, boiled	29
Soy milk	30
Apricots (dried)	31
Milk, skim	32
Chickpeas	33
Spaghetti, whole wheat	37
Apples	38
Pears	38
Plums	39
Carrots, cooked	39
Apple juice	41
Wheat kernels	41
Black-eyed beans	41
All-Bran	42
Peaches	42
Oranges	44
Macaroni	45
Rice, instant	46
Grapes	46
Grapefruit juice	48
Multigrain bread	48
Whole grain	50
Barley, cracked	50
Yam	51
Orange juice	52
Kiwifruit	53
Bananas	54
Sweet potato	54

Oat bran	55
Rice, brown	55
Fruit cocktail	55
Spaghetti, durum wheat	55

Some Medium-GI Foods (GI between 56 and 69) and Their Glycemic Index

Muesli	56
Mangoes	56
Potato, boiled	56
Pita bread, white	57
Rice, wild	57
Apricots	57
Potato, new	57
Rice, white	58
Danish pastry	59
Pizza, cheese	60
Hamburger bun	61
Muffin (unsweetened)	62
Rye-flour bread	64
Raisins	64
Cake, tart	65
Pineapple	66
Cake, angel	67
Croissant	67
Taco shell	68
Whole-meal bread	69
Shredded Wheat	69
Potato, mashed	70

Some High-GI Foods (GI 70 and Above) and Their Glycemic Index

White bread	71
Golden Grahams	71
Puffed Wheat	74

Potato chips	75
Waffles	76
Doughnut	76
Rice Krispies	82
Cornflakes	83
Potato, baked	85
Baguette	95
Parsnips	97

Looking down this list, we can begin to make some generalizations about the kinds of foods we should and should not be eating. Let's look at a couple of categories and some recommendations about them.

Fruits and Vegetables

With a few exceptions, fruits and vegetables are good choices for low-GI eating. A few fruits like pineapple and apricots have a medium GI and potatoes have a medium to high GI, but almost all others fall in the low category.

Legumes

Kidney beans, chickpeas, lentils, and other legumes typically fall into the low-GI category. They are great choices since the amount of fiber they have helps to slow down digestion and keep you from feeling hungry for a longer period of time. They also contain high-quality, fat-free protein, packing a lot of nutrition into the number of calories they contain.

Grains and Baked Goods

Here we get into an area where being choosy really pays off. White flour and processed grain products tend to be much higher in GI than comparable whole grain products. This is for two reasons. First, highly processed grains have a significant amount of their fiber removed, increasing their GI rating and contributing to faster digestion. Secondly, they are typically ground into much finer particles. This also makes them easier to digest, meaning their carbohydrates are converted into glucose more quickly, again raising the GI number and leaving you feeling hungry again sooner. You can see this not just with white bread, but also with the more highly processed breakfast cereals.

Sweets

There aren't a lot of these on the list, but they are pretty obviously an area where you want to be extra careful. They tend to be higher in GI, giving you that quick but short-lived lift. They also tend to have fewer nutrients to offer, providing empty calories that add to your weight but not to your health. I've included some recipes for low-GI desserts that you can eat in moderation, but you should consider having an apple or a container of yogurt rather than a candy bar when you really feel the need for something sweet.

Putting It All Together

So what should we really be doing to eat a more healthy, lower-GI diet? As a starting point, let's take a quick look at the U.S. Department of Agriculture Food Guide Pyramid below. It shows their recommendation for the number of servings per day of various types of food. The areas we want to look at are the two levels at the bottom of the pyramid. The lowest level shows six to eleven servings a day of bread, cereal, rice, and pasta. The next level up shows three to five servings of vegetables and two to four servings of fruit.

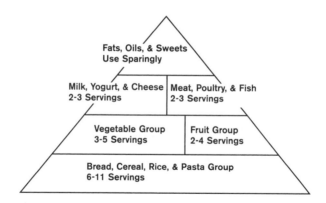

What I'm going to suggest is that we should reverse those two levels, resulting in the new pyramid shown on the next page. By doing this we've cut back in the higher-carbohydrate and -GI items and added more fruits and vegetables. I'm suggesting we set target goals of five to seven servings of vegetables, three to five servings of fruit, and limit the high-carb foods to three to eight servings. The next thing I'm going to suggest is that we try to eat foods that have gone through the least possible amount of processing. Here are a few examples:

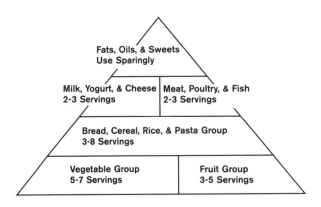

Fats, Oils, & Sweets
Use Sparingly

Milk, Yogurt, & Cheese | Meat, Poultry, & Fish
2-3 Servings | 2-3 Servings

Bread, Cereal, Rice, & Pasta Group
3-8 Servings

Vegetable Group
5-7 Servings

Fruit Group
3-5 Servings

- Choose whole grains over refined grains. Multigrain bread has a GI of 48, compared to 71 for white bread. Whole wheat spaghetti has a GI of 37, while regular durum wheat spaghetti has 55. And as I said, you'll find that whole grain products also have more flavor. It's a win-win situation.

- Choose raw fruits and vegetables over processed ones as much as possible. Raw fruit generally has more nutrients and a longer digestive cycle than canned fruit. Canned fruit has the same advantage over fruit juice. Raw vegetables are similarly better than cooked or canned ones. When you cook vegetables, steam or stir-fry them quickly until just crisp-tender to retain as much of the nutrition as possible.

Even though we're focusing here on carbohydrates and GI, be aware of other nutritional considerations. Meat does not contain enough carbohydrates to be an issue, but depending on the kind of meat and the cut it can contain a lot of saturated fat. Not only is that bad from a heart health and cholesterol standpoint, but if you're trying to maintain a healthy weight (and aren't we all), fat contains nearly twice the number of calories per gram as protein or carbs. Let's not get so focused on carbs that we don't remember the other things that make a diet healthy. In general, what many experts now think is the healthiest diet is one that is high in fiber and high in carbohydrates, but low in GI and low in fat. The bottom line in doing this is that just as all fats are not created equal and we have learned to cut down on saturated fats and trans fats, so all carbohydrates are not equal. We need to concentrate on choosing wisely. What we are looking for is not no carbs, but the right quantity of the right kind of carbs—those that are low on the glycemic index scale.

What about Artificial Sweeteners?

One question that often comes up when talking about carbohydrates is whether or not to use artificial sweeteners. Even with the newer sweeteners, which most experts feel are safe, a number of adamant people have raised questions. My personal opinion is that the closer we get to eating things that are natural and minimally processed, the better we are. But replacing sugar with a no-calorie, no-carbohydrate sweetener certainly has an appeal. In general I use natural sweeteners like sugar, brown sugar, and honey when the amount in the recipe is not a significant part of the overall nutritional values. However, I do use Splenda brand sucralose sweetener in some baked goods where sugar would represent a significant part of the calories. I've never had any problem from a recipe standpoint substituting Splenda one for one for sugar. You will find that it is called for in some of the baked goods in this book. In the end you will need to decide for yourself whether other potential issues outweigh the benefits.

Where's the Salt?

One question that may occur to some people looking over the recipes in this book is "Why is there no salt in any of the ingredient lists?" That's a fair question and deserves an answer. As I said in the introduction, I first got involved with heart-healthy cooking because my doctor put me on a low-sodium diet. It took some time and lots of experimentation, but I learned how to cook things that both taste good and are easy to prepare that are still low in sodium. Along the way we literally threw away our salt shaker. There's one shaker full of light salt, half salt and half salt substitute, on the table. My wife uses that occasionally. Two of my children have given up salt completely, not because they need to for medical reasons, but because they are convinced like I am that it's the healthy thing to do. When I started looking at creating healthy, low-glycemic-index recipes, going back to using salt wasn't even something I considered.

Most Americans get far more than the 2,400 mg of sodium a day recommended for a healthy adult. This happens without our even thinking about it. In creating these recipes, I was not as strict about the amount of sodium as I usually am. I didn't plan on people buying special sodium-free baking powder that is difficult to find except online. I didn't eliminate most cheeses except Swiss. But I also didn't add any salt. I think if you try the recipes you'll find that they taste good without it. If you are tempted to add some salt because you think it's needed, I'd suggest you check with your doctor first. I believe that most of them will agree that in the interest of total health, you are better off without the salt.

2

Sauces and Condiments

Sauces and condiments are not generally a big concern from a GI standpoint. Most contain few carbohydrates. But there are other concerns, like the amount of sodium that many contain. What I've included here are some ideas that may help you think healthy and are very low in GI. They include reduced-sodium soy and teriyaki sauces, some other sauces that you won't find on your grocer's shelves, and some condiments to go with your new healthy meals.

Dick's Reduced-Sodium Soy Sauce

Even though sodium is not a problem from a glycemic index standpoint, it is definitely connected to heart health and other medical problems. Soy sauce, even the reduced-sodium kinds, contains more sodium than many people's diet can stand. A teaspoonful often contains at least a quarter of the amount of sodium that is recommended for a healthy adult. If you have heart disease or are African American, the recommendation is even less. This sauce gives you real soy sauce flavor while holding the sodium to a level that should fit in most people's diet.

4 tablespoons (24 g) sodium-free beef bouillon

4 tablespoons (60 ml) cider vinegar

2 tablespoons (40 g) molasses

1½ cups (355 ml) water, boiling

⅛ teaspoon black pepper

⅛ teaspoon ginger

¼ teaspoon garlic powder

¼ cup (60 ml) reduced-sodium soy sauce

Combine ingredients, stirring to blend thoroughly. Pour into jars. Cover and seal tightly. This may be kept refrigerated indefinitely.

Yield: 48 servings

Each with: 10 g water; 6 calories (13% from fat, 11% from protein, 76% from carb); 0 g protein; 0 g total fat; 0 g saturated fat; 0 g monounsaturated fat; 0 g polyunsaturated fat; 1 g carb; 0 g fiber; 1 g sugar; 3 mg phosphorus; 4 mg calcium; 0 mg iron; 52 mg sodium; 19 mg potassium; 3 IU vitamin A; 0 mg vitamin C; 0 mg cholesterol

Glycemic Index: Low

Dick's Reduced-Sodium Teriyaki Sauce

The story on this recipe is the same as the soy sauce. In this case, you can sometimes find some commercial teriyaki sauces that aren't too high in sodium. But this one is much lower and to my mind tastes as good if not better.

1 cup (235 ml) Dick's Reduced-Sodium Soy Sauce (see recipe in this chapter)

1 tablespoon (15 ml) sesame oil

2 tablespoons (30 ml) mirin wine

½ cup (100 g) sugar

3 cloves garlic, crushed

2 slices gingerroot

Dash black pepper

TIP *You can substitute sherry or saki for the mirin, a sweet Japanese rice wine.*

Combine all ingredients in a saucepan and heat until sugar is dissolved. Store in the refrigerator.

Yield: 20 servings

Each with: 17 g water; 37 calories (2% from fat, 0% from protein, 98% from carb); 0 g protein; 1 g total fat; 0 g saturated fat; 0 g monounsaturated fat; 2 g polyunsaturated fat; 84 g carb; 0 g fiber; 7 g sugar; 10 mg phosphorus; 7 mg calcium; 0 mg iron; 83 mg sodium; 32 mg potassium; 5 IU vitamin A; 0 mg vitamin C; 0 mg cholesterol

Glycemic Index: Low

Chili Sauce

I've got to admit I've never been a really big fan of bottled chili sauce. The kids used it on hot dogs for a while, but I've always been a mustard and relish type of guy. Anyway, I much prefer the flavor of this chili sauce, which was adapted from a recipe from the American Heart Association to the kind found in stores. There are enough veggies in it to give it something more than a glorified ketchup taste. It keeps well in the refrigerator for weeks and you could freeze it if you wanted. The serving size for the nutritional calculation is 1 tablespoon.

1 can (14½ ounces or 410 g) no-salt-added tomatoes

1 can (8 ounces or 225 g) no-salt-added tomato sauce

½ cup (80 g) chopped onion

½ cup (100 g) sugar

½ cup (50 g) chopped celery

½ cup (75 g) chopped green pepper

1 tablespoon (15 ml) lemon juice

1 tablespoon (15 g) brown sugar

1 tablespoon (20 g) molasses

¼ teaspoon hot pepper sauce

⅛ teaspoon cloves

⅛ teaspoon cinnamon

⅛ teaspoon black pepper

⅛ teaspoon basil

⅛ teaspoon tarragon

½ cup (120 ml) cider vinegar

Combine all ingredients in a large saucepan. Bring to boil, reduce heat, and simmer uncovered 1½ hours or until mixture is reduced to half the original volume.

Yield: 48 servings

Each with: 12 calories (1% from fat, 1% from protein, 98% from carb); 0 g protein; 0 g total fat; 0 g saturated fat; 0 g monounsaturated fat; 3 g carb; 0 g fiber; 2 mg calcium; 0 mg iron; 2 mg sodium; 19 mg potassium; 12 IU vitamin A; 2 mg vitamin C; 0 mg cholesterol

Glycemic Index: Low

Spicy Barbecue Sauce

I like spicy food, but my wife doesn't. Every once in a while I'll mix up a batch of something like this sauce that has quite a nice kick to it and do dinner on separate sides of the grill. It starts with catsup, so it's really easy to make.

⅓ cups (80 ml) low-sodium catsup

¼ teaspoon cayenne pepper

½ teaspoon pepper

⅓ teaspoon garlic powder

½ teaspoon chili powder

Combine all 5 ingredients together in small bowl.

Yield: 3 servings

Each with: 19 g water; 29 calories (5% from fat, 7% from protein, 88% from carb); 1 g Protein; 0 g total fat; 0 g saturated fat; 0 g monounsaturated fat; 0 g polyunsaturated fat; 7 g carb; 0 g fiber; 6 g sugar; 12 mg phosphorous; 6 mg calcium; 0 mg iron; 10 mg sodium; 117 mg potassium; 450 IU vitamin A; 0 mg ATE vitamin E; 5 mg vitamin C; 0 mg cholesterol

Glycemic Index: Low

Sofrito

Sofrito is a Spanish condiment. It's flavorful, but not hot, and can be used to season any type of meat, sauce, rice, or soup.

½ cup (75 g) red peppers, not hot, chopped

½ cup (80 g) onions

¼ cup (15 g) fresh cilantro

½ cup (75 g) green peppers

1 cup (180 g) tomatoes

Put everything into blender and grind until finely chopped.

Yield: 20 servings

Each with: 18 g water; 5 calories (8% from fat, 13% from protein, 79% from carb); 0 g Protein; 0 g total fat; 0 g saturated fat; 0 g monounsaturated fat; 0 g polyunsaturated fat; 1 g carb; 0 g fiber; 0 g sugar; 5 mg phosphorous; 2 mg calcium; 0 mg iron; 1 mg sodium; 40 mg potassium; 212 IU vitamin A; 0 mg ATE vitamin E; 10 mg vitamin C; 0 mg cholesterol

Glycemic Index: Low

Cranberry Catsup

I know it sounds funny, but cranberry catsup is a good condiment served with any kind of poultry and a wonderful spread on cold turkey sandwiches as well as on hot turkey burgers.

½ pound (225 g) raw cranberries

½ cup (80 g) onion, chopped

¼ cup (60 ml) water

¼ cup (60 ml) apple juice concentrate unsweetened

¼ cup (60 ml) white vinegar

⅛ teaspoon cloves

½ teaspoon ground cinnamon

½ teaspoon ground allspice

⅛ teaspoon white pepper

Place cranberries and onions in small saucepan with the water and cook until tender. Stir every few minutes to keep it from burning. Pour into food processor with metal blade and blend until smooth. Place mixture back in saucepan and add remaining ingredients. Cook until thick, stirring while cooking, approximately 10 minutes.

Yield: 12 servings

Each with: 35 g water; 21 calories (3% from fat, 3% from protein, 94% from carb); 0 g Protein; 0 g total fat; 0 g saturated fat; 0 g monounsaturated fat; 0 g polyunsaturated fat; 5 g carb; 1 g fiber; 3 g sugar; 6 mg phosphorous; 6 mg calcium; 0 mg iron; 2 mg sodium; 52 mg potassium; 12 IU vitamin A; 0 mg ATE vitamin E; 7 mg vitamin C; 0 mg cholesterol

Glycemic Index: Low

Hollandaise Sauce

There is no way this can be considered good for you. But our version has less cholesterol and less fat than the traditional ones and no carbs. So maybe you'll want to splurge once a year for the first batch of fresh asparagus. This easy version can also be made in a blender.

¼ cup (60 ml) white vinegar

1 bay leaf

6 peppercorns

3 eggs

½ cup (112 g) unsalted butter, melted

Place the vinegar and spices in a small pan and boil until reduced to about a tablespoon of liquid. Remove spices and add vinegar to food processor container with eggs. Cover and turn on to high. Slowly add butter through feeder tube. Serve while warm.

Yield: 4 servings

Each with: 58 g water; 246 calories (90% from fat, 10% from protein, 1% from carb); 6 g protein; 25 g total fat; 15 g saturated fat; 6 g monounsaturated fat; 2 g polyunsaturated fat; 0 g carb; 0 g fiber; 0 g sugar; 65 mg phosphorus; 33 mg calcium; 1 mg iron; 87 mg sodium; 173 mg potassium; 879 IU vitamin A; 0 mg vitamin C; 61 mg cholesterol

Glycemic Index: Low

Horseradish Mustard Cream Sauce

This is a really simple sauce, but one that is great on roast beef (or a leftover roast beef sandwich). It's also good on ham, egg, or vegetable dishes.

½ cup (120 g) prepared horseradish, drained

½ teaspoon dry mustard

½ cup (120 ml) heavy cream, whipped

Combine horseradish and dry mustard. Let stand in refrigerator until meal time. Just before serving, whip cream and fold in horseradish mixture. Serve at once.

Yield: 8 servings

Each with: 17 g water; 33 calories (74% from fat, 4% from protein, 22% from carb); 0 g Protein; 3 g total fat; 2 g saturated fat; 1 g monounsaturated fat; 0 g polyunsaturated fat; 2 g carb; 0 g fiber; 1 g sugar; 9 mg phosphorous; 13 mg calcium; 0 mg iron; 50 mg sodium; 43 mg potassium; 110 IU vitamin A; 30 mg ATE vitamin E; 4 mg vitamin C; 10 mg cholesterol

Glycemic Index: Low

Hamburger Sauce

This is better than McDonald's thousand island dressing—Whoops, I mean secret sauce.

1 cup (240 ml) mayonnaise

⅓ cup (80 ml) French dressing

¼ cup (60 g) sweet pickle relish

1 teaspoon dry onion

1 tablespoon (13 g) sugar

1 teaspoon mustard

¼ teaspoon pepper

Mix everything together and store in the refrigerator until ready to use.

Yield: 16 servings

Each with: 7 g water; 131 calories (89% from fat, 1% from protein, 11% from carb); 0 g Protein; 13 g total fat; 2 g saturated fat; 3 g monounsaturated fat; 7 g polyunsaturated fat; 4 g carb; 0 g fiber; 2 g sugar; 5 mg phosphorous; 4 mg calcium; 0 mg iron; 153 mg sodium; 10 mg potassium; 96 IU vitamin A; 11 mg ATE vitamin E; 0 mg vitamin C; 5 mg cholesterol

Glycemic Index: Low

Quick Black Bean Salsa

Combine canned beans and canned salsa with some extra spices for a quick dip that's more than the sum of its parts.

1 cup (240 g) canned black beans, drained

12 ounces (340 g) salsa

¼ cup (4 g) chopped fresh cilantro

¼ teaspoon cumin

2 tablespoons (30 ml) lime juice

Roughly chop beans in food processor. Do not puree them. Stir in remaining ingredients. Serve immediately or refrigerate overnight. Serve with corn chips or raw vegetables.

Yield: 20 servings

Each with: 23 g water; 17 calories (4% from fat, 23% from protein, 73% from carb); 1 g protein; 0 g total fat; 0 g saturated fat; 0 g monounsaturated fat; 0 g polyunsaturated fat; 3 g carb; 1 g fiber; 1 g sugar; 18 mg phosphorus; 8 mg calcium; 0 mg iron; 40 mg sodium; 86 mg potassium; 87 IU vitamin A; 1 mg vitamin C; 0 mg cholesterol

Glycemic Index: Low

Black Bean Relish

This relish is a good way to use up some leftover black beans. It's not very spicy, but you can adjust the Tabasco to your own taste. It's good mixed into a little rice or on a salad.

⅔ cup (115 g) black beans, cooked until tender and drained

½ cup (8 g) cilantro, chopped

½ cup (82 g) corn

⅓ cup (50 g) red bell peppers, seeded and diced

2 tablespoons (30 ml) olive oil

3 tablespoons (45 ml) lime juice

2 dashes Tabasco sauce (or to taste)

¼ teaspoon pepper

In a medium bowl, place all of the ingredients and stir them together. Let the relish sit for 1 hour in the refrigerator before serving it.

Yield: 8 servings

Each with: 31 g water; 61 calories (50% from fat, 11% from protein, 40% from carb); 2 g Protein; 4 g total fat; 0 g saturated fat; 2 g monounsaturated fat; 0 g polyunsaturated fat; 6 g carb; 2 g fiber; 1 g sugar; 30 mg phosphorous; 7 mg calcium; 0 mg iron; 3 mg sodium; 101 mg potassium; 378 IU vitamin A; 0 mg ATE vitamin E; 11 mg vitamin C; 0 mg cholesterol

Glycemic Index: Low

Fresh Tomato Relish

This is a simple relish. It's good on sandwiches, salads, or as a fresh pasta sauce.

½ cup (80 g) onion, cut into pieces

½ cup (75 g) green bell pepper, cut into pieces

¼ cup (60 ml) vinegar

2 teaspoons (8.4 g) sugar

1 teaspoon celery seed

½ teaspoon salt

1 dash pepper

1 cup (180 g) tomatoes, cut up

Put the onion, green pepper, vinegar, sugar, celery seed, salt, and pepper in a blender container and blend until the pepper and onion are coarsely chopped. Add the tomatoes and blend until coarsely chopped. Chill and drain before serving.

Yield: 8 servings

Each with: 42 g water; 16 calories (8% from fat, 9% from protein, 82% from carb); 0 g Protein; 0 g total fat; 0 g saturated fat; 0 g monounsaturated fat; 0 g polyunsaturated fat; 3 g carb; 1 g fiber; 2 g sugar; 11 mg phosphorous; 10 mg calcium; 0 mg iron; 151 mg sodium; 82 mg potassium; 151 IU vitamin A; 0 mg ATE vitamin E; 13 mg vitamin C; 0 mg cholesterol

Glycemic Index: Low

Tomato Chutney

This makes a great-tasting chutney. It's pretty spicy, so you may want to adjust the number of jalapeños.

1 cup (235 ml) cider vinegar

½ cup (12 g) sugar substitute, such as Splenda

1½ pounds (680 g) cherry tomatoes, quartered

2 cups (320 g) chopped onion

4 jalapeño peppers, chopped

2 teaspoons (4 g) ginger

2 cloves garlic, minced

1 teaspoon cumin

½ teaspoon cinnamon

½ cup (75 g) golden raisins

Combine vinegar and sugar in nonaluminum saucepan. Bring to a boil, stirring to dissolve sugar. Add remaining ingredients. Bring to a boil, reduce heat, and simmer 30 to 45 minutes, or until most of the liquid has cooked off. Stir often to prevent sticking. Refrigerate for up to 2 weeks or separate into containers and freeze.

Yield: 16 servings

Each with: 37 g water; 63 calories (3% from fat, 6% from protein, 91% from carb); 1 g protein; 0 g total fat; 0 g saturated fat; 0 g monounsaturated fat; 0 g polyunsaturated fat; 15 g carb; 1 g fiber; 10 g sugar; 23 mg phosphorus; 17 mg calcium; 1 mg iron; 3 mg sodium; 230 mg potassium; 272 IU vitamin A; 11 mg vitamin C; 0 mg cholesterol

Glycemic Index: Low

Sun-Dried Tomato Pesto

Serve this as a spread or a dip. It's every bit as good with vegetables as with higher-carbohydrate dippers.

¼ cup (25 g) walnuts

½ cup (55 g) sun-dried tomatoes, oil-packed

¼ cup (25 g) grated Parmesan cheese

1 clove garlic

2 teaspoons (15 ml) olive oil

Black pepper, to taste

Preheat the oven to 375°F (190°C, gas mark 5). Toast the nuts for 7 to 8 minutes; cool. Drain the oil from the tomatoes. In a food processor, combine everything. Process until smooth.

Yield: 8 servings

Each with: 5 g water; 80 calories (79% from fat, 11% from protein, 10% from carb); 2 g protein; 7 g total fat; 1 g saturated fat; 4 g monounsaturated fat; 2 g polyunsaturated fat; 2 g carb; 1 g fiber; 0 g sugar; 38 mg calcium; 0 mg iron; 61 mg sodium; 132 mg potassium; 106 IU vitamin A; 7 mg vitamin C; 2 mg cholesterol

Glycemic Index: Low

Spinach Pesto Sauce

This is a delicious variation on pesto. It's a perfect sauce for whole wheat pasta.

10 ounces (280 g) frozen spinach, thawed and drained

½ teaspoon crushed garlic

¼ cup (25 g) grated Parmesan cheese

¼ cup (27 g) almonds

½ cup (30 g) fresh parsley

½ cup (120 ml) olive oil

¼ teaspoon black pepper, fresh ground

Process all the ingredients in food processor or blender. Serve over pasta.

Yield: 4 servings

Each with: 72 g water; 345 calories (85% from fat, 8% from protein, 7% from carb); 7 g protein; 34 g total fat; 5 g saturated fat; 23 g monounsaturated fat; 4 g polyunsaturated fat; 6 g carb; 4 g fiber; 1 g sugar; 130 mg phosphorus; 209 mg calcium; 2 mg iron; 172 mg sodium; 329 mg potassium; 9,209 IU vitamin A; 12 mg vitamin C; 6 mg cholesterol

Glycemic Index: Low

Broccoli Pesto

Pesto is an easy way to create a pasta sauce without having to cook and simmer. Just mix it in with warm pasta and you're done. Basil is the usual main ingredient, but here broccoli makes a nice variation.

¼ pound (113 g) broccoli florets

¼ cup (15 g) fresh parsley, chopped

⅛ teaspoon pepper

2 cloves garlic, minced

2 tablespoons (16 g) walnuts, chopped

2 tablespoons (12.5 g) Romano cheese, grated

2 tablespoons (30 ml) extra virgin olive oil

In a blender or a food processor fitted with the metal blade, place all ingredients and process to a puree.

Yield: 6 servings

Each with: 21 g water; 80 calories (79% from fat, 13% from protein, 8% from carb); 3 g Protein; 7 g total fat; 2 g saturated fat; 4 g monounsaturated fat; 1 g polyunsaturated fat; 2 g carb; 0 g fiber; 0 g sugar; 63 mg phosphorous; 64 mg calcium; 0 mg iron; 63 mg sodium; 93 mg potassium; 800 IU vitamin A; 4 mg ATE vitamin E; 21 mg vitamin C; 5 mg cholesterol

Glycemic Index: Low

Cilantro Pesto

Yes, I believe I did mention that I like pesto. This one features cilantro, which makes it good with Latin foods as well as Italian.

1½ cup (24 g) fresh cilantro, firm packed

½ cup (30 g) parsley, firmly packed

½ cup (50 g) parmesan cheese

½ cup (120 ml) vegetable oil

¼ teaspoon salt

3 cloves garlic

¼ cup (35 g) pine nuts

Place all ingredients in food processor work bowl fitted with steel blade or in a blender container; cover and process until well blended.

Yield: 4 servings

(continued on page 40)

Each with: 25 g water; 358 calories (90% from fat, 7% from protein, 3% from carb); 7 g Protein; 37 g total fat; 6 g saturated fat; 10 g monounsaturated fat; 18 g polyunsaturated fat; 3 g carb; 1 g fiber; 0 g sugar; 153 mg phosphorous; 162 mg calcium; 1 mg iron; 352 mg sodium; 196 mg potassium; 1747 IU vitamin A; 15 mg ATE vitamin E; 16 mg vitamin C; 11 mg cholesterol

Glycemic Index: Low

Baked Potato Topping

This is sort of like a baked potato bar all in one bowl. You can also use it over other vegetables. Feel free to add a little shredded cheese if you like.

1 cup (230 g) plain fat-free yogurt

½ teaspoon dill weed

⅛ teaspoon pepper

1½ teaspoons dried chives

2 teaspoons (5 g) imitation bacon bits

Combine all ingredients and mix well. Chill.

Yield: 8 servings

Each with: 26 g water; 20 calories (8% from fat, 40% from protein, 51% from carb); 2 g Protein; 0 g total fat; 0 g saturated fat; 0 g monounsaturated fat; 0 g polyunsaturated fat; 3 g carb; 0 g fiber; 2 g sugar; 49 mg phosphorous; 63 mg calcium; 0 mg iron; 38 mg sodium; 82 mg potassium; 16 IU vitamin A; 1 mg ATE vitamin E; 0 mg vitamin C; 1 mg cholesterol

Glycemic Index: Low

Roasted Garlic

Roasted garlic seems to be everywhere these days, from packaged mixes to restaurant menus. It adds a mild garlic flavor without being overpowering. And it's easy to make at home, even without one of the clay garlic roasters that you'll see advertised.

1 whole garlic pod
1 tablespoon (15 ml) olive oil

Hold pod of garlic on the side, take a sharp knife, and cut the pod about ¼ inch (½ cm) from the top all the way across, exposing the raw garlic cloves. Place on a baking sheet covered with aluminum foil. Pour and rub olive oil into the top of the garlic. Bake in a 325°F (170°C, gas mark 3) oven for about 45 minutes to an hour or until garlic is soft, remove, and let cool. Separate each garlic clove from the pod and pinch at the stem end to remove the garlic paste. Cover and refrigerate.

Yield: 8 servings

Each with: 0 g water; 15 calories (96% from fat, 1% from protein, 3% from carb); 0 g protein; 2 g total fat; 0 g saturated fat; 1 g monounsaturated fat; 0 g polyunsaturated fat; 0 g carb; 0 g fiber; 0 g sugar; 1 mg calcium; 0 mg iron; 0 mg sodium; 1 mg potassium; 0 IU vitamin A; 0 mg vitamin C; 0 mg cholesterol

Glycemic Index: Low

Roasted Peppers

Traditional Italian roasted peppers are made with a variety of pepper that isn't typically grown in the United States. I planted some this year in the garden, a variety named Carmen from Burpee Seeds, and they have done marvelously, growing lots of long red peppers. So I started looking for information on how to roast them and preserve them. Several websites suggested that they can be frozen, so that's what I've done. I haven't tried any of the frozen ones yet, but the fresh ones were great, much better than the canned ones. I also did some regular bell peppers and they worked just as well, so don't worry if you can't find the Italian ones.

6 red peppers

Preheat oven to 400°F (200°C, gas mark 6). Cover a baking sheet with foil. Lay the peppers on the sheet and place in the oven. Roast for 30 to 40 minutes until skin has begun to blacken and loosen from the flesh, turning every 10 minutes. Remove from oven and fold foil over peppers and seal, forming a packet. Allow to steam in the foil for 15 minutes. Remove from foil and allow to cool until they can be handled. Peel off skin, remove stem, cut open, and remove seeds. Store in the refrigerator for up to a week or freeze.

Yield: 12 servings

Each with: 69 g water; 19 calories (9% from fat, 13% from protein, 78% from carb); 1 g protein; 0 g total fat; 0 g saturated fat; 0 g monounsaturated fat; 0 g polyunsaturated fat; 4 g carb; 1 g fiber; 3 g sugar; 5 mg calcium; 0 mg iron; 1 mg sodium; 157 mg potassium; 2,333 IU vitamin A; 142 mg vitamin C; 0 mg cholesterol

Glycemic Index: Low

Pickled Banana Peppers

When the banana peppers in the garden have finally started to produce in quantity or you can get a good deal at the farmer's market, this is a good use for them. These make a nice addition to a sandwich or sub.

2 cups (248 g) banana peppers, sliced in thin rings
¾ cup (175 ml) white vinegar
½ cup (120 ml) water

2 tablespoons (26 g) sugar

1 tablespoon (3 g) mixed pickling spice

Tie spices in cheesecloth. Place ingredients in a small saucepan, bring to a boil, reduce heat, and simmer until peppers begin to soften. Cool, seal in a glass jar, and store in the refrigerator.

Yield: 16 servings

Each with: 12 calories (5% from fat, 7% from protein, 88% from carb); 0 g protein; 0 g total fat; 0 g saturated fat; 0 g monounsaturated fat; 3 g carb; 1 g fiber; 3 mg calcium; 0 mg iron; 2 mg sodium; 51 mg potassium; 53 IU vitamin A; 13 mg vitamin C; 0 mg cholesterol

Glycemic Index: Low

Pickled Cucumbers and Peppers

Scott sent along this recipe that he made for Thanksgiving. He reports that they came out very crunchy and tasted like a cross between a sweet and a dill pickle.

4 cucumbers, sliced

3 green bell peppers, sliced

1 quart (945 ml) cider vinegar

1 quart (945 ml) water

¼ cup (6 g) sugar substitute, such as Splenda

Slice cucumbers and peppers into thin slices and submerge in vinegar for 2 days. Pour off vinegar and rinse once with clean water, followed by further soaking for 2 days in solution of water and Splenda. Drain and serve.

Yield: 14 servings

Each with: 244 g water; 40 calories (3% from fat, 7% from protein, 90% from carb); 1 g protein; 0 g total fat; 0 g saturated fat; 0 g monounsaturated fat; 0 g polyunsaturated fat; 11 g carb; 1 g fiber; 6 g sugar; 22 mg calcium; 1 mg iron; 5 mg sodium; 251 mg potassium; 208 IU vitamin A; 28 mg vitamin C; 0 mg cholesterol

Glycemic Index: Low

3

Appetizers, Snacks, and Party Foods

When many people think of snacks, the first thing they think of is chips and crackers, which are not good GI choices. Instead, use the recipes in this chapter to think about veggies, bean dips, and high-protein snacks. Many of these are fancy enough and tasty enough to serve at any party. By why wait? They are also easy enough to make for everyday use.

Garlic Shrimp

These shrimp make a fancy appetizer or party food. They have just enough spiciness to be interesting.

1¾ pounds (800 g) shrimp, large

2 tablespoons (28 g) unsalted butter

1 tablespoon (15 ml) olive oil

1 tablespoon (10 g) garlic, finely minced

2 tablespoons (20 g) shallots, finely minced

¼ teaspoon (30 ml) black pepper, freshly ground

2 tablespoons (30 ml) lemon juice

2 tablespoons (6 g) fresh dill, finely chopped

Peel and devein shrimp. In a large skillet over low heat, melt butter with olive oil. Add garlic and shallots and sauté for 2 minutes without browning. Add shrimp, increase heat slightly, and cook shrimp for 3 minutes or until just done to taste. Add pepper to taste and toss well. Remove to a bowl, scraping in all the sauce. Add lemon juice and dill; toss together well. Cover and refrigerate 3 to 4 hours before serving. Serve on the ends of bamboo skewers as an appetizer.

Yield: 10 servings

Each with: 66 g water; 122 calories (38% from fat, 55% from protein, 7% from carb); 16 g Protein; 5 g total fat; 2 g saturated fat; 2 g monounsaturated fat; 1 g polyunsaturated fat; 2 g carb; 0 g fiber; 0 g sugar; 170 mg phosphorous; 56 mg calcium; 2 mg iron; 120 mg sodium; 183 mg potassium; 275 IU vitamin A; 62 mg ATE vitamin E; 4 mg vitamin C; 127 mg cholesterol

Glycemic Index: Low

Teriyaki Chicken Nibbles

These tasty little chicken fingers are always a hit as an appetizer or buffet item. The Asian flavor is a surprise, since they don't look any different from ordinary chicken fingers.

½ cup (120 ml) water

¾ cup (175 g) Dick's Reduced-Sodium Soy Sauce (see chapter 2)

¼ teaspoon garlic powder

1 teaspoon sugar

½ teaspoon ginger

1 pound (455 g) boneless skinless chicken breast

1½ cups (175 g) bread crumbs

TIP *The Asian dipping sauce in this chapter is great with these.*

Combine water, soy sauce, garlic powder, and ginger. Cut chicken into pieces approximately 2 x 1 x ½ inch (5 x 2½ x 1¼ cm). Marinate in soy sauce mixture for 2 hours. Drain. Coat pieces with bread crumbs. Deep fat fry in vegetable oil at 375°F (190°C) for about 1 minute. Drain on absorbent towels.

Yield: 6 servings

Each with: 78 g water; 193 calories (11% from fat, 45% from protein, 43% from carb); 21 g Protein; 2 g total fat; 1 g saturated fat; 1 g monounsaturated fat; 1 g polyunsaturated fat; 20 g carb; 1 g fiber; 2 g sugar; 193 mg phosphorous; 59 mg calcium; 2 mg iron; 50 mg sodium; 249 mg potassium; 16 IU vitamin A; 5 mg ATE vitamin E; 1 mg vitamin C; 44 mg cholesterol

Glycemic Index: Low

Japanese Chicken Wings

If you are looking for something different from Buffalo wings, try these tasty Asian flavored ones.

1 pound (455 g) chicken wings

⅓ cup (80 ml) sake or sherry

3 tablespoons (45 ml) Dick's Reduced-Sodium Soy Sauce (see chapter 2)

1 teaspoon gingerroot, grated

¼ cup (32 g) cornstarch

Cut chicken wings at joints. Discard the wing tips. In a bowl, combine sake or sherry, soy sauce, and gingerroot to make a marinade. Place chicken in a resealable plastic bag. Pour marinade over the chicken in the bag. Close the bag. Marinate in the refrigerator several hours or overnight, turning occasionally. Drain chicken; pat it dry with paper towels. Coat chicken wings with cornstarch. Fry, 3 or 4 pieces at a time, in deep hot fat (365°F[185°C]) for about 5 minutes. Drain on paper towels.

Yield: 4 servings

Each with: 86 g water; 174 calories (22% from fat, 60% from protein, 18% from carb); 25 g Protein; 4 g total fat; 1 g saturated fat; 1 g monounsaturated fat; 1 g polyunsaturated fat; 7 g carb; 0 g fiber; 0 g sugar; 177 mg phosphorous; 15 mg calcium; 1 mg iron; 93 mg sodium; 222 mg potassium; 67 IU vitamin A; 20 mg ATE vitamin E; 1 mg vitamin C; 65 mg cholesterol

Glycemic Index: Low

Southwestern Chicken Wings

This is a southwestern-flavored chicken wing recipe. It's not as hot as a typical Buffalo wing but still has plenty of spice and flavor.

½ cup (120 ml) lime juice

½ teaspoon garlic powder

½ teaspoon ginger

2 jalapeño peppers, seeded and chopped

12 chicken wings

Combine lime juice, garlic, ginger, and peppers in a glass bowl. Cut off chicken wing tips and discard. Cut wing at joint. Add to bowl and toss to coat. Cover and refrigerate at least 1 hour, turning occasionally. Remove from refrigerator and place in roasting pan. Cook in oven heated to 350°F (180°C, gas mark 4) until done, about 30 to 40 minutes, basting occasionally with any remaining sauce.

Yield: 4 servings

Each with: 59 g water; 90 calories (32% from fat, 54% from protein, 14% from carb); 12 g protein; 3 g total fat; 1 g saturated fat; 1 g monounsaturated fat; 1 g polyunsaturated fat; 3 g carb; 0 g fiber; 1 g sugar; 73 mg phosphorus; 11 mg calcium; 1 mg iron; 37 mg sodium; 137 mg potassium; 95 IU vitamin A; 12 mg vitamin C; 33 mg cholesterol

Glycemic Index: Low

Greek Chicken Drumettes

Here's one more chicken wing appetizer for you. My daughter made this one for her friends while they were watching the Super Bowl.

12 chicken wings

3 tablespoons (45 ml) lemon juice

2 tablespoons (30 ml) olive oil

2 tablespoons (40 g) honey

1 teaspoon oregano

1 garlic clove, minced

Separate chicken wings into sections. Discard wing tips. Combine all ingredients except chicken in a large resealable plastic bag. Mix well. Add chicken, seal, and turn to coat. Refrigerate 8 hours or overnight. Remove chicken from marinade and place in baking pan. Bake at 400°F (200°C, gas mark 6) for 30 to 40 minutes until golden brown.

Yield: 8 servings

Each with: 18 g water; 87 calories (51% from fat, 27% from protein, 22% from carb); 6 g protein; 5 g total fat; 1 g saturated fat; 3 g monounsaturated fat; 1 g polyunsaturated fat; 5 g carb; 0 g fiber; 4 g sugar; 33 mg phosphorus; 6 mg calcium; 0 mg iron; 18 mg sodium; 53 mg potassium; 22 IU vitamin A; 3 mg vitamin C; 17 mg cholesterol

Glycemic Index: Low

Carnitas Bites

Carnitas, flavorful pork that has been cooked and then crisped in the oven, is one of my favorite Mexican meals. Here a skillet version makes a great appetizer or snack.

1½ pounds (680 g) pork loin, cut into 1-inch (2½ cm) cubes.

2 tablespoons (28 g) brown sugar, packed

1 tablespoon (15 ml) tequila

1 tablespoon (15 ml) molasses

¼ teaspoon black pepper

2 cloves garlic, finely chopped

⅓ cup (80 g) water

¼ cup (25 g) green onion with top, sliced

Place pork cubes in single layer in 10-inch (25 cm) skillet. Top with remaining ingredients except green onion. Heat to boiling. Reduce heat and simmer uncovered, stirring occasionally, until the water has evaporated and the pork is slightly caramelized, about 35 minutes. Sprinkle with green onion and serve with wooden picks.

Yield: 10 servings

Each with: 59 g water; 107 calories (26% from fat, 57% from protein, 17% from carb); 14 g Protein; 3 g total fat; 1 g saturated fat; 1 g monounsaturated fat; 0 g polyunsaturated fat; 4 g carb; 0 g fiber; 4 g sugar; 150 mg phosphorous; 16 mg calcium; 1 mg iron; 37 mg sodium; 293 mg potassium; 5 IU vitamin A; 1 mg ATE vitamin E; 1 mg vitamin C; 43 mg cholesterol

Glycemic Index: Low

Scotch Eggs

These are a classic finger food. They can be served whole, halved, or quartered.

1½ pounds (675 g) sausage

12 eggs, hard cooked and peeled

1 egg, beaten

½ cup (60 g) dry bread crumbs

Preheat oven to 450°F (230°C, or gas mark 8). Divide sausage into 12 equal portions; shape into patties. Wrap each sausage patty completely around 1 hard cooked egg, pressing edges together to seal. Dip sausage wrapped eggs in beaten egg; roll in bread crumbs until completely coated. Place in ungreased 15 x 10-inch (38 x 25 cm) jelly roll pan. Bake at 450°F (230°C, or gas mark 8) for 30 minutes or until meat is thoroughly browned and cooked.

Yield: 12 servings

Each with: 73 g water; 300 calories (71% from fat, 23% from protein, 6% from carb); 17 g Protein; 24 g total fat; 8 g saturated fat; 11 g monounsaturated fat; 3 g polyunsaturated fat; 4 g carb; 0 g fiber; 1 g sugar; 212 mg phosphorous; 49 mg calcium; 2 mg iron; 560 mg sodium; 224 mg potassium; 301 IU vitamin A; 85 mg ATE vitamin E; 0 mg vitamin C; 298 mg cholesterol

Glycemic Index: Low

Tortilla Roll-Ups

These are tasty little tortilla snacks with just enough heat to be interesting.

8 ounces (225 g) cream cheese

4 ounces (115 g) black olives, chopped

4 ounces (115 g) diced green chiles

¼ teaspoon Tabasco sauce

8 whole wheat tortillas

Cream together cream cheese, olives, chiles, and Tabasco sauce. Spread approximately
2 tablespoons onto a tortilla, roll jelly-roll fashion, roll in plastic wrap, and chill. Before serving,
unwrap and cut into ¾-inch-wide (2 cm wide) pieces.

Yield: 16 servings

Each with: 25 g water; 105 calories (59% from fat, 9% from protein, 32% from carb); 2 g protein; 7 g total
fat; 3 g saturated fat; 3 g monounsaturated fat; 0 g polyunsaturated fat; 9 g carb; 2 g fiber; 0 g sugar; 34 mg
phosphorus; 37 mg calcium; 1 mg iron; 200 mg sodium; 41 mg potassium; 221 IU vitamin A; 0 mg vitamin C;
16 mg cholesterol

Glycemic Index: Low

Ranch Pinwheels

These little pinwheels make not only a good looking appetizer but a great tasting one.

8 ounces (225 g) cream cheese, softened

1 package ranch dressing mix

¼ cup (25 g) green onions, minced

2 flour tortillas, 12-inch (30 cm)

¼ cup (38 g) red bell peppers, diced

¼ cup (25 g) celery, diced

2 tablespoons (12.5 g) black olives, drained

Mix first 3 ingredients. Spread on tortillas. Sprinkle on remaining ingredients. Roll and wrap tightly in plastic wrap. Chill at least 2 hours. Cut into slices of about 1 inch (2½ cm).

Yield: 12 servings

Each with: 20 g water; 85 calories (74% from fat, 9% from protein, 17% from carb); 2 g Protein; 7 g total fat; 4 g saturated fat; 2 g monounsaturated fat; 0 g polyunsaturated fat; 4 g carb; 0 g fiber; 0 g sugar; 28 mg phosphorous; 25 mg calcium; 0 mg iron; 102 mg sodium; 48 mg potassium; 387 IU vitamin A; 68 mg ATE vitamin E; 4 mg vitamin C; 21 mg cholesterol

Glycemic Index: Low

Cheese Quesadillas

Quesadillas make a quick and easy appetizer or snack. They can also be grilled on a contact grill like the George Foreman models.

2 flour tortillas, 7-inch (18 cm))

¼ cup (25 g) black olives, drained

¼ cup (25 g) Monterey jack cheese shredded

2 tablespoons (32 g) salsa

¼ cup (4 g) fresh cilantro

Preheat oven to 425°F (220°C, or gas mark 7). Place tortilla flat on baking sheet. Combine olives, cheese and sauce in bowl. Add cilantro to cheese mixture. Evenly spread mixture over tortilla. Top with other tortilla; pressing down firmly. Bake 8–10 minutes or until tops are lightly browned. Remove from oven and cool 5 minutes. Cut quesadilla into 8 wedges.

Yield: 8 servings

Each with: 12 g water; 45 calories (45% from fat, 15% from protein, 39% from carb); 2 g Protein; 2 g total fat; 1 g saturated fat; 1 g monounsaturated fat; 0 g polyunsaturated fat; 4 g carb; 0 g fiber; 0 g sugar; 30 mg phosphorous; 46 mg calcium; 0 mg iron; 117 mg sodium; 35 mg potassium; 149 IU vitamin A; 8 mg ATE vitamin E; 1 mg vitamin C; 4 mg cholesterol

Glycemic Index: Low

Chili Tortilla Chips

Make lower fat and lower carbohydrate tortilla chips by baking flour tortilla wedges in the oven. You can vary the spices to suit your own taste. If you like spicy, add a little cayenne pepper. We prefer them with chili powder and cumin.

6 flour tortillas, 7-inch (18 cm)

2 tablespoons (15 g) chili powder

Preheat oven to 350°F (180°C, or gas mark 4). Lightly spray tortillas with nonstick cooking spray; sprinkle with chili powder. Turn tortillas over; repeat. Cut each tortilla into 8 wedges; place on cookie sheet. Bake 8 to 10 minutes until crisp and lightly browned.

Yield: 12 servings

Each with: 5 g water; 51 calories (24% from fat, 11% from protein, 65% from carb); 1 g Protein; 1 g total fat; 0 g saturated fat; 1 g monounsaturated fat; 0 g polyunsaturated fat; 8 g carb; 1 g fiber; 0 g sugar; 22 mg phosphorous; 23 mg calcium; 1 mg iron; 108 mg sodium; 47 mg potassium; 371 IU vitamin A; 0 mg ATE vitamin E; 1 mg vitamin C; 0 mg cholesterol

Glycemic Index: Low

Chicken Wontons

These tasty little chicken snacks are actually easier to make than they sound, and they are always a big hit.

8 ounces (225 g) ground chicken

½ cup (55 g) carrots, shredded

¼ cup (25 g) celery, finely chopped

1 tablespoon (15 g) Dick's Reduced-Sodium Soy Sauce

1 tablespoon (15 ml) sherry

2 teaspoons (5 g) cornstarch

2 teaspoons (4 g) ginger root

8 ounces (225 g) wonton wrappers

2 tablespoons (28 g) unsalted butter, melted

TIP *Serve these with plum or sweet and sour sauce or the Asian dipping sauce in this chapter.*

In a medium skillet cook and stir ground chicken until no pink remains; drain. Stir in carrots, celery, soy sauce, sherry, cornstarch, and ginger root; mix well. Spoon 1 rounded teaspoon of the filling atop a wonton wrapper. Lightly brush edges with water. To shape each wonton, carefully bring 2 opposite points of the square wrapper up over the filling and pinch together in the center. Carefully bring the 2 remaining opposite points to the center and pinch together. Pinch together edges to seal. Place wontons on a greased baking sheet. Brush the wontons with melted butter. Bake in a 375°F (190°C, or gas mark 5) oven for 8-10 minutes or until lightly brown and crisp.

Yield: 25 servings

Each with: 13 g water; 48 calories (23% from fat, 26% from protein, 51% from carb); 3 g Protein; 1 g total fat; 1 g saturated fat; 0 g monounsaturated fat; 0 g polyunsaturated fat; 6 g carb; 0 g fiber; 0 g sugar; 27 mg phosphorous; 7 mg calcium; 0 mg iron; 61 mg sodium; 43 mg potassium; 466 IU vitamin A; 9 mg ATE vitamin E; 0 mg vitamin C; 9 mg cholesterol

Glycemic Index: Low

Fried Cheese Cubes

You can also make this with fresh mozzarella, which is much lower in sodium than the regular kind.

1 pound (455 g) Swiss cheese

1½ cups (180 g) baking mix (such as Bisquick), divided

½ cup (120 ml) skim milk

1 egg

Cut cheese into ¾-inch (2 cm) cubes. Heat oil in deep fryer or saucepan to 375°F (190°C, gas mark 5). Beat 1 cup (120 g) baking mix, milk, and egg with hand beater (or fork) until smooth. Coat cheese cubes lightly with remaining baking mix and insert round wooden pick in each cube. Dip into batter, covering cheese completely. Fry several cubes at a time, turning carefully until golden brown (1 to 2 minutes). Drain on paper towels.

Yield: 9 servings

Each with: 18 g water; 151 calories (46% from fat, 10% from protein, 44% from carb); 4 g protein; 8 g total fat; 2 g saturated fat; 3 g monounsaturated fat; 17 g carb; 1 g fiber; 23 mg calcium; 0 mg iron; 22 mg sodium; 48 mg potassium; 178 IU vitamin A; 0 mg vitamin C; 0 mg cholesterol

Glycemic Index: Low

Spicy Potato Skins

These tasty potato skins are free of fat. They are baked instead of fried.

4 potatoes

1½ teaspoons coriander

½ teaspoon black pepper

1½ teaspoons chili powder

1½ teaspoons curry powder

Preheat the oven to 400°F (200°C, gas mark 6). Bake the potatoes for 1 hour. Remove the potatoes from the oven but keep the oven on. Slice the potatoes in half lengthwise and let them cool for 10 minutes. Scoop out most of the potato flesh, leaving about ¼ inch (½ cm) of flesh against the potato skin (you can save the potato flesh for another use, like mashed potatoes). Cut each potato half crosswise into 3 pieces. Coat with olive oil spray. Combine the spices and sprinkle the mixture over the potatoes. Bake the potato skins for 15 minutes or until they are crispy and brown.

Yield: 24 servings

Each with: 50 g water; 44 calories (3% from fat, 11% from protein, 87% from carb); 1 g protein; 0 g total fat; 0 g saturated fat; 0 g monounsaturated fat; 0 g polyunsaturated fat; 10 g carb; 1 g fiber; 1 g sugar; 39 mg phosphorus; 8 mg calcium; 1 mg iron; 5 mg sodium; 287 mg potassium; 54 IU vitamin A; 6 mg vitamin C; 0 mg cholesterol

Glycemic Index: Low

Stuffed Mushrooms

This makes a very nice appetizer for entertaining. It's fancy looking and tasting but still healthy.

¼ cup (25 g) minced scallions

2 teaspoons unsalted butter

1 can (4 ounces or 115 g) crabmeat, drained

2 tablespoons (8 g) minced fresh parsley

1 tablespoon (15 g) horseradish

2 cloves garlic, pressed

¼ teaspoon hot pepper sauce

2½ cups (145 g) mushroom caps (24), stems removed

Ground red pepper for garnish

Combine scallions and butter in 2-cup measure. Microwave on high 2 minutes; stir in crabmeat, parsley, horseradish, garlic, and pepper sauce. Stir well. Place half the mushrooms, stemmed sides up, in a 9-inch (23 cm) pie plate. Fill each mushroom cap with 1 teaspoon crab mixture. Microwave on high 3 to 4 minutes, turning plate once. Remove mushrooms to serving plate; repeat with remaining mushrooms and filling. Let stand 2 to 3 minutes before serving. To garnish, sprinkle with ground red pepper. Each serving contains 4 mushrooms.

Yield: 6 servings

Each with: 49 g water; 43 calories (33% from fat, 48% from protein, 19% from carb); 5 g protein; 2 g total fat; 1 g saturated fat; 0 g monounsaturated fat; 0 g polyunsaturated fat; 2 g carb; 1 g fiber; 1 g sugar; 20 mg calcium; 0 mg iron; 83 mg sodium; 198 mg potassium; 209 IU vitamin A; 5 mg vitamin C; 18 mg cholesterol

Glycemic Index: Low

Apple Cheese Snack

This is a simple snack or appetizer which can be prepared in only a few minutes. But everyone seems to like the flavor, and we seldom see people taking only the one slice serving.

1 apple

1 ounce (28 g) cheddar

1 teaspoon cinnamon sugar

Wash apple. Pat dry. Cut apple into quarters. Remove seeds. Cut quarters in half. Arrange apple slices on a plate to resemble a pinwheel. Sprinkle slices with cinnamon-sugar. Cut slice of cheese into 8 pieces. Place a piece of cheese on each apple slice. Warm in the microwave on high for 10–20 seconds until cheese melts.

Yield: 8 servings

Each with: 15 g water; 24 calories (43% from fat, 15% from protein, 42% from carb); 1 g Protein; 1 g total fat; 1 g saturated fat; 0 g monounsaturated fat; 0 g polyunsaturated fat; 3 g carb; 0 g fiber; 2 g sugar; 20 mg phosphorous; 26 mg calcium; 0 mg iron; 22 mg sodium; 18 mg potassium; 42 IU vitamin A; 9 mg ATE vitamin E; 1 mg vitamin C; 4 mg cholesterol

Glycemic Index: Low

Herbed Cheese

This is similar to commercial herbed cheeses but with reduced fat and sodium, making it a healthier choice.

8 ounces (225 g) cream cheese

¼ cup (60 ml) non fat evaporated milk

½ cup (32 g) minced parsley

2 cloves garlic, pressed

½ teaspoon basil

½ teaspoon oregano

TIP *To make a fancier presentation, mound the cheese on a serving plate and cover with sliced almonds.*

Mix all the ingredients together and let stand 1 day in refrigerator.

Yield: 8 servings

Each with: 25 g water; 107 calories (82% from fat, 11% from protein, 7% from carb); 3 g Protein; 10 g total fat; 6 g saturated fat; 3 g monounsaturated fat; 0 g polyunsaturated fat; 2 g carb; 0 g fiber; 1 g sugar; 48 mg phosphorous; 53 mg calcium; 1 mg iron; 95 mg sodium; 84 mg potassium; 737 IU vitamin A; 111 mg ATE vitamin E; 5 mg vitamin C; 32 mg cholesterol

Glycemic Index: Low

Veggie Cheese Ball

This recipe makes a little different type of appetizer, with carrots providing color and crunch.

1½ cups (165 g) shredded carrot

8 ounces (225 g) cream cheese, softened

2 cups (225 g) shredded Cheddar cheese

½ teaspoon minced garlic

1 teaspoon Worcestershire sauce

½ teaspoon Tabasco sauce

3 tablespoons (12 g) chopped fresh parsley

½ cup (55 g) chopped pecans

Press carrot between paper towels to remove excess moisture; set aside. Combine cream cheese and Cheddar cheese in a medium bowl; stir well. Add carrot and garlic; stir well. Cover and chill 1 hour. These ingredients may also be combined in a food processor and mixed. Shape cheese mixture into a ball; roll in parsley and pecans. Wrap in waxed paper and chill at least 1 hour.

Yield: 24 servings

Each with: 17 g water; 97 calories (78% from fat, 15% from protein, 6% from carb); 4 g protein; 9 g total fat; 5 g saturated fat; 3 g monounsaturated fat; 1 g polyunsaturated fat; 2 g carb; 1 g fiber; 1 g sugar; 76 mg phosphorus; 92 mg calcium; 0 mg iron; 105 mg sodium; 62 mg potassium; 1625 IU vitamin A; 2 mg vitamin C; 22 mg cholesterol

Glycemic Index: Low

Vegetable and Nut Pâté

This veggie and nut spread makes a great dip for raw vegetables. You can also spread it on pita bread triangles or crackers.

½ cup (55 g) pecans

½ cup (60 g) walnuts

½ cup (73 g) sunflower seeds

⅓ cup (55 g) onions, chopped

1 tablespoon (12 g) no-salt-added seasoning blend

1 cup (235 ml) water

¼ cup (4 g) fresh cilantro, chopped

¼ cup (15 g) fresh parsley, chopped

¼ cup (28 g) carrots, grated

¼ cup (31 g) zucchini, grated

¼ cup (38 g) red bell pepper, finely chopped

TIP *Serve this on bed of lettuce surrounded by vegetables for dipping.*

Place nuts, sunflower seeds, onions, seasoning, and water in food processor. Process 25 to 30 seconds until smooth. Pour mixture into medium-sized bowl. Stir in next 5 ingredients and chill 1 to 2 hours.

Yield: 16 servings

Each with: 25 g water; 75 calories (76% from fat, 11% from protein, 13% from carb); 2 g Protein; 7 g total fat; 1 g saturated fat; 2 g monounsaturated fat; 3 g polyunsaturated fat; 3 g carb; 1 g fiber; 1 g sugar; 80 mg phosphorous; 12 mg calcium; 0 mg iron; 3 mg sodium; 99 mg potassium; 540 IU vitamin A; 0 mg ATE vitamin E; 5 mg vitamin C; 0 mg cholesterol

Glycemic Index: Low

Curried Cheese Spread

Curry powder gives this cheese spread a different flavor. We like it with broccoli and cauliflower.

¼ cup (40 g) onions, chopped

1 tablespoon (15 ml) olive oil

6 ounces (170 g) cream cheese

1 cup (115 g) cheddar cheese, shredded

2 tablespoons (30 g) tomato chutney (see recipe in chapter 2)

1 teaspoon curry powder

1 tablespoon (15 ml) sherry

TIP *You can also heat the mixture until the cheese melts and use it as a dip.*

Sauté onions in oil until softened. Mix all ingredients and chill.

Yield: 10 servings

Each with: 19 g water; 129 calories (82% from fat, 14% from protein, 4% from carb); 5 g Protein; 12 g total fat; 7 g saturated fat; 4 g monounsaturated fat; 0 g polyunsaturated fat; 1 g carb; 0 g fiber; 0 g sugar; 87 mg phosphorous; 111 mg calcium; 0 mg iron; 133 mg sodium; 44 mg potassium; 363 IU vitamin A; 95 mg ATE vitamin E; 0 mg vitamin C; 33 mg cholesterol

Glycemic Index: Low

Roasted Red Pepper Spread

This spread can be used as a dip or can be served over pasta for a different kind of sauce.

1 slice whole wheat bread, crusts trimmed

12 ounces (340 g) roasted red peppers, drained

1 garlic clove

2 tablespoons (30 ml) olive oil

In a covered food processor container, process bread until crumbly; set aside. Add red peppers and garlic to container. Cover and process until smooth. With the processor running, gradually add oil through feed tube. Add reserved bread crumbs; cover and process until smooth. Transfer to small bowl. Serve chilled or at room temperature with crackers or toasted bread.

Yield: 6 servings

Each with: 54 g water; 66 calories (63% from fat, 6% from protein, 31% from carb); 1 g Protein; 5 g total fat; 1 g saturated fat; 3 g monounsaturated fat; 1 g polyunsaturated fat; 5 g carb; 1 g fiber; 3 g sugar; 21 mg phosphorous; 10 mg calcium; 0 mg iron; 24 mg sodium; 127 mg potassium; 1775 IU vitamin A; 0 mg ATE vitamin E; 72 mg vitamin C; 0 mg cholesterol

Glycemic Index: Low

Chicken Liver Pâté

Here's another appetizer spread. This one uses chicken livers.

4 tablespoons (60 ml) olive oil

4 slices low-sodium bacon

½ cup (80 g) finely chopped onion

1 clove minced garlic

10 ounces (280 g) chicken livers

4 tablespoons (7 g) fresh rosemary

2 ounces (60 ml) sherry

⅛ teaspoon nutmeg

2 ounces (60 ml) milk

Add olive oil, bacon, and onion to a large sauté pan. Cook for 4 minutes on low heat and add the garlic and liver. Cook on medium heat for about 15 minutes. Add the rosemary and sherry and let simmer about 15 minutes or until the liver is done all the way through. Add a dash of pepper and the nutmeg and let cool. Puree in a food processor until mixture is smooth. Slowly stir in the milk and pulse till blended. Spread on crostini.

Yield: 10 servings

Each with: 128 calories (64% from fat, 28% from protein, 8% from carb); 8 g protein; 9 g total fat; 2 g saturated fat; 5 g monounsaturated fat; 1 g polyunsaturated fat; 2 g carb; 0 g fiber; 1 g sugar; 16 mg calcium; 3 mg iron; 51 mg sodium; 124 mg potassium; 9 mg vitamin C; 163 mg cholesterol

Glycemic Index: Low

Apple Pecan Log

This makes a different type party snack. Serve it with crackers or slices of firm fruit like apples.

8 ounces (225 g) cream cheese, softened

1 tablespoon (15 ml) apple juice

½ teaspoon ground nutmeg

1 teaspoon fresh lemon juice

1 cup (125 g) apple, chopped

1 cup (110 g) pecans, chopped

Combine cream cheese, apple juice, and nutmeg in mixer bowl and blend until smooth. Pour lemon juice over chopped apples and add to the creamed cheese mixture. Gently fold in ¾ cup (83 g) of the pecans and then shape into a 6-inch (15 cm) log and roll in the remaining chopped nuts. Wrap it in plastic and refrigerate until ready to serve.

Yield: 8 servings

Each with: 30 g water; 202 calories (84% from fat, 7% from protein, 9% from carb); 3 g Protein; 20 g total fat; 7 g saturated fat; 8 g monounsaturated fat; 3 g polyunsaturated fat; 5 g carb; 2 g fiber; 2 g sugar; 69 mg phosphorous; 33 mg calcium; 1 mg iron; 84 mg sodium; 106 mg potassium; 395 IU vitamin A; 102 mg ATE vitamin E; 1 mg vitamin C; 31 mg cholesterol

Glycemic Index: Low

Chile Con Queso

This is a popular dip in our house, and you can usually find some left in the refrigerator. It gives you something to nibble on with fresh vegetables when you need a little snack but don't want something with a lot of calories or carbohydrates.

1 cup (115 g) cheddar cheese, shredded

4 ounces (115 g) green chilies, chopped

¼ cup (60 ml) half-and-half

2 tablespoons (20 g) onion, finely chopped

2 teaspoons (5 g) cumin, ground

Heat all ingredients over low heat, stirring constantly, until the cheese is melted. Serve warm with tortilla chips or vegetables.

Yield: 12 servings

Each with: 18 g water; 55 calories (70% from fat, 22% from protein, 8% from carb); 3 g Protein; 4 g total fat; 3 g saturated fat; 1 g monounsaturated fat; 0 g polyunsaturated fat; 1 g carb; 0 g fiber; 0 g sugar; 65 mg phosphorous; 89 mg calcium; 0 mg iron; 182 mg sodium; 43 mg potassium; 200 IU vitamin A; 33 mg ATE vitamin E; 7 mg vitamin C; 13 mg cholesterol

Glycemic Index: Low

Green Onion Dip

This is not at all like the packaged onion dip mixes, but it's still very tasty. It has a little more tang and is great to dip veggies in.

1 cup (225 g) cottage cheese

¼ cup (25 g) chopped green onion

2 teaspoons (10 ml) lemon juice

Combine ingredients in a blender or food processor and process until smooth. Refrigerate for at least an hour to give the flavors time to develop.

Yield: 8 servings

Each with: 18 g water; 17 calories (5% from fat, 79% from protein, 17% from carb); 3 g protein; 0 g total fat; 0 g saturated fat; 0 g monounsaturated fat; 0 g polyunsaturated fat; 1 g carb; 0 g fiber; 0 g sugar; 20 mg phosphorus; 8 mg calcium; 0 mg iron; 3 mg sodium; 16 mg potassium; 37 IU vitamin A; 1 mg vitamin C; 1 mg cholesterol

Glycemic Index: Low

Hummus

Hummus is a traditional Middle Eastern dip. I usually cook my own dried chickpeas, which you should be able to find with the other dried beans in most large markets. They are lower in sodium than the canned ones.

1 cup (164 g) cooked chickpeas

3 cloves garlic

3 tablespoons (45 ml) lemon juice

¼ cup (60 ml) water

¼ cup (60 g) tahini

1 teaspoon cumin

½ teaspoon paprika

1 tablespoon (15 ml) olive oil

Place the cooked chickpeas in the food processor along with the garlic, lemon juice, and water. Process for about a minute until smooth. If it's too thick, add more water. Stir in the tahini and spices, taste, and add more lemon juice/tahini/cumin/paprika as desired. Spread into a shallow bowl; drizzle with olive oil. Serve chilled.

Yield: 8 servings

Each with: 16 g water; 155 calories (41% from fat, 15% from protein, 44% from carb); 6 g protein; 7 g total fat; 1 g saturated fat; 3 g monounsaturated fat; 3 g polyunsaturated fat; 18 g carb; 5 g fiber; 3 g sugar; 63 mg calcium; 2 mg iron; 16 mg sodium; 269 mg potassium; 102 IU vitamin A; 4 mg vitamin C; 0 mg cholesterol

Glycemic Index: Low

Bean Dip

This makes a great bean and cheese dip that not only tastes better than commercial ones but is healthier besides.

2 tablespoons (30 ml) olive oil

½ teaspoon crushed garlic

1 cup (160 g) finely chopped onion

1 jalapeño pepper, finely chopped

1 teaspoon chili powder

2 cups (200 g) cooked kidney beans

½ cup (58 g) shredded Cheddar cheese

Heat oil in a skillet. Add garlic, onion, jalapeño, and chili powder and cook gently 4 minutes. Drain kidney beans, reserving juice. Process beans in a blender or food processor to a puree. Add to onion mixture and stir in 2 tablespoons (30 ml) of reserved bean liquid; mix well. Stir in cheese. Cook gently about 2 minutes, stirring until cheese melts. If mixture becomes too thick, add a little more reserved bean liquid. Spoon into serving dish and serve warm with tortilla chips.

Yield: 12 servings

(continued on page 70)

Each with: 19 g water; 151 calories (26% from fat, 23% from protein, 52% from carb); 9 g protein; 4 g total fat; 2 g saturated fat; 1 g monounsaturated fat; 1 g polyunsaturated fat; 20 g carb; 8 g fiber; 1 g sugar; 158 mg phosphorus; 87 mg calcium; 3 mg iron; 44 mg sodium; 463 mg potassium; 126 IU vitamin A; 3 mg vitamin c; 6 mg cholesterol

Glycemic Index: Low

Guacamole Dip

This recipe makes a lighter version of guacamole. It is a molded dip made with lemon gelatin.

1 small lemon flavor sugar-free gelatin

1 cup (235 ml) boiling water

¼ cup (60 ml) lemon juice

16 ounces (455 g) fat free cottage cheese

2 cloves garlic

2 teaspoons (5.2 g) chili powder

1 cup (146 g) avocado

¼ cup (45 g) tomatoes, finely chopped

½ cup (50 g) green onion, chopped, divided

4 pitted ripe olives, sliced

¼ cup (34 g) pickled jalapeno pepper

Completely dissolve gelatin in boiling water; pour into blender container. Add cottage cheese, avocado, half of the green onions, the jalapeno peppers, lemon juice, garlic, and chili powder. Cover and blend on low speed, scraping down sides occasionally, about 2 minutes or until mixture is smooth. Pour into shallow 5-cup (1.2 L) serving dish; smooth top. Chill until set, about 4 hours. When ready to serve, top guacamole with the remaining ¼ cup (25 g) chopped green onion, the tomatoes, and olives. Serve as a dip with chips or vegetables.

Yield: 10 servings

Each with: 93 g water; 80 calories (46% from fat, 30% from protein, 24% from carb); 6 g Protein; 4 g total fat; 1 g saturated fat; 3 g monounsaturated fat; 0 g polyunsaturated fat; 5 g carb; 2 g fiber; 2 g sugar; 86 mg phosphorous; 39 mg calcium; 0 mg iron; 214 mg sodium; 196 mg potassium; 290 IU vitamin A; 5 mg ATE vitamin E; 7 mg vitamin C; 2 mg cholesterol

Glycemic Index: Low

Tofu Avocado Dip

When you have an avocado and you are tired of guacamole, try this flavorful dip. The taste is vaguely Middle Eastern or Asian, but it really isn't quite like any other dip I've ever had. It can also be used as is for a tasty vegetarian sandwich filling.

8 ounces (225 g) tofu

½ cup (23 g) avocado

2 garlic cloves, chopped

2 teaspoons (4 g) minced fresh ginger

½ cup (30 g) fresh parsley leaves

2 tablespoons (30 ml) lemon juice

1 tablespoon (16 g) peanut butter

1 tablespoon (15 g) applesauce

Blend all ingredients in a food processor until very smooth.

Yield: 8 servings

Each with: 41 g water; 54 calories (63% from fat, 15% from protein, 22% from carb); 2 g Protein; 4 g total fat; 1 g saturated fat; 2 g monounsaturated fat; 1 g polyunsaturated fat; 3 g carb; 1 g fiber; 1 g sugar; 32 mg phosphorous; 12 mg calcium; 0 mg iron; 3 mg sodium; 145 mg potassium; 22 IU vitamin A; 0 mg ATE vitamin E; 3 mg vitamin C; 0 mg cholesterol

Glycemic Index: Low

Hominy Dip

I'd be willing to bet no one will guess what the main ingredient of this flavorful dip is. The corn and cumin give it a southwestern taste, but the hominy is not at all obvious.

14.5 ounces (411 g) hominy

½ teaspoon ground cumin

8 ounces (225 g) creamed corn

¼ teaspoon cayenne

2 tablespoons (30 ml) lemon juice

1 clove garlic

¼ cup (29 g) radishes, chopped

Drain the hominy. In a food processor or a blender, combine the hominy, creamed corn, lemon juice, garlic, cumin, and cayenne. Blend until smooth. Mound into a bowl. Sprinkle with chopped radishes and offer crisp raw vegetables to scoop up the mixture.

Yield: 10 servings

Each with: 28 g water; 161 calories (4% from fat, 9% from protein, 87% from carb); 4 g Protein; 1 g total fat; 0 g saturated fat; 0 g monounsaturated fat; 0 g polyunsaturated fat; 37 g carb; 2 g fiber; 1 g sugar; 81 mg phosphorous; 4 mg calcium; 2 mg iron; 3 mg sodium; 104 mg potassium; 37 IU vitamin A; 0 mg ATE vitamin E; 3 mg vitamin C; 0 mg cholesterol

Glycemic Index: Low

White Bean Dip

This tasty appetizer is good either warm or cold.

1 cup (250 g) dried navy beans

½ cup (80 g) chopped onion

¾ teaspoon minced garlic

1 tablespoon (15 g) Dijon mustard

¼ cup (25 g) chopped green onion

2 tablespoons (30 ml) lime juice

1 teaspoon tarragon

Bring beans to a boil for 1 minute and remove from heat to soak for 1 hour. Rinse well. Add onion and cook beans until tender, about 1 hour. Drain beans and rinse well. In a food processor, place mustard, green onions, lime juice, and tarragon. Pulse to combine. Add beans and blend until smooth.

Yield: 8 servings

Each with: 40 g water; 45 calories (5% from fat, 24% from protein, 72% from carb); 3 g protein; 0 g total fat; 0 g saturated fat; 0 g monounsaturated fat; 0 g polyunsaturated fat; 8 g carb; 2 g fiber; 1 g sugar; 51 mg phosphorus; 23 mg calcium; 1 mg iron; 169 mg sodium; 128 mg potassium; 38 IU vitamin A; 3 mg vitamin C; 0 mg cholesterol

Glycemic Index: Low

Spicy Cheese Dip

This dip is a little on the spicy side. You can add or decrease the jalapeños to make it suit your own desired heat.

3 ounces (85 g) cream cheese, room temperature

3 ounces (85 g) blue cheese, room temperature

8 ounces (225 g) sour cream

2½ teaspoons (5.8 g) unflavored gelatin

¼ cup (60 ml) water

2 tablespoons (30 ml) vinegar

2 jalapeño peppers, minced

1¼ cups (125 g) pecans, toasted, chopped

2 ounces (55 g) pimento, drained and minced

Mix cheeses with sour cream until smooth. Add gelatin that has been softened in water and heated to dissolve. Add vinegar and let stand until slightly thickened. Add jalapeños, pecans, and pimentos. Pour into mold that has been coated with nonstick vegetable oil spray and chill.

Yield: 12 servings

Each with: 36 g water; 156 calories (83% from fat, 9% from protein, 8% from carb); 4 g protein; 15 g total fat; 5 g saturated fat; 7 g monounsaturated fat; 3 g polyunsaturated fat; 3 g carb; 1 g fiber; 1 g sugar; 86 mg phosphorus; 72 mg calcium; 1 mg iron; 129 mg sodium; 112 mg potassium; 370 IU vitamin A; 5 mg vitamin C; 20 mg cholesterol

Glycemic Index: Low

Easy Clam Dip

We originally made this clam dip to serve with crackers, but it's just as good with vegetables if you are watching your carbs.

1 can (15 ounces or 425 g) condensed clam chowder

1 medium clove garlic, minced

½ teaspoon Worcestershire sauce

8 ounces (225 g) cream cheese, softened

With electric mixer or food processor, gradually blend soup, garlic, and Worcestershire into cream cheese; beat until just smooth. Chill.

Yield: 12 servings

Each with: 31 g water; 84 calories (75% from fat, 12% from protein, 13% from carb); 3 g Protein; 7 g total fat; 4 g saturated fat; 2 g monounsaturated fat; 0 g polyunsaturated fat; 3 g carb; 0 g fiber; 0 g sugar; 29 mg phosphorous; 24 mg calcium; 1 mg iron; 247 mg sodium; 47 mg potassium; 267 IU vitamin A; 72 mg ATE vitamin E; 1 mg vitamin C; 22 mg cholesterol

Glycemic Index: Low

Bread Bowl Dip

This one is really easy to make. When the interior pieces are finished, break off pieces of the "bowl" itself to continue dipping.

1 round bread loaf, homemade

1 cup (225 g) mayonnaise

½ cup (50 g) chopped green onion

½ cup (30 g) chopped fresh parsley

¼ cup (60 g) plain yogurt

Slice off the top of the loaf and scoop out as much of the interior of the loaf as possible while leaving about ½ inch (1 cm) of the crust. Slice the top and the interior into bite-size pieces. Combine the rest of the ingredients in a large bowl and mix together. Spoon the mixture into the hollowed loaf and arrange the bread pieces around.

Yield: 8 servings

Each with: 21 g water; 216 calories (91% from fat, 2% from protein, 7% from carb); 1 g protein; 22 g total fat; 3 g saturated fat; 6 g monounsaturated fat; 10 g polyunsaturated fat; 4 g carb; 0 g fiber; 1 g sugar; 27 mg phosphorus; 32 mg calcium; 1 mg iron; 39 mg sodium; 69 mg potassium; 459 IU vitamin A; 6 mg vitamin C; 17 mg cholesterol

Glycemic Index: Low

Asian Dipping Sauce

This sauce can be used as a dip for fresh vegetables, but it is also really great with cubes of chicken or beef as either an appetizer or main dish.

1 tablespoon (15 ml) Dick's Reduced-Sodium Soy Sauce (see chapter 2)

1 teaspoon sesame oil

1 teaspoon rice vinegar

¼ teaspoon chili oil

¼ teaspoon honey

1 tablespoon (15 ml) water

Combine all ingredients in a jar with a lid. Shake to combine. This will keep indefinitely if stored in the refrigerator.

Yield: 4 servings

Each with: 5 g water; 12 calories (87% from fat, 0% from protein, 13% from carb); 0 g Protein; 1 g total fat; 0 g saturated fat; 0 g monounsaturated fat; 0 g polyunsaturated fat; 0 g carb; 0 g fiber; 0 g sugar; 0 mg phosphorous; 0 mg calcium; 0 mg iron; 0 mg sodium; 1 mg potassium; 0 IU vitamin A; 0 mg ATE vitamin E; 0 mg vitamin C; 0 mg cholesterol

Glycemic Index: Low

Chili Horseradish Dip

This is a flavorful dip for vegetables. We also like it as a salad dressing.

1 cup (230 g) plain fat-free yogurt

2 tablespoons (30 ml) chili sauce, see recipe in chapter 2

2 tablespoons (10 g) horseradish

Mix all ingredients; cover and refrigerate at least 1 hour.

Yield: 6 servings

Each with: 44 g water; 27 calories (4% from fat, 36% from protein, 60% from carb); 2 g Protein; 0 g total fat; 0 g saturated fat; 0 g monounsaturated fat; 0 g polyunsaturated fat; 4 g carb; 0 g fiber; 4 g sugar; 66 mg phosphorous; 85 mg calcium; 0 mg iron; 81 mg sodium; 116 mg potassium; 87 IU vitamin A; 1 mg ATE vitamin E; 3 mg vitamin C; 1 mg cholesterol

Glycemic Index: Low

Crab Dip

This crab dip has become a standard part of our Thanksgiving meal, giving people something to nibble on while dinner is being finished.

1 cup (230 g) sour cream

8 ounces (225 g) cream cheese

1 pound (455 g) crab meat

1 teaspoon dry mustard

¼ teaspoon garlic powder

¼ cup (60 g) mayonnaise

1 teaspoon old bay seasoning

1 cup (120 g) grated cheddar cheese

Cream all ingredients except crab meat and half of the cheese. Add crab meat and stir gently to combine. Sprinkle reserved cheese on top. Bake at 325°F (170°C, or gas mark 3) for 20 minutes.

Yield: 10 servings

Each with: 73 g water; 245 calories (74% from fat, 23% from protein, 3% from carb); 14 g Protein; 20 g total fat; 10 g saturated fat; 5 g monounsaturated fat; 3 g polyunsaturated fat; 2 g carb; 0 g fiber; 0 g sugar; 220 mg phosphorous; 180 mg calcium; 1 mg iron; 323 mg sodium; 224 mg potassium; 546 IU vitamin A; 145 mg ATE vitamin E; 2 mg vitamin C; 86 mg cholesterol

Glycemic Index: Low

Dried Beef Appetizer Dip

I don't use dried chipped beef very often because of the high sodium content. But for your guests who aren't watching their sodium, this is an excellent choice with a lot of flavor.

8 ounces (225 g) cream cheese, softened

2 tablespoons (30 ml) milk

2½ ounces (70 g) sliced dried beef, finely snipped

2 tablespoons (20 g) minced onion

2 tablespoons (19 g) green pepper, finely chopped

⅛ teaspoon pepper

½ cup (115 g) sour cream

¼ cup (30 g) walnuts, coarsely chopped

Blend cream cheese and milk. Stir in dried beef, onion, green pepper, and pepper; mix well. Stir in sour cream. Spoon into 8-inch (20 cm) pie plate or small shallow baking dish. Sprinkle walnuts over top. Bake at 350°F (180°C, or gas mark 4) for 15 minutes. Serve hot with assorted crackers.

Yield: 12 servings

Each with: 27 g water; 107 calories (78% from fat, 16% from protein, 6% from carb); 4 g Protein; 9 g total fat; 5 g saturated fat; 3 g monounsaturated fat; 1 g polyunsaturated fat; 2 g carb; 0 g fiber; 0 g sugar; 58 mg phosphorous; 31 mg calcium; 0 mg iron; 226 mg sodium; 76 mg potassium; 305 IU vitamin A; 79 mg ATE vitamin E; 2 mg vitamin C; 29 mg cholesterol

Glycemic Index: Low

Amaretto Fruit Dip

This slightly sweet dip is perfect with fruit. Apples are our favorite, but you can use whatever appeals to you.

8 ounces (225 g) cream cheese, softened

½ cup (8 g) brown sugar substitute, like Splenda

2 tablespoons (30 ml) vanilla

2 tablespoons (30 ml) skim milk

4 tablespoons (60 ml) Amaretto

Mix cream cheese, sugar, vanilla, milk, and Amaretto in blender. Serve with fruit of your choice.

Yield: 9 servings

Each with: 19 g water; 128 calories (76% from fat, 7% from protein, 17% from carb); 2 g Protein; 10 g total fat; 6 g saturated fat; 3 g monounsaturated fat; 0 g polyunsaturated fat; 5 g carb; 0 g fiber; 4 g sugar; 30 mg phosphorous; 22 mg calcium; 0 mg iron; 81 mg sodium; 37 mg potassium; 382 IU vitamin A; 102 mg ATE vitamin E; 0 mg vitamin C; 32 mg cholesterol

Glycemic Index: Low

Parmesan Garlic Pita Toasts

Use these flavorful pita crisps for any of the spreads or dips in the book. Or you can just nibble on them for a healthier-than-usual snack option.

3 tablespoons (42 g) unsalted butter

1 teaspoon minced garlic

2 whole wheat pitas, cut into 8 triangles

½ teaspoon black pepper, fresh ground

¼ cup (25 g) grated Parmesan cheese

Salt to taste

Melt butter and cook garlic in butter over low heat, stirring occasionally for 5 minutes. Brush mixture lightly on rough side of pita triangles. Arrange butter side up in 1 layer on baking sheet. Sprinkle salt to taste, pepper, and Parmesan cheese. Bake in preheated oven, 350°F (180°C, gas mark 4) for 12 to 15 minutes until crisp and light brown. Cool on racks and store in airtight container in dry place.

Yield: 8 servings

Each with: 7 g water; 95 calories (51% from fat, 12% from protein, 37% from carb); 3 g protein; 6 g total fat; 3 g saturated fat; 1 g monounsaturated fat; 0 g polyunsaturated fat; 9 g carb; 1 g fiber; 0 g sugar; 54 mg phosphorus; 40 mg calcium; 1 mg iron; 134 mg sodium; 35 mg potassium; 147 IU vitamin A; 0 mg vitamin C; 14 mg cholesterol

Glycemic Index: Low

4

Breakfast

Breakfast can be a carbohydrate nightmare, with pancakes, waffles, and white bread toast. This chapter includes some lower-GI ideas. There are breakfast skillet and casserole dishes that feature mostly eggs, meat, and vegetables. There are grab-and-go ideas wrapped in tortillas rather than bread. And there are high-protein, low-carb smoothies that will keep you satisfied throughout the morning.

Sun-Dried Tomato Scrambled Eggs

Sun dried tomatoes turn ordinary scrambled eggs into a different taste treat. This recipe is perfect for those mornings when you want something a little different, but you don't know what.

4 eggs

¼ cup (60 ml) skim milk

½ teaspoon dried parsley

¼ cup (30 g) cheddar cheese, shredded

½ cup (27 g) sun-dried tomatoes

If using dried tomatoes, boil water in pot. Turn off heat and place tomatoes in water for about 3 minutes until soft. Cut up tomatoes in small pieces. Beat together eggs and milk. Place egg mixture in greased skillet. Add tomato pieces, cheese, and parsley. Scramble until done.

Yield: 4 servings

Each with: 67 g water; 148 calories (61% from fat, 27% from protein, 12% from carb); 10 g Protein; 10 g total fat; 4 g saturated fat; 4 g monounsaturated fat; 1 g polyunsaturated fat; 5 g carb; 1 g fiber; 1 g sugar; 184 mg phosphorous; 115 mg calcium; 1 mg iron; 173 mg sodium; 323 mg potassium; 577 IU vitamin A; 108 mg ATE vitamin E; 14 mg vitamin C; 246 mg cholesterol

Glycemic Index: Low

Creamy Egg Bake

This is an unusual looking dish with eggs baked to a poached egg consistency in a flavorful, cheesy mixture.

½ cup (58 g) cheddar cheese, shredded

4 eggs

½ cup (115 g) sour cream

3 tablespoons (45 ml) skim milk

1½ teaspoons flour

½ teaspoon prepared mustard

¼ teaspoon Worcestershire sauce

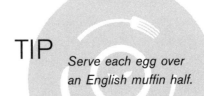

TIP *Serve each egg over an English muffin half.*

Sprinkle half the cheese evenly over the bottom of greased 8 x 8-inch (20 x 20 cm) baking dish. Break and slip eggs onto cheese in dish. Beat together remaining ingredients except remaining cheese. Pour over eggs and sprinkle with remaining cheese. Bake in a 325°F (170°C, gas mark 3) oven until whites are set and yolks are soft, about 25 to 30 minutes.

Yield: 4 servings

Each with: 83 g water; 196 calories (68% from fat, 26% from protein, 7% from carb); 13 g Protein; 15 g total fat; 7 g saturated fat; 5 g monounsaturated fat; 1 g polyunsaturated fat; 3 g carb; 0 g fiber; 1 g sugar; 233 mg phosphorous; 195 mg calcium; 1 mg iron; 201 mg sodium; 153 mg potassium; 575 IU vitamin A; 158 mg ATE vitamin E; 1 mg vitamin C; 266 mg cholesterol

Glycemic Index: Low

Mexican Egg Bake

Cheese and chilies add a fresh taste to these eggs.

½ cup (112 g) unsalted butter

10 eggs

½ cup (63 g) flour

1 teaspoon baking powder

4 ounces (115 g) canned chilies, chopped

2 cups (450 g) cottage cheese

1 cup (115 g) Monterey jack cheese shredded

TIP *Top with a little sour cream and salsa for even more flavor.*

Melt butter. Beat eggs; add flour and baking powder. Add butter and then add chilies, cottage cheese, and Monterey Jack. Pour into 9 x 13-inch (23 x 33 cm) pan. Bake at 400°F (200°C, or gas mark 6) for 15 minutes. Reduce heat to 250°F (130°C, or gas mark ½) and bake an additional 35 minutes.

Yield: 6 servings

Each with: 123 g water; 431 calories (66% from fat, 25% from protein, 9% from carb); 27 g Protein; 32 g total fat; 17 g saturated fat; 10 g monounsaturated fat; 2 g polyunsaturated fat; 10 g carb; 0 g fiber; 2 g sugar; 359 mg phosphorous; 280 mg calcium; 3 mg iron; 338 mg sodium; 174 mg potassium; 1111 IU vitamin A; 303 mg ATE vitamin E; 0 mg vitamin C; 458 mg cholesterol

Glycemic Index: Low

Three Cheese Quiche

This is one of the easiest quiches you'll find, but it's one that makes a great breakfast to serve either family or overnight guests.

1 pie crust

1 cup (225 g) cottage cheese

8 ounces (110 g) Swiss cheese, shredded

¼ cup (25 g) parmesan cheese, grated

4 eggs, beaten

Bake pie crust for 5 minutes at 425°F (220°C, or gas mark 7). Decrease temperature to 350°F (180°C). Mix ingredients and pour into pie crust. Bake at 350°F (180°C, or gas mark 4) for 45–50 minutes or until knife comes out clean.

Yield: 6 servings

Each with: 69 g water; 386 calories (59% from fat, 24% from protein, 17% from carb); 23 g Protein; 25 g total fat; 11 g saturated fat; 9 g monounsaturated fat; 4 g polyunsaturated fat; 16 g carb; 1 g fiber; 1 g sugar; 375 mg phosphorous; 440 mg calcium; 2 mg iron; 129 mg sodium; 124 mg potassium; 517 IU vitamin A; 139 mg ATE vitamin E; 0 mg vitamin C; 198 mg cholesterol

Glycemic Index: Low

Crustless Quiche

Cut back on the carbs even more with this crustless quiche. Two kinds of cheese team with ham and mushrooms to give it great flavor.

1 cup (235 ml) skim milk

1 cup (125 g) flour

6 eggs

16 ounces (450 g) cottage cheese

1 cup (115 g) Monterey jack cheese shredded

⅓ cup (75 g) unsalted butter

½ cup (75 g) ham, chopped

½ cup (35 g) mushrooms, sliced

Preheat oven to 350°F (180°C, or gas mark 4). Mix all ingredients thoroughly except butter. Melt butter and pour half of it into an 8 x 12-inch (20 x 30 cm) glass pan. Pour remaining butter into batter and pour batter into pan. Bake for 50 minutes.

Yield: 6 servings

Each with: 167 g water; 427 calories (51% from fat, 30% from protein, 19% from carb); 32 g Protein; 24 g total fat; 13 g saturated fat; 7 g monounsaturated fat; 2 g polyunsaturated fat; 20 g carb; 1 g fiber; 4 g sugar; 381 mg phosphorous; 276 mg calcium; 2 mg iron; 350 mg sodium; 266 mg potassium; 863 IU vitamin A; 236 mg ATE vitamin E; 0 mg vitamin C; 294 mg cholesterol

Glycemic Index: Low

Apple and Sausage Quiche

Apples and sausage are a great combination, but it may not be one that we think about for breakfast. This crustless quiche will cure that. It can also be used for dinner.

½ cup (115 g) mayonnaise

½ cup (120 ml) skim milk

2 tablespoons (16 g) flour

2 eggs

2 apples, peeled, cored and sliced

1 cup (110 g) Swiss cheese, shredded

8 ounces (225 g) sausage links, cooked and thinly sliced

Preheat oven to 350°F (180°C, or gas mark 4). Combine mayonnaise, milk, flour, and eggs in bowl. Stir in apples, cheeses, and sausage. Pour the ingredients into pie pan. Bake 60 minutes or until top is nicely browned. Cool in pan for 10 minutes before serving.

(continued on page 88)

Yield: 6 servings

Each with: 100 g water; 408 calories (74% from fat, 16% from protein, 10% from carb); 16 g Protein; 34 g total fat; 11 g saturated fat; 12 g monounsaturated fat; 10 g polyunsaturated fat; 10 g carb; 1 g fiber; 6 g sugar; 262 mg phosphorous; 259 mg calcium; 1 mg iron; 458 mg sodium; 219 mg potassium; 380 IU vitamin A; 100 mg ATE vitamin E; 2 mg vitamin C; 136 mg cholesterol

Glycemic Index: Low

Breakfast Pockets

This is a quick little alternative to the traditional breakfast sandwich. It's good for a grab and go type of morning on the run.

1 slice bacon

2 eggs

¼ cup (30 g) cheddar cheese, shredded

1 pita bread

Dice bacon. Brown in frying pan. Add eggs to pan and scramble. Turn off heat and add cheese until melted. Soften pita bread in microwave for 15 seconds. Open up the pocket and fill with scrambled egg mixture.

Yield: 2 servings

Each with: 59 g water; 251 calories (47% from fat, 25% from protein, 28% from carb); 15 g Protein; 13 g total fat; 6 g saturated fat; 4 g monounsaturated fat; 1 g polyunsaturated fat; 17 g carb; 1 g fiber; 1 g sugar; 242 mg phosphorous; 175 mg calcium; 2 mg iron; 434 mg sodium; 150 mg potassium; 440 IU vitamin A; 121 mg ATE vitamin E; 0 mg vitamin C; 259 mg cholesterol

Glycemic Index: Low

Breakfast Wraps

Use this recipe on those days when you want a little something different for breakfast. This is similar to the breakfast burritos served at several fast food restaurants but with a lot less fat.

½ pound (225 g) turkey sausage

½ cup (80 g) onion, chopped

1 teaspoon chili powder

¼ teaspoon cayenne pepper

4 eggs

6 flour tortillas

½ cup (58 g) shredded low-fat Cheddar cheese

Brown sausage in frying pan; add chopped onion, chili powder, and cayenne pepper. Cook for 10 minutes. Drain and discard any fat. Add eggs. Stir until eggs are set. Spoon mixture into center of warmed tortilla, top with shredded cheese, and roll up tortilla.

Yield: 6 servings

Each with: 52 g water; 209 calories (44% from fat, 22% from protein, 34% from carb); 11 g protein; 10 g total fat; 4 g saturated fat; 3 g monounsaturated fat; 2 g polyunsaturated fat; 18 g carb; 1 g fiber; 1 g sugar; 166 mg phosphorus; 101 mg calcium; 2 mg iron; 485 mg sodium; 157 mg potassium; 177 IU vitamin A; 13 mg vitamin C; 25 mg cholesterol

Glycemic Index: Low

Basque Breakfast Skillet

This is an entire breakfast in a pan.

4 slices bacon

2 potatoes, shredded

2 teaspoons sliced green onion (tops)

1 tablespoon (4 g) snipped parsley

1/8 teaspoon crushed dried thyme

3/4 teaspoon salt

1/4 teaspoon pepper

4 large eggs

1/2 cup (120 ml) milk

Fry the bacon in a heavy skillet over medium-high heat until crisp. Remove the bacon and crumble. Pour off all but 2 tablespoons (30 ml) of the drippings. Return the skillet to the stove and reduce heat to low. Add the potatoes, onion, parsley, thyme, salt, and pepper to the skillet, cover, and cook until the potatoes are just tender (about 8 minutes), stirring occasionally. Beat together the eggs and milk and pour over the potato mixture. Cover and continue cooking until the mixture is set to your liking (about 10 minutes). Serve with sour cream and the bacon bits sprinkled over the top. (A splash of Tabasco will get your morning off on the right foot too!)

Yield: 4 servings

Each with: 125 g water; 201 calories (43% from fat, 25% from protein, 32% from carb); 13 g protein; 10 g total fat; 3 g saturated fat; 4 g monounsaturated fat; 1 g polyunsaturated fat; 16 g carb; 1 g fiber; 3 g sugar; 215 mg phosphorus; 81 mg calcium; 2 mg iron; 727 mg sodium; 444 mg potassium; 370 IU vitamin A; 11 mg vitamin C; 248 mg cholesterol

Glycemic Index: Low

Italian Breakfast Casserole

I probably should say "Italian flavored." Something like this has most likely never been seen in Italy, but it seemed like a good idea when I created it. And everyone liked it, so I'm sure we'll have it again.

1 pound (455 g) Italian sausage, casings removed

1 tablespoon (14 g) butter

4 ounces (115 g) mushrooms, sliced

1 cup (160 g) red onion, chopped

12 eggs, beaten

1 cup (235 ml) milk

8 ounces (115 g) mozzarella cheese, shredded

1 cup (180 g) tomatoes, peeled and chopped

½ teaspoon freshly ground pepper

½ teaspoon oregano, crumbled

Sauté crumbled sausage until no longer pink. Drain and put aside in bowl. Sauté onion and mushrooms in butter until soft but not brown. Stir into sausage. Blend in remaining ingredients and mix well. Pour into greased 9 x 13-inch (23 x 33 cm) pan and bake at 400°F (200°C, or gas mark 6) for 30 to 35 minutes or until knife inserted in center comes out clean.

Yield: 8 servings

Each with: 183 g water; 440 calories (70% from fat, 24% from protein, 6% from carb); 27 g Protein; 34 g total fat; 14 g saturated fat; 14 g monounsaturated fat; 4 g polyunsaturated fat; 6 g carb; 1 g fiber; 4 g sugar; 395 mg phosphorous; 244 mg calcium; 3 mg iron; 736 mg sodium; 444 mg potassium; 829 IU vitamin A; 197 mg ATE vitamin E; 8 mg vitamin C; 425 mg cholesterol

Glycemic Index: Low

Hash Brown Omelet

This is more like a frittata than an omelet really. The potatoes and veggies are browned, and then eggs are pored over and cooked until they are set without stirring.

4 slices bacon

2 cups (420 g) frozen hash brown potatoes

¼ cup (40 g) onion, chopped

¼ cup (38 g) green pepper, chopped

4 eggs

¼ cup (60 ml) skim milk

1 cup (115 g) cheddar, shredded

¼ teaspoon pepper

TIP *Make it even easier on yourself and get the frozen O'Brien potatoes, which have the onions and peppers already added.*

In a 10 or 12-inch (25 or 30 cm) skillet, cook bacon until crisp. Leave some drippings and remove bacon. Brown potatoes, onion, and green pepper and pat down into bottom of pan. Blend eggs, milk, and pepper and pour over potatoes. Top with cheese and crumbled bacon. Cover and cook over low heat until

egg is set.

Yield: 6 servings

Each with: 113 g water; 236 calories (52% from fat, 24% from protein, 24% from carb); 14 g Protein; 14 g total fat; 7 g saturated fat; 4 g monounsaturated fat; 1 g polyunsaturated fat; 14 g carb; 1 g fiber; 1 g sugar; 259 mg phosphorous; 201 mg calcium; 2 mg iron; 333 mg sodium; 338 mg potassium; 448 IU vitamin A; 115 mg ATE vitamin E; 11 mg vitamin C; 187 mg cholesterol

Glycemic Index: Low

Cinnamon Apple Omelet

This is a little different version of an omelet. I remember years ago there were often recipes for omelets with jelly or other sweet fillings, but you don't see them much anymore. This one makes me think they are still a good idea.

1 tablespoon (14 g) unsalted butter, divided

1 apple, peeled and sliced thin

½ teaspoon cinnamon

1 tablespoon (15 g) brown sugar

3 eggs

1 tablespoon (15 ml) cream

1 tablespoon (15 g) sour cream

Melt 2 teaspoons (10 g) butter in a skillet. Add apple, cinnamon, and brown sugar. Sauté until tender. Set aside. Whip eggs and cream until fluffy; set aside. Clean the skillet. Melt remaining butter; pour in egg mixture. Cook as you would for omelet. When eggs are ready to flip, turn them. Add the sour cream to the center of the eggs and top it with, the apple mixture. Fold the omelet onto a plate.

Yield: 2 servings

Each with: 129 g water; 252 calories (57% from fat, 17% from protein, 25% from carb); 11 g protein; 16 g total fat; 8 g saturated fat; 5 g monounsaturated fat; 1 g polyunsaturated fat; 16 g carb; 1 g fiber; 14 g sugar; 181 mg phosphorus; 73 mg calcium; 2 mg iron; 126 mg sodium; 211 mg potassium; 695 IU vitamin A; 3 mg vitamin C; 379 mg cholesterol

Glycemic Index: Low

Veggie Frittata

A frittata is an Italian-style omelet with the filling mixed in with the eggs. It's cooked without turning, and then the top is set under the broiler. This version does not have any of the meat and potatoes that they often have, providing you with a filling weekend breakfast low in sodium, fat, and carbohydrates.

½ cup (75 g) chopped red bell pepper

½ cup (80 g) chopped onion

1 cup (71 g) broccoli florets

8 ounces (225 g) sliced mushrooms

1 cup (113 g) sliced zucchini

6 eggs

1 tablespoon (4 g) parsley

¼ teaspoon black pepper

2 ounces (55 g) Swiss cheese, shredded

Coat a large ovenproof skillet with nonstick vegetable oil spray. Stir-fry the bell pepper, onion, and broccoli until crisp-tender. Add the mushrooms and zucchini and stir-fry 1 to 2 minutes more. Stir together the eggs, parsley, and black pepper and pour over vegetable mixture, spreading to cover. Cover and cook over medium heat 10 to 12 minutes or until eggs are nearly set. Sprinkle cheese over top. Place the skillet under broiler until eggs are set and cheese is melted.

Yield: 4 servings

Each with: 220 g water; 140 calories (26% from fat, 51% from protein, 22% from carb); 18 g protein; 4 g total fat; 1 g saturated fat; 1 g monounsaturated fat; 2 g polyunsaturated fat; 8 g carb; 2 g fiber; 4 g sugar; 283 mg phosphorus; 209 mg calcium; 3 mg iron; 216 mg sodium; 721 mg potassium; 1,618 IU vitamin A; 50 mg vitamin C; 66 mg cholesterol

Glycemic Index: Low

Cottage Cheese Pancakes

These pancakes are lighter than most, thanks to the addition of cottage cheese.

3 eggs

¼ cup (6 g) Splenda

¼ teaspoon salt

1 cup (225 g) cottage cheese

¼ cup (60 ml) skim milk

1 cup (125 g) flour

2 tablespoons (28 g) butter, melted

Beat the eggs with Splenda and salt. Add cottage cheese and milk and beat well. Gradually add flour and beat until smooth. Stir in melted butter. Pour spoonfuls on greased griddle. Turn when lightly browned and brown on other side.

Yield: 4 servings

Each with: 80 g water; 270 calories (35% from fat, 23% from protein, 42% from carb); 15 g Protein; 10 g total fat; 5 g saturated fat; 3 g monounsaturated fat; 1 g polyunsaturated fat; 28 g carb; 1 g fiber; 4 g sugar; 169 mg phosphorous; 59 mg calcium; 2 mg iron; 111 mg sodium; 127 mg potassium; 424 IU vitamin A; 119 mg ATE vitamin E; 0 mg vitamin C; 196 mg cholesterol

Glycemic Index: Low

Cornmeal Pancakes

This is another of those old-fashioned breakfast meals. Do you suppose I keep saying that because people ate more healthy food in the good old days?

1 cup (235 ml) boiling water

¾ cup (105 g) cornmeal

1¼ cups (295 ml) buttermilk

2 eggs

1 cup (120 g) whole wheat pastry flour

1 tablespoon (14 g) baking powder

¼ teaspoon baking soda

¼ cup (60 ml) canola oil

Pour water over cornmeal; stir until thick. Add buttermilk; beat in eggs. Mix flour, baking powder, and baking soda. Add to cornmeal mixture. Stir in canola oil. Bake on hot griddle.

Yield: 7 servings

Each with: 89 g water; 233 calories (40% from fat, 12% from protein, 48% from carb); 7 g protein; 11 g total fat; 1 g saturated fat; 6 g monounsaturated fat; 3 g polyunsaturated fat; 29 g carb; 3 g fiber; 3 g sugar; 190 mg phosphorus; 182 mg calcium; 2 mg iron; 280 mg sodium; 184 mg potassium; 127 IU vitamin A; 0 mg vitamin C; 69 mg cholesterol

Glycemic Index: Low

Cranberry Apricot Waffles

Sweet, fruity sauce makes these waffles special.

½ cup (63 g) flour

½ teaspoon baking powder

4 egg yolks

1 cup (225 g) cottage cheese

1 tablespoon (14 g) unsalted butter, melted

4 egg whites, stiffly beaten

16 ounces (455 g) apricot halves

3 tablespoons (39 g) sugar

2 tablespoons (16 g) cornstarch

1 cup (235 ml) cranberry juice

¼ teaspoon almond extract

Sift together flour and baking powder. In blender, combine next 3 ingredients and flour mixture. Blend until smooth. Fold whites into batter. Bake in preheated waffle baker. Drain and cut up apricots, reserving juice. In saucepan, combine sugar and cornstarch. Stir in apricot juice and cranberry juice. Cook and stir until thick and bubbly. Stir in extract and apricots. Serve warm over waffles.

Yield: 2 servings

Each with: 490 g water; 725 calories (26% from fat, 20% from protein, 54% from carb); 37 g Protein; 21 g total fat; 8 g saturated fat; 7 g monounsaturated fat; 3 g polyunsaturated fat; 99 g carb; 5 g fiber; 46 g sugar; 385 mg phosphorous; 190 mg calcium; 4 mg iron; 445 mg sodium; 696 mg potassium; 4717 IU vitamin A; 232 mg ATE vitamin E; 23 mg vitamin C; 441 mg cholesterol

Glycemic Index: Low

Apple and Banana Fritters

A search for something for breakfast that would use up some overripe bananas was rewarded with this recipe. They are incredibly light and very tasty.

1 cup (120 g) whole wheat pastry flour

1 tablespoon (1½ g) sugar substitute, such as Splenda

1 tablespoon (14 g) baking powder

½ cup (120 ml) skim milk

1 egg

1 tablespoon (15 ml) canola oil

½ cup (75 g) chopped banana

½ cup (63 g) chopped apple

½ teaspoon nutmeg

Stir together flour, sugar substitute, and baking powder. Combine the milk, egg, and oil. Add banana, apple, and nutmeg. Stir into dry ingredients, stirring until just moistened. Drop by tablespoonfuls into hot oil. Fry for 2 to 3 minutes on a side until golden brown. Drain on paper towels before serving.

Yield: 4 servings

Each with: 74 g water; 212 calories (23% from fat, 13% from protein, 64% from carb); 7 g protein; 6 g total fat; 1 g saturated fat; 3 g monounsaturated fat; 1 g polyunsaturated fat; 36 g carb; 5 g fiber; 8 g sugar; 249 mg phosphorus; 267 mg calcium; 2 mg iron; 405 mg sodium; 311 mg potassium; 157 IU vitamin A; 3 mg vitamin C; 60 mg cholesterol

Glycemic Index: Low

Orange Smoothie

Buttermilk and orange juice concentrate provide the flavor here. And a great flavor it is.

1½ cup (355 ml) buttermilk

⅓ cup (83 g) orange juice concentrate

2 tablespoons (30 g) brown sugar

1 teaspoon vanilla

2 ice cubes

In a blender container, combine buttermilk, orange juice concentrate, brown sugar, and vanilla. Cover and blend until smooth. With blender running, add ice cubes one at a time, through opening in lid. Blend until smooth and frothy.

Yield: 1 serving

Each with: 389 g water; 414 calories (7% from fat, 14% from protein, 79% from carb); 14 g Protein; 3 g total fat; 2 g saturated fat; 1 g monounsaturated fat; 0 g polyunsaturated fat; 81 g carb; 1 g fiber; 80 g sugar; 387 mg phosphorous; 480 mg calcium; 1 mg iron; 400 mg sodium; 1295 mg potassium; 454 IU vitamin A; 26 mg ATE vitamin E; 134 mg vitamin C; 15 mg cholesterol

Glycemic Index: Low

Mixed Fruit Smoothie

Smoothies make a quick and easy breakfast, and they are packed with nutrition.

2 cups (460 g) low-fat peach yogurt

1 cup (145 g) blueberries

2 cups (300 g) sliced banana

Mix all ingredients in a blender and then serve.

Yield: 2 servings

Each with: 415 g water; 485 calories (7% from fat, 10% from protein, 83% from carb); 13 g protein; 4 g total fat; 2 g saturated fat; 1 g monounsaturated fat; 0 g polyunsaturated fat; 108 g carb; 8 g fiber; 81 g sugar; 325 mg phosphorus; 354 mg calcium; 1 mg iron; 133 mg sodium; 1,296 mg potassium; 282 IU vitamin A; 28 mg vitamin C; 12 mg cholesterol

Glycemic Index: Low

Banana Smoothie

Smoothies make a great tasting, quick breakfast. I find that having a breakfast that contains protein keeps me from getting hungry as soon, and the milk and yogurt make this a good choice.

1 cup (235 ml) skim milk

2 tablespoons (30 g) yogurt (any flavor)

1 banana, broken in pieces

1 teaspoon honey

Put all ingredients in blender. Whip for 1 minute until smooth. Add ice cubes into blender to thicken, if desired

Yield: 1 serving

Each with: 413 g water; 353 calories (4% from fat, 14% from protein, 82% from carb); 13 g Protein; 2 g total fat; 1 g saturated fat; 0 g monounsaturated fat; 0 g polyunsaturated fat; 77 g carb; 6 g fiber; 39 g sugar; 359 mg phosphorous; 406 mg calcium; 1 mg iron; 164 mg sodium; 1311 mg potassium; 656 IU vitamin A; 153 mg ATE vitamin E; 23 mg vitamin C; 6 mg cholesterol

Glycemic Index: Low

Strawberry Pineapple Smoothie

There's nothing fancy about this smoothie, just great strawberry taste with a little pineapple juice added for sweetness.

½ cup (113 g) frozen strawberries

½ cup (115 g) plain yogurt

¼ cup (60 ml) unsweetened pineapple juice

¼ cup (30 g) nonfat dry milk

Blend all ingredients together in a blender.

Yield: 1 serving

Each with: 216 g water; 240 calories (7% from fat, 19% from protein, 74% from carb); 12 g Protein; 2 g total fat; 1 g saturated fat; 0 g monounsaturated fat; 0 g polyunsaturated fat; 46 g carb; 2 g fiber; 42 g sugar; 324 mg phosphorous; 399 mg calcium; 1 mg iron; 160 mg sodium; 704 mg potassium; 463 IU vitamin A; 134 mg ATE vitamin E; 53 mg vitamin C; 9 mg cholesterol

Glycemic Index: Low

Oat Baked Apple

The cheese gives these baked apples that special touch. They are good for dessert as well as breakfast.

4 ounces (115 g) cheddar cheese

3 tablespoons (15 g) quick cooking oats

2 tablespoons (30 g) brown sugar

1 tablespoon (6 g) oat bran

1 tablespoon (7 g) pecans, coarsely chopped

1 tablespoon (9 g) raisins

¼ teaspoon cinnamon

4 apples, cored

½ cup (120 ml) cold water

Preheat oven to 375°F (190°C, or gas mark 5). Cut half of cheese into small cubes; shred remainder. Mix cheese cubes, oats, brown sugar, oat bran, pecans, raisins, and cinnamon until well blended. Place baking apples in 8 x 8-inch (20 x 20 cm) square pan; fill with oat mixture. Pour water in bottom of pan. Cover with foil; bake 30 minutes. Uncover and continue baking 15 minutes or until tender. Sprinkle with shredded cheese and continue baking until cheese is melted.

Yield: 4 servings

Each with: 152 g water; 239 calories (40% from fat, 13% from protein, 46% from carb); 8 g Protein; 11 g total fat; 6 g saturated fat; 3 g monounsaturated fat; 1 g polyunsaturated fat; 29 g carb; 2 g fiber; 21 g sugar; 190 mg phosphorous; 225 mg calcium; 1 mg iron; 183 mg sodium; 211 mg potassium; 341 IU vitamin A; 75 mg ATE vitamin E; 5 mg vitamin C; 30 mg cholesterol

Glycemic Index: Low

Pineapple Boats

Are you looking for a breakfast meal that's fancy enough to serve guests but doesn't take a long time to fix? These pineapple boats will definitely do the trick.

2 pineapples

1 cup (150 g) seedless green grapes

2 cups (450 g) bananas, sliced

2 tablespoons (30 g) brown sugar

1 teaspoon poppy seeds

½ pound (225 g) ham, thinly sliced

¼ pound (115 g) Swiss cheese, cubed

Slice pineapple lengthwise in half, crown to stem. Leave leafy crown on. Remove tough core. Loosen fruit by cutting to rind; cut in bite size pieces. Place in large bowl. Peel bananas; slice. Cut grapes in half and add to pineapple. Toss with brown sugar and poppy seeds. Line pineapple shells with ham. Spoon fruit mixture on top. Top with cheese.

Yield: 4 servings

Each with: 356 g water; 460 calories (25% from fat, 19% from protein, 56% from carb); 23 g Protein; 14 g total fat; 7 g saturated fat; 4 g monounsaturated fat; 1 g polyunsaturated fat; 68 g carb; 7 g fiber; 46 g sugar; 350 mg phosphorous; 332 mg calcium; 2 mg iron; 616 mg sodium; 977 mg potassium; 459 IU vitamin A; 60 mg ATE vitamin E; 96 mg vitamin C; 49 mg cholesterol

Glycemic Index: Low

5

Main Dishes:
Vegetarian

Vegetarian meals are a great way to up the number of vegetable servings you are eating and get some high-quality protein without either the high-GI carbs or the fat that meat dishes often contain. We have here a selection of quiches and omelets, tofu and portobello mushroom dishes, and soups that will satisfy even the people who think they have to have meat at every meal.

Frittata O'Brien

This sounds like more work than it really is. Once it goes in the oven you are free to do other things. It could also be used for breakfast, where it would serve 8 to 10 people.

½ cup (120 ml) olive oil

2 large potatoes, peeled and thinly sliced

1 cup (160 g) onion, peeled and thinly sliced

1 cup (113 g) zucchini, thinly sliced

½ cup (75 g) red bell pepper, diced

½ cup (75 g) green bell pepper, diced

12 eggs

Pepper to taste

2 tablespoons (8 g) chopped fresh parsley

Preheat oven to 450°F (230°C, or gas mark 8). Pour oil into 12-inch (30 cm) square or round baking dish. Heat oil in oven for 5 minutes, then remove. Place potatoes and onions over bottom of dish and bake until potatoes are just tender, about 20 minutes. Arrange zucchini slices over potatoes and onions and then sprinkle peppers over all. Beat eggs and season with salt and pepper. Add chopped parsley to eggs. Pour eggs over vegetables. Bake until eggs are set and sides are "puffy," about 25 minutes. Top should be golden brown. Serve hot or at room temperature.

Yield: 6 servings

Each with: 252 g water; 426 calories (61% from fat, 16% from protein, 23% from carb); 17 g protein; 29 g total fat; 6 g saturated fat; 17 g monounsaturated fat; 4 g polyunsaturated fat; 25 g carb; 3 g fiber; 4 g sugar; 311 mg phosphorous; 85 mg calcium; 3 mg iron; 169 mg sodium; 858 mg potassium; 1136 IU vitamin A; 156 mg ATE vitamin E; 44 mg vitamin C; 474 mg cholesterol

Glycemic Index: Low

Ricotta Omelet

This makes a nice summer dinner with a salad and bread. You could also add some vegetables if you like.

4 eggs

¼ teaspoon garlic powder

¼ teaspoon black pepper

½ cup (125 g) low-fat ricotta cheese

2 tablespoons (30 ml) olive oil

Beat the eggs with the garlic powder, pepper, and cheese. Heat the oil in a skillet or omelet pan. Add the eggs; swirl to distribute evenly. Cook until nearly set, lifting edge to allow uncooked egg to run underneath. Fold over, cover, and cook until done.

Yield: 2 servings

Each with: 150 g water; 311 calories (66% from fat, 29% from protein, 6% from carb); 22 g protein; 23 g total fat; 6 g saturated fat; 12 g monounsaturated fat; 4 g polyunsaturated fat; 4 g carb; 0 g fiber; 1 g sugar; 266 mg phosphorus; 235 mg calcium; 3 mg iron; 299 mg sodium; 498 mg potassium; 689 IU vitamin A; 0 mg vitamin C; 20 mg cholesterol

Glycemic Index: Low

Mushroom and Pepper Quiche

If you believe that quiche has to include eggs, think again. In this one tofu takes their place, providing the base for a flavorful vegetable mixture.

2 teaspoons (10 ml) olive oil

1 cup (160 g) onion, chopped

¾ cup (113 g) green bell pepper, chopped

2 cups (140 g) mushroom, sliced

2 cloves garlic, minced

2 pounds (900 g) tofu

Sliced tomatoes for garnish

Heat oil in a medium-sized skillet. Sauté vegetables and garlic until soft. In a large bowl, crumble or mash tofu. Add sautéed vegetables. Preheat oven to 350°F (180°C, or gas mark 4). Spread tofu mixture evenly into a 9 or 10-inch (23 x 25 cm) quiche pan. Bake 30 to 40 minutes until the edges of the tofu start to brown. Garnish with tomatoes.

Yield: 6 servings

Each with: 197 g water; 116 calories (43% from fat, 28% from protein, 29% from carb); 8 g Protein; 6 g total fat; 1 g saturated fat; 2 g monounsaturated fat; 3 g polyunsaturated fat; 9 g carb; 1 g fiber; 4 g sugar; 125 mg phosphorous; 56 mg calcium; 1 mg iron; 10 mg sodium; 418 mg potassium; 69 IU vitamin A; 0 mg ATE vitamin E; 17 mg vitamin C; 0 mg cholesterol

Glycemic Index: Low

Onion Pie

There's an old saying around our house that you can never have too many onions, so you can probably guess that this pie is popular.

2 tablespoons (30 ml) olive oil

3 cups (480 g) onions, finely diced

1 cup (235 ml) skim milk

8 ounces (225 g) tofu, crushed by hand

¼ teaspoon black pepper

⅛ teaspoon nutmeg

2 tablespoons (16 g) flour

1 pie crust

Sauté onions in oil until translucent and mostly soft. Blend the milk, tofu, pepper, nutmeg, and flour until smooth. Then combine the onions and the milk mixture. Pour into the prepared pie shell. Bake in a preheated oven at 350°F (180°C, or gas mark 4) for about 30 minutes.

Yield: 6 servings

Each with: 149 g water; 268 calories (52% from fat, 9% from protein, 39% from carb); 6 g Protein; 16 g total fat; 3 g saturated fat; 8 g monounsaturated fat; 4 g polyunsaturated fat; 26 g carb; 3 g fiber; 6 g sugar; 110 mg phosphorous; 85 mg calcium; 1 mg iron; 27 mg sodium; 272 mg potassium; 85 IU vitamin A; 25 mg ATE vitamin E; 6 mg vitamin C; 1 mg cholesterol

Glycemic Index: Low

Cheese Pie

This is an ideal vegetarian main dish, needing only a salad to make it a complete meal.

¼ pound (115 g) feta cheese

16 ounces (455 g) low-fat ricotta cheese

4 eggs

¼ cup (32 g) flour

¾ cup (175 ml) skim milk

¼ teaspoon black pepper

Preheat oven to 375°F (190°C, gas mark 5). Coat an ovenproof skillet or glass baking dish with nonstick vegetable oil spray. Mix the cheeses together and then stir in the eggs, flour, milk, and pepper. Pour the batter into the prepared pan. Bake until golden and set, about 40 minutes. Cut into wedges.

Yield: 4 servings

Each with: 194 g water; 332 calories (47% from fat, 33% from protein, 20% from carb); 27 g protein; 17 g total fat; 10 g saturated fat; 5 g monounsaturated fat; 2 g polyunsaturated fat; 16 g carb; 0 g fiber; 2 g sugar; 439 mg phosphorus; 549 mg calcium; 2 mg iron; 597 mg sodium; 460 mg potassium; 875 IU vitamin A; 1 mg vitamin C; 62 mg cholesterol

Glycemic Index: Low

Eggplant Lasagna

This is truly vegetarian version of lasagna with a flavor that will please even the meat lovers in your family.

1 medium eggplant

2 tablespoons (30 ml) lemon juice

¼ cup (31 g) flour

¼ cup (35 g) cornmeal

½ teaspoon oregano

½ teaspoon garlic powder

⅛ teaspoon black pepper

2 tablespoons (30 ml) oil

Filling

1½ pounds (680 g) firm tofu

¼ cup (60 ml) lemon juice

2 teaspoons (2.8 g) dried basil

1 garlic clove

1½ cup (368 g) tomato sauce

Wash, peel, and slice eggplant into ¼-inch (½ cm) pieces. Spread slices out on racks or paper towels and then sprinkle with lemon juice. Let stand 5–10 minutes and then wipe off with paper towels. While eggplant is standing, mix flour, cornmeal, oregano, garlic powder, and black pepper together in a bowl. Preheat oven to 350°F (180°C, or gas mark 4). Dredge eggplant slices in flour-cornmeal mix. Lay on cookie sheet spread with the oil. Oven-fry slices for 8–10 minutes on each side or until golden brown. While the eggplant slices are baking, prepare the tofu filling. Process the tofu, lemon juice, basil, and garlic in food processor to a fine grainy texture like ricotta cheese. Cover bottom of 8 x 8-inch (20 x 20 cm) pan with ⅓ of the tomato sauce. Use half the oven fried eggplant slices to cover the bottom of the pan. Then spread the tofu filling over, reserving ½ cup (125 g) for the top. Next, cover the tofu filling with the rest of the eggplant slices and pour the remaining tomato sauce over the top. Arrange reserved tofu mix in small dollops over the top. Bake about 45 minutes or until dollops are slightly browned.

(continued on page 110)

Yield: 6 servings

Each with: 241 g water; 192 calories (36% from fat, 21% from protein, 43% from carb); 11 g Protein; 8 g total fat; 1 g saturated fat; 2 g monounsaturated fat; 4 g polyunsaturated fat; 21 g carb; 4 g fiber; 6 g sugar; 153 mg phosphorous; 60 mg calcium; 3 mg iron; 364 mg sodium; 645 mg potassium; 279 IU vitamin A; 0 mg ATE vitamin E; 13 mg vitamin C; 0 mg cholesterol

Glycemic Index: Low

Vegetable "Lasagna"

You could use this as a side dish with something like a grilled chicken breast or just serve it as a vegetarian main dish. I used a George Foreman grill to grill the vegetables, but you could also use a regular grill or roast them in the oven.

4 cups (452 g) zucchini, sliced lengthwise

1 eggplant, sliced

8 ounces (225 g) mushrooms, sliced

1 onion, sliced

2 cups (500 g) spaghetti sauce

1 cup (115 g) shredded mozzarella cheese

Slice vegetables and coat with olive oil spray. Grill until crisp-tender. Place a small amount of sauce in an 8 × 12-inch (20 × 30 cm) baking dish. Layer zucchini, eggplant, more sauce, onion and mushroom, sauce, eggplant, and zucchini. Top with remaining sauce and sprinkle with cheese. Bake at 400°F (200°C, gas mark 6) until cheese is melted and starts to brown, about 15 minutes.

Yield: 6 servings

285 g water; 158 calories (32% from fat, 25% from protein, 43% from carb); 10 g protein; 6 g total fat; 3 g saturated fat; 2 g monounsaturated fat; 1 g polyunsaturated fat; 18 g carb; 6 g fiber; 10 g sugar; 204 mg calcium; 1 mg iron; 40 mg sodium; 807 mg potassium; 912 IU vitamin A; 25 mg vitamin C; 12 mg cholesterol

Glycemic Index: Low

Spinach Rolls

There's something special about anything that has phyllo pastry in it and these rolls are no exception. They are a bit of work to assemble, but they are worth the effort.

2 pounds (900 g) spinach

1 cup (160 g) onion, chopped

1 cup (104 g) leek, chopped

1 cup (100 g) green onion, sliced

⅓ cup (80 ml) olive oil

½ cup (30 g) chopped fresh parsley

3 teaspoons (4 g) chopped fresh dill

¼ teaspoon ground nutmeg

¼ teaspoon freshly ground black pepper

8 phyllo pastry sheets

2 tablespoons (30 ml) olive oil

Wash spinach well and cut off any coarse stems. Chop coarsely and put into a large pan. Cover and place over heat for 7–8 minutes, shaking pan now and then or turning spinach with a fork. Heat just long enough to wilt spinach so that juices can run out freely. Drain well in colander, pressing occasionally with a spoon. Gently fry onions in olive oil for 10 minutes; add chopped leek and green onions and fry gently for 5 minutes until transparent. Place well-drained spinach in a mixing bowl and add oil and onion mixture, herbs, nutmeg, and pepper. Blend thoroughly. Place a sheet of phyllo pastry on work surface and brush lightly with olive oil. Top with 3 more sheets of pastry, brushing each with oil. Brush top layer lightly with oil and place half the spinach mixture along the length of the pastry towards one edge and leaving 1½ inches (3½ cm) clear on each side. Fold bottom edge of pastry over filling, roll once, fold in sides, and then roll up. Place a hand at each end of roll and push it in gently. Repeat with remaining pastry and filling. Place rolls in an oiled baking dish, leaving space between rolls. Brush tops lightly with oil and bake in a moderate oven for 30 minutes until golden. Serve hot, cut into portions.

Yield: 8 servings

(continued on page 112)

Each with: 149 g water; 245 calories (54% from fat, 11% from protein, 35% from carb); 7 g Protein; 16 g total fat; 3 g saturated fat; 10 g monounsaturated fat; 2 g polyunsaturated fat; 23 g carb; 6 g fiber; 3 g sugar; 98 mg phosphorous; 216 mg calcium; 4 mg iron; 211 mg sodium; 489 mg potassium; 14331 IU vitamin A; 0 mg ATE vitamin E; 13 mg vitamin C; 0 mg cholesterol

Glycemic Index: Low

Stuffed Portobellos

We recently discovered the joys of portobello mushrooms. This has become one of our favorite recipes.

2/3 cup (120 g) chopped plum tomato

2 ounces (55 g) part-skim mozzarella cheese, shredded

1 teaspoon olive oil, divided

½ teaspoon fresh rosemary

⅛ teaspoon black pepper, coarse ground

¼ teaspoon crushed garlic

4 portobello mushroom caps, about 4 to 5 inches (10 to 13 cm)

2 tablespoons (30 ml) lemon juice

2 teaspoons (2.6 g) fresh parsley

Prepare grill. Combine the tomato, cheese, ½ teaspoon oil, rosemary, pepper, and garlic in a small bowl. Remove brown gills from the undersides of mushroom caps using a spoon and discard gills. Remove stems and discard. Combine remaining ½ teaspoon oil and lemon juice in a small bowl. Brush over both sides of mushroom caps. Place the mushroom caps, stem sides down, on grill rack coated with nonstick vegetable oil spray and grill for 5 minutes on each side or until soft. Spoon ¼ cup tomato mixture into each mushroom cap. Cover and grill 3 minutes or until cheese is melted. Sprinkle with parsley.

Yield: 4 servings

Each with: 115 g water; 75 calories (40% from fat, 29% from protein, 32% from carb); 6 g protein; 4 g total fat; 2 g saturated fat; 1 g monounsaturated fat; 0 g polyunsaturated fat; 6 g carb; 2 g fiber; 3 g sugar; 181 mg phosphorus; 122 mg calcium; 1 mg iron; 95 mg sodium; 490 mg potassium; 331 IU vitamin A; 8 mg vitamin C; 9 mg cholesterol

Glycemic Index: Low

Vegetable Burgers

Many people think of veggie burgers as being dry and tasteless. These will change their minds.

1 pound (455 g) tofu, mashed

1 cup (80 g) quick cooking oats

½ cup (56 g) wheat germ

1 cup (160 g) onion, finely minced

2 tablespoons (30 ml) Dick's Reduced-Sodium Soy Sauce (see chapter 2)

½ teaspoon basil

½ teaspoon oregano

½ teaspoon garlic powder

⅛ teaspoon black pepper

Mix ingredients together. Knead for a few minutes. Shape into six patties. Oven fry on cookie sheet sprayed with nonstick oil spray at 325°F (170°C, or gas mark 3) for 25 minutes.

Yield: 4 servings

Each with: 139 g water; 212 calories (24% from fat, 24% from protein, 51% from carb); 13 g Protein; 6 g total fat; 1 g saturated fat; 1 g monounsaturated fat; 3 g polyunsaturated fat; 28 g carb; 5 g fiber; 5 g sugar; 342 mg phosphorous; 66 mg calcium; 3 mg iron; 9 mg sodium; 477 mg potassium; 32 IU vitamin A; 0 mg ATE vitamin E; 4 mg vitamin C; 0 mg cholesterol

Glycemic Index: Low

Black Bean Quesadillas

I usually add a bit more cilantro because I like the flavor (and I'm the cook so I can). Use mild or hot salsa according to your own taste.

15 ounces (420 g) black beans, drained

¼ cup (45 g) chopped tomato

3 tablespoons (4 g) chopped cilantro

12 black olives, pitted, sliced

8 whole wheat tortillas, 6-inch (15 cm)

4 ounces (58 g) pepper jack cheese, shredded

1 cup (30 g) spinach leaves, shredded

4 tablespoons (65 g) salsa

Mash beans. Stir in tomato, cilantro, and olives. Spread evenly onto 4 tortillas. Sprinkle with cheese, spinach, and salsa. Top with remaining tortillas. Preheat oven to 350°F (180°C, or gas mark 4). Bake tortillas on ungreased cookie sheet for 12 minutes. Cut into wedges and serve.

Yield: 4 servings

Each with: 142 g water; 457 calories (30% from fat, 19% from protein, 51% from carb); 22 g Protein; 15 g total fat; 7 g saturated fat; 6 g monounsaturated fat; 2 g polyunsaturated fat; 59 g carb; 12 g fiber; 2 g sugar; 362 mg phosphorous; 344 mg calcium; 5 mg iron; 696 mg sodium; 618 mg potassium; 1238 IU vitamin A; 54 mg ATE vitamin E; 4 mg vitamin C; 25 mg cholesterol

Glycemic Index: Low

Beans and Barley

This hearty main dish cooks in the slow cooker while you are gone.

1 cup (215 g) white beans, uncooked

1 cup (193 g) pinto beans, uncooked

¾ cup (120 g) onion, chopped

1 cup (130 g) carrot, chopped

½ cup (35 g) mushrooms, chopped

4 cups (940 g) low-sodium vegetable broth

½ teaspoon prepared mustard

2 tablespoons (8 g) fresh parsley, minced

½ cup (113 g) split peas, dried

¼ cup (50 g) pearl barley

¼ cup (48 g) lentils, dried

Soak white beans and pinto beans overnight. Sauté onion, mushrooms, and carrots in
1 tablespoon (15 ml) of vegetable stock until tender. To sautéed vegetables, add drained
beans, vegetable stock, mustard, and parsley. Bring to boil. Reduce heat, cover, and simmer
45 minutes. Add split peas, lentils, and barley. Transfer all ingredients to a big slow cooker
set on low for 12–14 hours.

Yield: 4 servings

Each with: 337 g water; 487 calories (6% from fat, 26% from protein, 68% from carb); 33 g Protein; 3 g
total fat; 1 g saturated fat; 1 g monounsaturated fat; 1 g polyunsaturated fat; 84 g carb; 22 g fiber; 6 g
sugar; 529 mg phosphorous; 279 mg calcium; 10 mg iron; 181 mg sodium; 2160 mg potassium; 5554 IU
vitamin A; 2 mg ATE vitamin E; 10 mg vitamin C; 0 mg cholesterol

Glycemic Index: Low

Vegetarian Vegetable Soup

This is a good cold-weather meal that makes use of the best late fall and winter vegetables.

6 cups (1.4 L) water

1 onion, chopped

1 teaspoon black pepper

1 teaspoon salt-free seasoning

1 teaspoon basil

2 cups (360 g) chopped tomato

3 potatoes, peeled and diced

2 turnips, peeled and diced

3 carrots, peeled and sliced

½ cup (50 g) sliced celery

12 ounces (340 g) frozen mixed vegetables

2 cups (140 g) shredded cabbage

TIP *Feel free to vary the veggies to meet availability and individual likes.*

Place all ingredients in a large pot. Simmer until vegetables are done.

Yield: 8 servings

Each with: 435 g water; 367 calories (43% from fat, 20% from protein, 37% from carb); 19 g protein; 17 g total fat; 7 g saturated fat; 8 g monounsaturated fat; 1 g polyunsaturated fat; 34 g carb; 6 g fiber; 6 g sugar; 65 mg calcium; 3 mg iron; 122 mg sodium; 858 mg potassium; 84 IU vitamin A; 28 mg vitamin C; 61 mg cholesterol

Glycemic Index: Low

Vegetable Chowder

This quick soup provides a hearty meal in a bowl. Serve with bread and a salad if desired.

1 tablespoon (15 g) olive oil

¼ cup (40 g) onion, chopped

¼ cup (38 g) green pepper, chopped

¼ cup (25 g) celery, chopped

¼ cup (33 g) carrots, chopped

1 clove garlic, minced

⅔ cup (150 g) fat-free cottage cheese

10 ounces (280 g) tomatoes

½ cup (120 ml) water

⅛ teaspoon dried thyme

½ teaspoon dried oregano

¼ teaspoon dried basil

1 cup (195 g) brown rice, cooked

Heat oil in saucepan. Cook onion, pepper, celery, carrots, and garlic until lightly browned. In blender combine cottage cheese, tomatoes, water, and spices. Blend until smooth and add to vegetables. Stir in rice and cook, stirring until heated through. Do not boil.

Yield: 4 servings

Each with: 193 g water; 137 calories (29% from fat, 20% from protein, 51% from carb); 7 g Protein; 5 g total fat; 1 g saturated fat; 3 g monounsaturated fat; 1 g polyunsaturated fat; 18 g carb; 2 g fiber; 2 g sugar; 118 mg phosphorous; 44 mg calcium; 1 mg iron; 174 mg sodium; 288 mg potassium; 1879 IU vitamin A; 4 mg ATE vitamin E; 27 mg vitamin C; 2 mg cholesterol

Glycemic Index: Low

Curried Lentil Stew

We don't have lentils as often as we probably should. When I make something like this tasty stew, I wonder why.

2 tablespoons (30 ml) olive oil

1 cup (160 g) onion, chopped

2 garlic cloves, chopped

1 medium potato, diced

½ cup (65 g) carrot, sliced

½ cup (75 g) green bell peppers, diced

1 tablespoon (6 g) coriander

1 teaspoon cumin

1 teaspoon ginger

1 teaspoon turmeric

1 cup (192 g) lentils

2 cups (475 ml) water

2 tablespoons (32 g) tomato paste

In a large pot, heat oil. Fry onion and garlic for a couple of minutes. Add potatoes, carrots and bell pepper and continue to fry for a few more minutes, stirring occasionally. Add spices and stir-fry for a couple of seconds. Add lentils and tomato paste, stir quickly, and add water. Cover, raise heat and bring to a boil. Reduce heat and simmer gently for 30 minutes. Check the water levels and lentil consistency. Cook for another 15 minutes if lentils are not cooked. Remove from heat and let cool slightly. The mixture should be moist but not overly thin.

Yield: 8 servings

Each with: 142 g water; 112 calories (29% from fat, 13% from protein, 58% from carb); 4 g Protein; 4 g total fat; 1 g saturated fat; 3 g monounsaturated fat; 0 g polyunsaturated fat; 17 g carb; 4 g fiber; 3 g sugar; 89 mg phosphorous; 25 mg calcium; 2 mg iron; 47 mg sodium; 433 mg potassium; 1465 IU vitamin A; 0 mg ATE vitamin E; 17 mg vitamin C; 0 mg cholesterol

Glycemic Index: Low

Split Pea Soup

I'm not sure what I like best about this soup, the great taste or the fact that it cooks while you are away.

1 pound (455 g) dried green split peas, rinsed

1½ cups (195 g) carrots, peeled and sliced

1 cup (160 g) chopped onion

½ cup (50 g) chopped celery

½ teaspoon minced garlic

1 bay leaf

¼ cup (15 g) chopped fresh parsley

½ teaspoon black pepper

1½ quarts (1.4 L) water

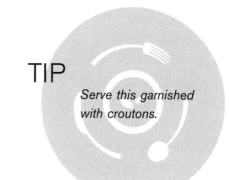

TIP

Serve this garnished with croutons.

Layer ingredients in slow cooker; pour in water. Do not stir. Cover and cook on high 4 to 5 hours or on low 8 to 10 hours until peas are very soft. Remove bay leaf before serving.

Yield: 6 servings

Each with: 338 g water; 363 calories (12% from fat, 32% from protein, 56% from carb); 29 g Protein; 5 g total fat; 1 g saturated fat; 2 g monounsaturated fat; 1 g polyunsaturated fat; 52 g carb; 21 g fiber; 9 g sugar; 403 mg phosphorus; 77 mg calcium; 4 mg iron; 548 mg sodium; 1,088 mg potassium; 5742 IU vitamin A; 9 mg vitamin C; 19 mg cholesterol

Glycemic Index: Low

Apple and Barley Stew

Apple cider gives this stew a unique flavor. When fall comes and the days start getting cooler, this is one of the first recipes we pull out.

2 cups (320 g) onion, thinly sliced

2 tablespoons (30 ml) olive oil

3½ cup (825 ml) low-sodium vegetable broth

1½ cups (355 ml) apple cider

⅓ cup (67 g) pearl barley

1 cup (130 g) carrot, diced

1 teaspoon thyme

¼ teaspoon dried marjoram

1 bay leaf

2 cups (250 g) apples, unpeeled, chopped

¼ cup (15 g) fresh parsley, minced

1 tablespoon (15 ml) lemon juice

In a small soup pot, sauté onions in oil over medium heat for 5 minutes, stirring constantly. Reduce heat, cover, and cook, stirring frequently for 10 minutes more until onions are browned. Add stock, cider, barley, carrots, thyme, marjoram, and bay leaf. Cover and cook for one hour or until barley is tender. Add apples, parsley, and lemon juice. Cook for 5 minutes or until apples are slightly soft. Discard bay leaf and serve.

Yield: 6 servings

Each with: 295 g water; 178 calories (29% from fat, 11% from protein, 60% from carb); 5 g Protein; 6 g total fat; 1 g saturated fat; 4 g monounsaturated fat; 1 g polyunsaturated fat; 28 g carb; 4 g fiber; 14 g sugar; 103 mg phosphorous; 79 mg calcium; 2 mg iron; 103 mg sodium; 440 mg potassium; 3829 IU vitamin A; 1 mg ATE vitamin E; 12 mg vitamin C; 0 mg cholesterol

Glycemic Index: Low

Italian Chickpea Sauce

Can a pasta sauce be made with chickpeas? Yes, and you won't believe how good it is until you try it.

1½ cup (360 g) dried chick peas, soaked

1 tablespoon (15 ml) olive oil

¾ cup (120 g) onion, chopped

2 garlic cloves, crushed

14 ounces (400 g) no-salt-added tomatoes, chopped

6 ounces (170 g) no-salt-added tomato paste

1 teaspoon basil

1 teaspoon oregano

1 dash cinnamon

2 tablespoons (8 g) fresh parsley

Rinse chickpeas, place in fresh water, and cook for 50 minutes or until tender. Heat oil in large pot and sauté onions and garlic for a few minutes. Add the tomatoes and tomato paste. Bring to a boil, lower heat, and add the rest of the ingredients. Simmer for about 10 minutes or until the sauce has thickened.

Yield: 4 servings

Each with: 190 g water; 196 calories (23% from fat, 16% from protein, 61% from carb); 8 g Protein; 5 g total fat; 1 g saturated fat; 3 g monounsaturated fat; 1 g polyunsaturated fat; 32 g carb; 8 g fiber; 12 g sugar; 169 mg phosphorous; 93 mg calcium; 4 mg iron; 61 mg sodium; 861 mg potassium; 973 IU vitamin A; 0 mg ATE vitamin E; 24 mg vitamin C; 0 mg cholesterol

Glycemic Index: Low

6

Main Dishes:
Fish and Seafood

Like vegetarian meals, fish and seafood are low in fat and lend themselves to dishes that feature vegetables and not the higher-GI carbohydrates. Tuna and salmon feature prominently here, but there are also lots of other fish and seafood—all in a variety of flavors from Maryland to Italy to Southeast Asia.

Grilled Salmon Fillets

You can use a whole salmon fillet for this recipe. It makes an impressive display, but it can be difficult to turn. I usually cut the fillet into serving-size pieces, but then you need to be careful not to overcook them and dry them out. The sweetness of the sauce goes well with the salmon.

¼ cup (60 g) brown sugar

2 tablespoons (30 ml) cider vinegar

2 tablespoons (40 g) honey

¼ teaspoon liquid smoke

¼ teaspoon black pepper

¼ teaspoon crushed garlic

2 pounds (900 g) salmon fillets

Preheat the grill. In a small mixing bowl, combine sauce ingredients. Mix well. Brush one side of the salmon with the basting sauce and then place the salmon (basted side down) on the grill. When the salmon is half finished cooking, baste the top portion of the salmon and flip the fillet so the fresh basting sauce is on the grill. When the fish is almost finished cooking, apply the basting sauce and flip the salmon again. Baste and flip the salmon once more and serve. Be careful not to overcook the salmon, as it will lose its juices and flavor if cooked too long.

Yield: 6 servings

Each with: 110 g water; 334 calories (45% from fat, 37% from protein, 18% from carb); 30 g protein; 16 g total fat; 3 g saturated fat; 6 g monounsaturated fat; 6 g polyunsaturated fat; 15 g carb; 0 g fiber; 15 g sugar; 355 mg phosphorus; 27 mg calcium; 1 mg iron; 93 mg sodium; 587 mg potassium; 76 IU vitamin A; 6 mg vitamin C; 89 mg cholesterol

Glycemic Index: Low

Sweet and Spicy Salmon

This is one of our favorite ways to cook fish. The sweet and spicy sauce is reminiscent of the sauce on General Tso's chicken.

2 pounds (900 g) salmon fillets

2 tablespoons (40 g) honey

¼ cup (60 ml) Dick's Reduce-Sodium Soy Sauce (see chapter 2)

1 tablespoon (15 ml) lemon juice

1 tablespoon (15 ml) sesame oil

¼ teaspoon crushed red pepper flakes

Place fish in glass or ceramic baking dish. Combine honey and remaining ingredients and pour over fish to coat. Cover with plastic wrap and marinate 30 minutes before cooking. Light barbecue grill. When coals are ready, oil grill with oil or cooking spray and put in place. Place fish on grill, skin side down if not skinless. Cover and cook 5 minutes. Drizzle fish with marinade and cook 3 minutes more or until fish turns opaque.

Yield: 6 servings

Each with: 108 g water; 319 calories (54% from fat, 39% from protein, 8% from carb); 30 g Protein; 19 g total fat; 4 g saturated fat; 7 g monounsaturated fat; 7 g polyunsaturated fat; 6 g carb; 0 g fiber; 6 g sugar; 353 mg phosphorous; 19 mg calcium; 1 mg iron; 90 mg sodium; 556 mg potassium; 107 IU vitamin A; 23 mg ATE vitamin E; 7 mg vitamin C; 89 mg cholesterol

Glycemic Index: Low

Blackened Salmon

This is salmon blackened the Cajun way. It's one of the more spicy recipes here. You could reduce the amount of cayenne to suit your taste buds.

2 tablespoons (14 g) paprika

1 tablespoon (5 g) cayenne pepper

1 tablespoon (7 g) onion powder

½ teaspoon white pepper

½ teaspoon black pepper

¼ teaspoon thyme

¼ teaspoon basil

¼ teaspoon oregano

1 pound (455 g) salmon fillets

2 tablespoons (30 ml) olive oil

In a small bowl, mix paprika, cayenne pepper, onion powder, white pepper, black pepper, thyme, basil, and oregano. Brush salmon fillets on both sides with oil and sprinkle evenly with the cayenne pepper mixture. Drizzle 1 side of each fillet with half of the remaining oil. In a large, heavy skillet over high heat, cook salmon oiled side down until blackened, 2 to 5 minutes. Turn fillets, drizzle with remaining oil, and continue cooking until blackened and fish is easily flaked with a fork.

Yield: 4 servings

Each with: 79 g water; 289 calories (61% from fat, 32% from protein, 6% from carb); 23 g protein; 20 g total fat; 4 g saturated fat; 9 g monounsaturated fat; 6 g polyunsaturated fat; 5 g carb; 2 g fiber; 1 g sugar; 287 mg phosphorus; 33 mg calcium; 2 mg iron; 70 mg sodium; 541 mg potassium; 2,439 IU vitamin A; 8 mg vitamin C; 67 mg cholesterol

Glycemic Index: Low

Salmon Casserole

This recipe turned up one night during a fairly desperate search for something different to do with fish.

1 pound (455 g) potatoes, peeled and sliced

1½ pounds (680 g) salmon fillets

1 tablespoon (4 g) chopped fresh dill

¼ cup (60 ml) oil, heated

½ cup (120 ml) white wine

¼ cup (60 ml) sherry

½ cup (115 g) fat-free sour cream

2 tablespoons (30 g) grated horseradish

Boil potatoes until almost done, about 10 to 15 minutes. Layer in a large ovenproof casserole. Place the salmon on top. Sprinkle with the dill. Cover and cook at 350°F (180°C, gas mark 4) for 25 minutes. Remove from the oven and pour the heated oil, wine, and sherry over. Continue to cook uncovered until salmon is done. Stir together sour cream and horseradish and pour over top.

Yield: 6 servings

Each with: 162 g water; 346 calories (58% from fat, 23% from protein, 19% from carb); 19 g protein; 21 g total fat; 4 g saturated fat; 6 g monounsaturated fat; 8 g polyunsaturated fat; 16 g carb; 2 g fiber; 2 g sugar; 265 mg phosphorus; 53 mg calcium; 1 mg iron; 80 mg sodium; 719 mg potassium; 152 IU vitamin A; 11 mg vitamin C; 56 mg cholesterol

Glycemic Index: Low

Salmon Hash

When I was growing up canned salmon was cheaper than tuna and we had it fairly often. The recipe is similar to one my mother used to make, really just a simple mixture of salmon and potatoes with a few additions for flavor.

1 tablespoon (15 ml) vegetable oil

½ cup (80 g) chopped onion

½ cup (75 g) green bell peppers, chopped

½ cup (75 g) red bell peppers, chopped

⅛ teaspoon pepper

1 clove garlic, crushed

2 medium potatoes, diced and cooked

16 ounces (455 g) salmon

Heat oil in 10-inch (25 cm) nonstick skillet over medium-high heat. Sauté onion, bell peppers, pepper, and garlic in oil. Stir in potatoes and salmon. Cook uncovered, stirring frequently, until hot.

Yield: 4 servings

Each with: 282 g water; 336 calories (27% from fat, 34% from protein, 39% from carb); 28 g Protein; 10 g total fat; 2 g saturated fat; 3 g monounsaturated fat; 4 g polyunsaturated fat; 33 g carb; 4 g fiber; 4 g sugar; 528 mg phosphorous; 309 mg calcium; 2 mg iron; 98 mg sodium; 1281 mg potassium; 738 IU vitamin A; 20 mg ATE vitamin E; 56 mg vitamin C; 44 mg cholesterol

Glycemic Index: Low

Grilled Tuna with Honey Mustard

These tuna steaks can be grilled or broiled. If it's not good weather for outdoor grilling, they also work well on a contact grill like the George Foreman models.

⅓ cup (80 ml) red wine vinegar

1 tablespoon (11 g) spicy brown mustard

1 tablespoon (20 g) honey

3 tablespoons (45 ml) extra virgin olive oil

1 pound (455 g) tuna steaks

Combine the first 4 ingredients in a jar or covered container; shake to mix well. Put tuna in a food storage bag; add the mustard mixture. Seal the bag and let marinate for about 20 minutes. Heat the grill. Remove the tuna from the marinade and pour the marinade in a small saucepan. Bring marinade to a boil; remove from heat and set aside. Grill the tuna over high heat for about 2 minutes on each side or until done as desired. Drizzle with the hot marinade.

Yield: 4 servings

Each with: 100 g water; 275 calories (53% from fat, 40% from protein, 7% from carb); 27 g protein; 16 g total fat; 3 g saturated fat; 9 g monounsaturated fat; 3 g polyunsaturated fat; 5 g carb; 0 g fiber; 4 g sugar; 294 mg phosphorus; 13 mg calcium; 1 mg iron; 89 mg sodium; 302 mg potassium; 2,478 IU vitamin A; 0 mg vitamin C; 43 mg cholesterol

Glycemic Index: Low

Tuna Steaks

If you get them on sale, tuna steaks are one of the cheaper fish products you can buy. The key to cooking them is not to overcook them and dry them out. It's all right for them to be medium or even medium rare. Soaking them in a simple marinade also helps to keep them moist and flavorful.

6 ounces (170 g) tuna steaks

2 tablespoons (30 ml) olive oil

2 tablespoons (30 ml) lemon juice

½ teaspoon black pepper, fresh ground

Combine the olive oil and lemon juice. Marinate the steaks in the mixture at least 30 minutes, turning occasionally. Heat a skillet over high heat. Add the steaks and cook 2 minutes. Sprinkle with pepper, turn over, and cook 2 minutes longer.

Yield: 2 servings

Each with: 72 g water; 247 calories (65% from fat, 33% from protein, 3% from carb); 20 g protein; 1 8 g total fat; 3 g saturated fat; 11 g monounsaturated fat; 3 g polyunsaturated fat; 2 g carb; 0 g fiber; 0 g sugar; 10 mg calcium; 1 mg iron; 34 mg sodium; 240 mg potassium; 1,861 IU vitamin A; 7 mg vitamin C; 32 mg cholesterol

Glycemic Index: Low

Tuna Burger

These burgers are good either in a sandwich or just on their own. The nutritional counts are based on reduced-sodium tuna packed in water and bread crumbs without salt.

2 cans (5 ounces or 162 g each) tuna, low-sodium and packed in water

½ cup (60 g) bread crumbs

2 eggs

2 tablespoons (20 g) minced onion

¼ teaspoon garlic powder

½ teaspoon dry mustard

Drain tuna. Combine with bread crumbs, eggs, and spices. Form into 4 patties. Grill or fry until browned, turn, and continue cooking until done.

Yield: 4 servings

Each with: 185 calories (13% from fat, 60% from protein, 27% from carb); 27 g protein; 2 g total fat; 1 g saturated fat; 1 g monounsaturated fat; 1 g polyunsaturated fat; 12 g carb; 1 g fiber; 63 mg calcium; 3 mg iron; 98 mg sodium; 373 mg potassium; 725 IU vitamin A; 2 mg vitamin C; 25 mg cholesterol

Glycemic Index: Low

Dilly Tuna Salad

This recipe is easy to make and has the great taste of dill that goes so well with fish. You'll wonder why you never thought of adding dill to tuna salad before. This recipe works great either for sandwiches or as a salad with lettuce and whatever other veggies you want to add.

1 cup (284 g) light tuna, in water, drained

¼ cup (25 g) celery, chopped

2 tablespoons (28 g) low-fat mayonnaise

3 tablespoons (12 g) fresh dill, chopped

2 tablespoons (20 g) white onions, diced

Pepper to taste

Mix all ingredients well.

Yield: 2 servings

Each with: 26 g water; 66 calories (66% from fat, 7% from protein, 27% from carb); 1 g Protein; 5 g total fat; 1 g saturated fat; 0 g monounsaturated fat; 0 g polyunsaturated fat; 5 g carb; 1 g fiber; 1 g sugar; 39 mg phosphorous; 93 mg calcium; 2 mg iron; 140 mg sodium; 212 mg potassium; 419 IU vitamin A; 0 mg ATE vitamin E; 4 mg vitamin C; 5 mg cholesterol

Glycemic Index: Low

Parmesan Crusted Catfish

Catfish is one of our favorite fish and this crunchy presentation is one of our favorite ways to prepare it. It's perfect with just a steamed fresh vegetable.

8 catfish fillets

1 cup (115 g) bread crumbs

¾ cup (75 g) parmesan cheese, grated

¼ cup (15 g) fresh parsley, chopped

1 teaspoon paprika

½ teaspoon oregano

¼ teaspoon basil

½ teaspoon pepper

½ cup (112 g) melted butter

Pat fish dry. Combine bread crumbs, cheese, and seasonings; stir well. Dip catfish in butter and roll each in crumb mixture. Arrange fish in well-greased 13 x 9 x 2-inch (33 x 23 x 5 cm) baking dish. Bake at 375°F (190°C, or gas mark 4) about 25 minutes or until fish flakes easily when tested with a fork.

Yield: 8 servings

Each with: 127 g water; 412 calories (60% from fat, 30% from protein, 10% from carb); 30 g Protein; 27 g total fat; 12 g saturated fat; 10 g monounsaturated fat; 3 g polyunsaturated fat; 10 g carb; 1 g fiber; 1 g sugar; 418 mg phosphorous; 151 mg calcium; 2 mg iron; 311 mg sodium; 536 mg potassium; 797 IU vitamin A; 130 mg ATE vitamin E; 4 mg vitamin C; 113 mg cholesterol

Glycemic Index: Low

Swordfish Kabobs

This recipe is simplicity itself. Swordfish and veggies are grilled on skewers, with just a little lemon juice added. The nice thing about swordfish is that it has firm enough flesh to let you do this without worrying about it falling apart.

1 pound (455 g) swordfish steak portions cut in 2-inch (5 cm) pieces

2 red bell peppers, cut in 2-inch (5 cm) pieces

2 yellow bell peppers, cut in 2-inch (5 cm) pieces

1 onion, quartered

1 tablespoon (15 ml) lemon juice

On 8 skewers, alternate fish with peppers and onion. Sprinkle with lemon juice. Grill over medium grill. Cook until fish turns opaque and flesh flakes.

Yield: 4 servings

Each with: 279 g water; 199 calories (22% from fat, 49% from protein, 29% from carb); 25 g Protein; 5 g total fat; 1 g saturated fat; 2 g monounsaturated fat; 1 g polyunsaturated fat; 14 g carb; 3 g fiber; 5 g sugar; 352 mg phosphorous; 29 mg calcium; 2 mg iron; 109 mg sodium; 744 mg potassium; 2656 IU vitamin A; 41 mg ATE vitamin E; 272 mg vitamin C; 44 mg cholesterol

Glycemic Index: Low

Tropical Mahi Mahi

Citrus juice and just a little honey give this recipe a refreshing flavor. We often grill the fish rather than broiling.

1 pound (455 g) mahi mahi

⅓ cups (80 ml) orange juice

3 tablespoons (45 ml) lime juice

1 tablespoon (21 g) honey

1 clove garlic, crushed

Cut fish steaks into 4 serving pieces. Place in ungreased square baking dish, 8 x 8 x 2 inches (20 x 20 x 5 cm). Mix remaining ingredients and pour over fish. Cover and refrigerate at least 1 hour but no longer than 6 hours, turning once. Set oven control to broil. Spray broiler pan rack with nonstick cooking spray. Remove fish from marinade; reserve marinade. Place fish on rack in broiler pan. Broil with tops about 4 inches (10 cm) from heat for 12 to 15 minutes, turning and brushing with marinade after 6 minutes, until fish flakes easily with fork.

Yield: 4 servings

Each with: 110 g water; 152 calories (7% from fat, 73% from protein, 20% from carb); 27 g Protein; 1 g total fat; 0 g saturated fat; 0 g monounsaturated fat; 0 g polyunsaturated fat; 7 g carb; 0 g fiber; 5 g sugar; 212 mg phosphorous; 26 mg calcium; 2 mg iron; 129 mg sodium; 660 mg potassium; 258 IU vitamin A; 70 mg ATE vitamin E; 10 mg vitamin C; 107 mg cholesterol

Glycemic Index: Low

Chilean Sea Bass, Pan-Seared with Lime

This may be a simple preparation, but it has great flavor.

2 Chilean sea bass fillets (8 ounces or 225 g each)

½ teaspoon black pepper

2 tablespoons (16 g) flour

2 tablespoons (30 ml) olive oil

1 lime, zested and juiced

½ cup (120 ml) white wine

Sprinkle the fillets with pepper and then dust with flour and set aside. In a large sauté pan or skillet over medium-high heat, cook the seasoned fillets in olive oil for 3 minutes or until the undersides are golden brown. Turn the fillets and add lime zest, lime juice, and white wine. Gently shake the pan to distribute the juices and then cover, reduce heat to medium-low, and cook 3 minutes or until the fish is just cooked through. Transfer the fillets to warm plates and drizzle pan juices over each serving.

Yield: 2 servings

Each with: 208 g water; 529 calories (46% from fat, 47% from protein, 7% from carb); 56 g protein; 24 g total fat; 4 g saturated fat; 14 g monounsaturated fat; 5 g polyunsaturated fat; 8 g carb; 0 g fiber; 1 g sugar; 601 mg phosphorus; 243 mg calcium; 5 mg iron; 797 mg sodium; 1,091 mg potassium; 262 IU vitamin A; 5 mg vitamin C; 197 mg cholesterol

Glycemic Index: Low

Baked Fish

The use of lime instead of lemon juice gives these fish fillets a little different flavor. And that can be a good thing when you are trying to increase the number of heart healthy fish meals you eat.

1 pound (455 g) halibut fillets

2 tablespoons (30 ml) olive oil, divided

2 garlic cloves, finely chopped

¼ teaspoon ground black pepper

1 cup (160 g) onion, finely chopped

2 bay leaves

2 tablespoons (30 ml) lime juice

Preheat oven to 325°F (170°C, or gas mark 4). In 9 x 13-inch (23 x 33 cm) baking pan, spread 1 teaspoon (15 ml) olive oil; top with fillets. Over fillets, spread garlic, pepper, onion, and bay leaves. Sprinkle with lime juice and the remaining tablespoon olive oil. Cover and bake until fish is opaque and starts to flake, about 25 to 30 minutes. Remove bay leaves and garnish with lime wedges, if desired.

Yield: 4 servings

Each with: 131 g water; 203 calories (43% from fat, 48% from protein, 9% from carb); 24 g Protein; 9 g total fat; 1 g saturated fat; 6 g monounsaturated fat; 2 g polyunsaturated fat; 4 g carb; 1 g fiber; 2 g sugar; 265 mg phosphorous; 64 mg calcium; 1 mg iron; 63 mg sodium; 579 mg potassium; 183 IU vitamin A; 53 mg ATE vitamin E; 5 mg vitamin C; 36 mg cholesterol

Glycemic Index: Low

Grilled Hawaiian Fish Fillets

This is a really simple recipe with pineapple juice and bottled steak sauce providing lots of flavor. This is great with steamed broccoli and a little rice to soak up the extra sauce.

2 pounds (900 g) fish fillets

½ cup (120 ml) pineapple juice

¼ cup (60 ml) steak sauce

Dash of pepper

TIP *Use the chili sauce in chapter 2 as a lower sodium replacement for the steak sauce.*

Place fish in single layer in shallow baking dish. Combine remaining ingredients and pour over fish. Let stand 30 minutes; turn once. Remove fish, reserving sauce for basting. Place fish on broiler pan sprayed with nonstick vegetable oil spray. Broil about 4 minutes, brushing with sauce. Turn carefully and brush with sauce. Broil until fish flakes when tested with fork. Garnish with lime wedges or pineapple if desired.

Yield: 6 servings

Each with: 138 g water; 236 calories (45% from fat, 41% from protein, 13% from carb); 24 g Protein; 12 g total fat; 3 g saturated fat; 5 g monounsaturated fat; 2 g polyunsaturated fat; 8 g carb; 0 g fiber; 6 g sugar; 307 mg phosphorous; 16 mg calcium; 1 mg iron; 181 mg sodium; 479 mg potassium; 77 IU vitamin A; 23 mg ATE vitamin E; 3 mg vitamin C; 71 mg cholesterol

Glycemic Index: Low

Deviled Fish Broil

A spicy mustard sauce lifts these fish fillets out of the ordinary and makes them a great choice when you are looking for something a little different for dinner.

1 teaspoon onion flakes

¼ teaspoon Tabasco

½ teaspoon Worcestershire sauce

½ teaspoon Dick's Reduced-Sodium Soy Sauce (see chapter 2)

1 tablespoon prepared mustard

½ teaspoon parsley, fresh, minced

8 ounces (225 g) tilapia fillets

Combine all ingredients except fish. Mix well. Brush on both sides of fish. Broil until fish flakes easily with fork.

Yield: 2 servings

Each with: 90 g water; 136 calories (21% from fat, 75% from protein, 4% from carb); 24 g Protein; 3 g total fat; 0 g saturated fat; 1 g monounsaturated fat; 1 g polyunsaturated fat; 1 g carb; 0 g fiber; 0 g sugar; 256 mg phosphorous; 61 mg calcium; 1 mg iron; 78 mg sodium; 550 mg potassium; 221 IU vitamin A; 53 mg ATE vitamin E; 3 mg vitamin C; 36 mg cholesterol

Glycemic Index: Low

Barbecued Fish

This easy barbecue sauce starts with catsup that's spiced for a bit zing. We usually use catfish, but you can use whatever kind of fish you prefer and it will still be good

1 pound (455 g) catfish

¼ cup (60 ml) low-sodium catsup

3 tablespoons (45 ml) lemon juice

1 tablespoon (15 ml) Worcestershire sauce

2 teaspoons (10 g) instant minced onion

Dash Tabasco

Place fish fillets in ungreased 13 x 9 x 2-inch (33 x 23 x 5 cm) baking pan. Mix catsup, lemon juice, Worcestershire sauce, sugar, onion, and pepper sauce. Pour on fish; turn until both sides are coated. Cover and refrigerate 30 minutes. Heat oven to 400°F (200°C, or gas mark 6). Bake, uncovered, until fish flakes easily with fork, 15 to 20 minutes.

Yield: 3 servings

Each with: 143 g water; 235 calories (45% from fat, 41% from protein, 14% from carb); 24 g Protein; 12 g total fat; 3 g saturated fat; 5 g monounsaturated fat; 2 g polyunsaturated fat; 8 g carb; 0 g fiber; 5 g sugar; 322 mg phosphorous; 21 mg calcium; 1 mg iron; 134 mg sodium; 605 mg potassium; 271 IU vitamin A; 23 mg ATE vitamin E; 21 mg vitamin C; 71 mg cholesterol

Glycemic Index: Low

Honey Mustard Fish

Mustard with just a little honey can give a great flavor to just about any kind of fish.

¾ pounds (340 g) fish, such as bass

2 tablespoons (22 g) Dijon mustard

1 tablespoon (11 g) grainy mustard

2 teaspoons (5 g) ground cumin

1 tablespoon (21 g) honey

Preheat oven to 400°F (200°C, or gas mark 6). Line a baking sheet with foil and lightly spray with cooking spray. In a small bowl, stir together the mustards, cumin, and honey. Rinse fish and pat dry. Spoon mustard coating on both sides of fish and place on prepared baking sheet. For fish 1½ inches thick, bake 20 minutes. Place fish on individual plates and pour pan juices over top.

Yield: 2 servings

(continued on page 140)

Each with: 149 g water; 249 calories (28% from fat, 54% from protein, 18% from carb); 33 g Protein; 8 g total fat; 1 g saturated fat; 3 g monounsaturated fat; 2 g polyunsaturated fat; 11 g carb; 1 g fiber; 9 g sugar; 374 mg phosphorous; 168 mg calcium; 4 mg iron; 378 mg sodium; 678 mg potassium; 211 IU vitamin A; 51 mg ATE vitamin E; 4 mg vitamin C; 116 mg cholesterol

Glycemic Index: Low

Fish with Mayo Coating

Yes, I know it sounds strange, but it works, making the fish moist as well as adding flavor. We used bluefish that my daughter caught out on the Chesapeake Bay, but perch, orange roughy, or any other fish would work well too.

¾ pound (340 g) bluefish fillets

¼ cup (60 g) low-sodium mayonnaise

1 teaspoon dill

½ teaspoon onion powder

½ teaspoon lemon pepper

Place fish is ovenproof dish. Mix remaining ingredients and spread over fish. Bake at 350°F (180°C, gas mark 4) until fish flakes easily, about 10 to 15 minutes.

Yield: 2 servings

Each with: 45 g water; 272 calories (80% from fat, 17% from protein, 3% from carb); 12 g protein; 24 g total fat; 4 g saturated fat; 7 g monounsaturated fat; 11 g polyunsaturated fat; 2 g carb; 0 g fiber; 0 g sugar; 141 mg phosphorus; 23 mg calcium; 1 mg iron; 44 mg sodium; 248 mg potassium; 333 IU vitamin A; 0 mg vitamin C; 49 mg cholesterol

Glycemic Index: Low

Herbed Fish

Here's a simple baked fish made flavorful by a combination of herbs and spices.

2 pounds (900 g) perch, or other firm white fish

1 tablespoon (15 ml) olive oil

½ teaspoon garlic powder

½ teaspoon marjoram

⅓ teaspoon thyme

⅛ teaspoon white pepper

2 bay leaves

½ cup (80 g) chopped onion

½ cup (120 ml) white wine

Preheat oven to 350°F (180°C, gas mark 4). Wash fish, pat dry, and place in dish. Combine oil with and herbs and spices. Dribble over fish. Top with bay leaves and onion. Pour wine over all. Bake, uncovered, for 20 to 30 minutes or until fish flakes easily with a fork. Remove bay leaves before serving.

Yield: 6 servings

Each with: 148 g water; 185 calories (26% from fat, 69% from protein, 5% from carb); 28 g protein; 5 g total fat; 1 g saturated fat; 3 g monounsaturated fat; 1 g polyunsaturated fat; 2 g carb; 0 g fiber; 1 g sugar; 335 mg phosphorus; 169 mg calcium; 2 mg iron; 115 mg sodium; 450 mg potassium; 67 IU vitamin A; 2 mg vitamin C; 64 mg cholesterol

Glycemic Index: Low

Italian Baked Fish

This dish uses ingredients that I don't use very often, like capers and anchovies. Maybe that's why the flavor pleases me so much, because it's not an everyday sort of taste.

1 pound (455 g) bluefish, or other firm white fish

¼ cup (60 ml) dry red wine

2 tablespoons (13 g) ripe olives, chopped

1 tablespoon (8.6 g) capers

4 anchovy fillets, chopped

2 cloves garlic, crushed

28 ounces (795 g) plum tomato, chopped

Preheat oven to 350°F (180°C, or gas mark 4). Cut fish fillets into 4 serving pieces. Place in ungreased square baking dish, 8 X 8 X 2 inches (20 x 20 x 5 cm). Mix remaining ingredients; pour over fish. Bake uncovered about 40 minutes or until fish flakes easily with fork.

Yield: 4 servings

Each with: 288 g water; 203 calories (28% from fat, 54% from protein, 18% from carb); 26 g Protein; 6 g total fat; 1 g saturated fat; 3 g monounsaturated fat; 2 g polyunsaturated fat; 9 g carb; 3 g fiber; 5 g sugar; 319 mg phosphorous; 43 mg calcium; 2 mg iron; 326 mg sodium; 934 mg potassium; 2126 IU vitamin A; 137 mg ATE vitamin E; 25 mg vitamin C; 70 mg cholesterol

Glycemic Index: Low

Oven-Poached Fish

This is a really easy recipe that gives you fish that is a joy to eat, perfectly cooked, and subtly flavored.

4 halibut fillets, 1-inch (2½ cm) thick

¼ cup (16 g) fresh dill

4 slices lemon

2 tablespoons (10 g) black peppercorns

¼ cup (60 ml) dry white wine

Salt

Preheat oven to 450°F (230°C, or gas mark 8).. Place fish steaks in ungreased rectangular baking dish, 12 x 7 x 2 inches (30 x 18 x 5 cm). Sprinkle with salt. Place dill weed sprigs and lemon slice on each. Top with peppercorns. Pour wine over fish. Bake uncovered 20 to 25 minutes or until fish flakes easily.

Yield: 4 servings

Each with: 383 g water; 486 calories (19% from fat, 74% from protein, 7% from càrb); 86 g Protein; 10 g total fat; 1 g saturated fat; 3 g monounsaturated fat; 3 g polyunsaturated fat; 8 g carb; 2 g fiber; 2 g sugar; 924 mg phosphorous; 223 mg calcium; 5 mg iron; 224 mg sodium; 1971 mg potassium; 706 IU vitamin A; 192 mg ATE vitamin E; 32 mg vitamin C; 131 mg cholesterol

Glycemic Index: Low

Fish Fritters

Light, puffy balls of fish are deep fried to make these tasty morsels. They are great for an appetizer, but they also work well as a starting point for dinner.

1 pound (455 g) cod

3 eggs, separated

3 tablespoons (24 g) flour

1/8 teaspoon pepper

1/8 teaspoon garlic powder

1 tablespoon (4 g) fresh parsley, minced

Cook fish, remove skin and bones, and mash. Beat egg yolks until light and thick; then add flour, pepper, garlic, parsley, and fish. Fold in whites of eggs beaten until stiff. Drop by tablespoons into hot deep fat and fry until golden brown.

Yield: 4 servings

Each with: 126 g water; 175 calories (27% from fat, 62% from protein, 12% from carb); 26 g Protein; 5 g total fat; 1 g saturated fat; 2 g monounsaturated fat; 1 g polyunsaturated fat; 5 g carb; 0 g fiber; 0 g sugar; 318 mg phosphorous; 43 mg calcium; 2 mg iron; 121 mg sodium; 537 mg potassium; 332 IU vitamin A; 72 mg ATE vitamin E; 3 mg vitamin C; 226 mg cholesterol

Glycemic Index: Low

Shrimp Kabobs

These shrimp and veggies marinate in an unusual sauce containing mayonnaise and fresh cilantro. The resulting flavor is different, but it's different in a very good way.

⅓ cup (80 ml) Worcestershire sauce

½ cup (115 g) low-fat mayonnaise

½ cup (120 ml) lemon juice

2 cups (475 ml) clam juice

1 tablespoon (15 g) brown sugar

¼ cup (4 g) fresh chopped cilantro

1½ pounds (680 g) shrimp, peeled

1 cup (150 g) green bell pepper, cut in 1-inch (2½ cm) cubes

1 cup (150 g) red bell pepper, cut in 1-inch (2½ cm) cubes

1 onion, peeled and quartered

12 mushrooms

In oblong baking dish long enough to contain skewers, combine Worcestershire sauce, mayonnaise, lemon juice, clam juice, brown sugar, and cilantro, stirring briskly with fork to blend. On 6 long or 12 small skewers, arrange shrimp alternately with vegetables, ending with a mushroom to anchor (use 2 mushrooms if using long skewers, one at each end). Place skewers in pan with marinade, cover, and let stand 20 minutes or refrigerate overnight, turning often to coat all sides. Heat grill to medium. Remove kabobs from marinade and drain, reserving marinade. Cook kabobs over grill, about 4 minutes on each side, until seafood is cooked but still tender and vegetables are lightly browned. Heat remaining marinade to boiling in small saucepan and spoon over skewers before serving.

Yield: 6 servings

Each with: 226 g water; 242 calories (33% from fat, 42% from protein, 26% from carb); 25 g Protein; 9 g total fat; 1 g saturated fat; 0 g monounsaturated fat; 1 g polyunsaturated fat; 16 g carb; 2 g fiber; 7 g sugar; 313 mg phosphorous; 76 mg calcium; 4 mg iron; 465 mg sodium; 625 mg potassium; 1247 IU vitamin A; 61 mg ATE vitamin E; 91 mg vitamin C; 179 mg cholesterol

Glycemic Index: Low

Shrimp Scampi

Shrimp scampi is one of those dishes that seems to say "fancy", but it is really very easy to make. This recipe is ready to eat in only about 5 minutes.

1 teaspoon unsalted butter

2 teaspoons (10 ml) olive oil

3 garlic cloves, minced

1 pound (455 g) shrimp, peeled

¼ cup (60 ml) white wine

1 teaspoon lemon juice

¼ teaspoon ground black pepper

In sauté pan, melt butter and oil. Add garlic; sauté 1 minute. Add shrimp; sauté 1 minute. Add wine, lemon juice, and pepper. Sauté quickly until sauce reduces and shrimp turns pink, about 3 minutes. Do not overcook.

Yield: 6 servings

Each with: 67 g water; 108 calories (32% from fat, 64% from protein, 4% from carb); 15 g Protein; 3 g total fat; 1 g saturated fat; 1 g monounsaturated fat; 1 g polyunsaturated fat; 1 g carb; 0 g fiber; 0 g sugar; 157 mg phosphorous; 41 mg calcium; 2 mg iron; 113 mg sodium; 149 mg potassium; 156 IU vitamin A; 46 mg ATE vitamin E; 2 mg vitamin C; 117 mg cholesterol

Glycemic Index: Low

Fluffy Shrimp Omelet

Omelets are great because they can be used either for breakfast or dinner. I generally use a cast iron skillet for this one, which starts cooking on the stove and then gets transferred to the oven to set the top without turning.

8 ounces (225 g) shrimp, cooked

6 eggs, separated

3 tablespoons (42 g) unsalted butter, divided

½ cup (35 g) mushrooms

½ cup (55 g) Swiss cheese, grated

Pepper to taste

Preheat oven to 350°F (180°C, or gas mark 4). Sauté mushrooms and green onions in 2 tablespoons (28 g) butter. Beat egg whites until stiff. In a separate bowl, beat egg yolks and pepper. Fold into the beaten egg whites. Then add mushrooms, onions, grated cheese, and shrimp. Fold together gently. Melt remaining 1 tablespoon (14 g) butter in a heavy, ovenproof skillet. Pour omelet mixture into the skillet and spread evenly. Cook over low heat 3–5 minutes to brown the bottom. Then bake at 350°F (180°C, or gas mark 4) for 5–10 minutes until a knife inserted in the center comes out clean.

Yield: 4 servings

Each with: 123 g water; 320 calories (63% from fat, 34% from protein, 3% from carb); 27 g Protein; 23 g total fat; 11 g saturated fat; 7 g monounsaturated fat; 2 g polyunsaturated fat; 2 g carb; 0 g fiber; 1 g sugar; 387 mg phosphorous; 235 mg calcium; 3 mg iron; 205 mg sodium; 266 mg potassium; 912 IU vitamin A; 254 mg ATE vitamin E; 1 mg vitamin C; 480 mg cholesterol

Tip: You can use salmon or any other seafood in place of the shrimp.

Glycemic Index: Low

Garlic Scallops

These scallops are so simple to make and taste so great that you'll want to have them often. I stock up when scallops are on sale just so we always have some in the freezer.

3 tablespoons (24 g) flour

Pepper to taste

1 pound (455 g) scallops

2 tablespoons (42 g) unsalted butter

3 cloves garlic, minced

2 tablespoons (2.6 g) dried parsley flakes

2 tablespoons (30 ml) lemon juice

In a shallow bowl, combine flour and pepper. Add scallops and toss to coat. Melt butter in skillet. Add garlic and cook two minutes, stirring frequently. Add scallops and cook, turning frequently, until cooked through, about 5 minutes. Sprinkle with parsley and lemon juice.

Yield: 4 servings

Each with: 98 g water; 176 calories (35% from fat, 46% from protein, 19% from carb); 20 g Protein; 7 g total fat; 4 g saturated fat; 2 g monounsaturated fat; 1 g polyunsaturated fat; 8 g carb; 0 g fiber; 0 g sugar; 259 mg phosphorous; 41 mg calcium; 1 mg iron; 187 mg sodium; 410 mg potassium; 309 IU vitamin A; 65 mg ATE vitamin E; 8 mg vitamin C; 53 mg cholesterol

Glycemic Index: Low

Cioppino

Cioppino is a traditional fisherman's stew made from a combination of whatever the catch was that day. Our version contains fish, shrimp, and clams, but feel free to add crab or other seafood or to use multiple varieties of fish.

1 pound (455 g) catfish

½ cup (75 g) green bell pepper, cut into ½-inch (1 cm) squares

2 tablespoons (20 g) onion, finely chopped

1 clove garlic, minced

1 tablespoon (15 ml) cooking oil

6 ounces (170 g) tomatoes, cut up

8 ounces (225 g) no-salt-added tomato sauce

½ cup (120 ml) dry white wine

3 tablespoons (12 g) fresh parsley

¼ teaspoon oregano, crushed

¼ teaspoon basil, crushed

Dash of pepper

12 ounces (340 g) shrimp, frozen or fresh

7 ounces (200 g) minced clams

Cut fillets into 1-inch (1 cm) pieces; set aside. In a 3 quart saucepan, cook green pepper, onion, and garlic in hot oil until onion is tender, not brown. Add undrained tomatoes, tomato sauce, wine, parsley, oregano, basil, and pepper. Bring to a boil. Reduce heat. Cover; simmer 20 minutes. Add fish pieces, shrimp, and undrained clams. Bring just to boiling. Reduce heat; cover and simmer 5 to 7 minutes or until fish and shrimp are done.

Yield: 6 servings

Each with: 215 g water; 272 calories (35% from fat, 52% from protein, 13% from carb); 33 g Protein; 10 g total fat; 2 g saturated fat; 4 g monounsaturated fat; 3 g polyunsaturated fat; 8 g carb; 1 g fiber; 2 g sugar; 408 mg phosphorous; 81 mg calcium; 12 mg iron; 170 mg sodium; 794 mg potassium; 846 IU vitamin A; 99 mg ATE vitamin E; 34 mg vitamin C; 144 mg cholesterol

Glycemic Index: Low

Maryland Crab Soup

This soup is a typical Maryland crab soup. It's full of crabmeat, tomatoes, and a generous amount of pepper.

1 pound (455 g) crabmeat

2 cups (475 ml) low-sodium chicken broth

2 cups (480 g) diced no-salt-added canned tomatoes

½ cup (82 g) frozen corn

½ cup (65 g) no-salt-added frozen peas

1½ teaspoons seafood seasoning (Old Bay is traditional)

½ teaspoon black pepper

½ teaspoon cayenne pepper

Place all ingredients in a large saucepan and simmer until the crabmeat and vegetables are cooked.

Yield: 4 servings

Each with: 292 g water; 105 calories (7% from fat, 44% from protein, 49% from carb); 12 g protein; 1 g total fat; 0 g saturated fat; 0 g monounsaturated fat; 0 g polyunsaturated fat; 14 g carb; 3 g fiber; 5 g sugar; 60 mg calcium; 2 mg iron; 108 mg sodium; 612 mg potassium; 733 IU vitamin A; 22 mg vitamin C; 20 mg cholesterol

Glycemic Index: Low

Salmon Bisque

This is a quick and easy salmon bisque using canned salmon that can be put together in only a few minutes. It's great as a first course, or increase the serving size and make it dinner.

½ cup (80 g) onion, chopped

½ cup (50 g) celery, chopped

2 tablespoons (28 g) unsalted butter

3 tablespoons (24 g) flour

1 teaspoon dill

¼ teaspoon garlic powder

¼ teaspoon Worcestershire sauce

⅛ teaspoon pepper

4 cups (950 ml) skim milk

8 ounces (225 g) salmon

In saucepan, cook onion and celery in butter until tender, not brown. Stir in flour, dill weed, garlic powder, Worcestershire sauce, and pepper. Add milk; cook and stir until thickened and bubbly. Drain salmon. Remove bones and skin and flake. Stir into milk mixture; heat thoroughly.

Yield: 4 servings

Each with: 295 g water; 247 calories (34% from fat, 35% from protein, 31% from carb); 21 g Protein; 9 g total fat; 5 g saturated fat; 3 g monounsaturated fat; 1 g polyunsaturated fat; 19 g carb; 1 g fiber; 14 g sugar; 468 mg phosphorous; 464 mg calcium; 1 mg iron; 161 mg sodium; 636 mg potassium; 787 IU vitamin A; 207 mg ATE vitamin E; 3 mg vitamin C; 42 mg cholesterol

Glycemic Index: Low

Scallop Soup

This simple soup of scallops and vegetables makes a great first course for any fancy dinner, or it's just a nice way to start a family meal.

1 cup (235 ml) dry white wine

1 cup (235 ml) low-sodium vegetable broth

¼ cup (33 g) carrots, julienne strips

¼ cup (38 g) turnips, julienne strips

¼ cup (26 g) leeks, julienne strips

White pepper to taste

½ pound (225 g) scallops

TIP *If you have any fish stock, use that in place of the broth for even deeper flavor.*

In a medium saucepan, bring wine, broth, and vegetables to a boil; season with pepper to taste. Reduce heat and simmer 5 minutes or until vegetables are tender-crisp. Add scallops and simmer 1 to 2 minutes more until scallops are opaque.

Yield: 2 servings

Each with: 350 g water; 235 calories (10% from fat, 61% from protein, 29% from carb); 22 g Protein; 2 g total fat; 0 g saturated fat; 0 g monounsaturated fat; 1 g polyunsaturated fat; 10 g carb; 1 g fiber; 3 g sugar; 321 mg phosphorous; 93 mg calcium; 1 mg iron; 275 mg sodium; 659 mg potassium; 2937 IU vitamin A; 18 mg ATE vitamin E; 8 mg vitamin C; 37 mg cholesterol

Glycemic Index: Low

Sicilian Fish Soup

This is a soup to warm you on a cold night.

4 ounces (115 g) orzo, or other small pasta

½ cup (80 g) chopped onion

2 cloves minced garlic

1 teaspoon fennel seed

4 cups (1 kg) no-salt-added stewed tomatoes

2 cups (475 ml) low-sodium chicken broth

1 tablespoon (4 g) parsley

½ teaspoon black pepper

¼ teaspoon turmeric

12 ounces (340 g) fish, cut in 1-inch (2 ½-cm) cubes

Cook pasta according to package directions. Drain and set aside. In a large nonstick saucepan coated with nonstick vegetable oil spray, cook onion, garlic, and fennel seed until onion is tender. Add tomatoes, broth, and spices. Reduce heat and simmer for 10 minutes. Add fish and simmer until fish is cooked through, about 5 minutes. Divide pasta among 4 bowls. Ladle soup over pasta.

Yield: 4 servings

Each with: 445 g water; 192 calories (7% from fat, 46% from protein, 47% from carb); 23 g protein; 2 g total fat; 0 g saturated fat; 0 g monounsaturated fat; 0 g polyunsaturated fat; 23 g carb; 3 g fiber; 8 g sugar; 115 mg calcium; 2 mg iron; 144 mg sodium; 1,020 mg potassium; 423 IU vitamin A; 39 mg vitamin C; 41 mg cholesterol

Glycemic Index: Low

Fish Stew

This is a great fish stew that's full of vegetables and delicious. You can substitute any other white fish for the haddock.

6 slices low-sodium bacon, chopped

2 cups (320 g) onion, sliced

1½ pounds (680 g) haddock, cut in 2½-inch (7½ cm) pieces

1 pound (455 g) potatoes, cut in ¾-inch (2 cm) cubes

1 cup (130 g) carrot, cut in ¾-inch cubes

½ teaspoon celery seeds

¼ cup (38 g) green pepper, diced

½ teaspoon pepper

3 cups (705 ml) water

28 ounces (800 g) crushed tomatoes

2 tablespoons (8 g) fresh parsley

In a deep kettle or Dutch oven, sauté bacon until lightly browned; remove bacon and set aside. In same kettle, sauté onions until tender. Add fish, potatoes, celery seeds, carrots, green peppers, pepper, and water. Simmer, covered, until vegetables are tender, about 25 minutes. Add tomatoes; heat. Garnish with parsley and crumbled bacon bits.

Yield: 6 servings

Each with: 469 g water; 255 calories (17% from fat, 43% from protein, 40% from carb); 28 g Protein; 5 g total fat; 1 g saturated fat; 2 g monounsaturated fat; 1 g polyunsaturated fat; 26 g carb; 4 g fiber; 4 g sugar; 360 mg phosphorous; 81 mg calcium; 3 mg iron; 175 mg sodium; 1204 mg potassium; 4621 IU vitamin A; 20 mg ATE vitamin E; 53 mg vitamin C; 73 mg cholesterol

Glycemic Index: Low

7

Main Dishes:
Chicken and Turkey

Most recent dietary recommendations include less red meat. This chapter will make it easy to do. We have chicken and turkey recipes from literally all around the world, the Caribbean to Mexico to China to India to Italy to Spain, as well as some good old-fashioned recipes from the United States. There should be something here for everyone; probably a number of things.

Rotisserie Chicken

This recipe is equally good cooked in the oven or in a rotisserie if you have one. Be forewarned that the honey will give you a *very* brown skin.

1 teaspoon paprika

1 teaspoon onion powder

½ teaspoon black pepper

½ teaspoon thyme

¼ teaspoon garlic powder

¼ cup (85 g) honey

1 large roasting chicken (6 to 7 pounds or 2¾ to 3 kg)

Mix spices into honey. Brush onto chicken. Roast at 325°F (170°C, gas mark 3) until done, basting occasionally with pan juices.

Yield: 8 servings

Each with: 16 g water; 71 calories (18% from fat, 30% from protein, 51% from carb); 5 g protein; 1 g total fat; 0 g saturated fat; 1 g monounsaturated fat; 0 g polyunsaturated fat; 9 g carb; 0 g fiber; 9 g sugar; 7 mg calcium; 0 mg iron; 17 mg sodium; 67 mg potassium; 163 IU vitamin A; 0 mg vitamin C; 16 mg cholesterol

Glycemic Index: Low

Grilled Roasting Chicken

If you cook a large chicken on the weekend, you can have a great meal and lots of leftovers to use during the week. This one has a smoky flavor but not so much as to overpower other recipes.

1 large roasting chicken, 5 to 6 pounds (2 to 2¾ kg)

2 tablespoons (30 ml) olive oil

1 teaspoon paprika

1 teaspoon onion powder

½ teaspoon black pepper

½ teaspoon thyme

¼ teaspoon garlic powder

1 teaspoon liquid smoke

Split chicken in half along the backbone and breastbone. Mix together remaining ingredients and rub into both sides of chicken halves. Grill over indirect heat, turning occasionally, until done, 1½ to 2 hours. Place over low heat for the last 15 minutes to brown skin.

Yield: 12 servings

Each with: 0 g water; 289 calories (69% from fat, 30% from protein, 1% from carb); 22 g protein; 22 g total fat; 6 g saturated fat; 9 g monounsaturated fat; 4 g polyunsaturated fat; 1 g carb; 0 g fiber; 0 g sugar; 2 mg phosphorus; 15 mg calcium; 2 mg iron; 0 mg sodium; 255 mg potassium; 209 IU vitamin A; 3 mg vitamin C; 113 mg cholesterol

Glycemic Index: Low

Oven Barbecued Chicken

If you'd like a little barbecued chicken but don't really want to mess with the grill, this could be just the recipe you are looking for.

1 whole chicken, cut into pieces

¼ cup (60 ml) water

¼ cup (60 ml) vinegar

3 tablespoons (45 ml) vegetable oil

½ cup (140 g) chili sauce, see recipe in chapter 2

3 tablespoons (45 ml) Worcestershire sauce

1 teaspoon dry mustard

½ teaspoon pepper

2 tablespoons (20 g) onion, chopped

Preheat oven to 350°F (180°C, or gas mark 4). Combine all ingredients except chicken in saucepan, place over heat, and simmer for 5–10 minutes. Place chicken in a large baking pan. Pour half of the barbecue sauce over chicken and bake, uncovered, for about 45–60 minutes. Baste with remaining barbecue sauce every 15 minutes during cooking.

Yield: 4 servings

Each with: 101 g water; 177 calories (62% from fat, 26% from protein, 12% from carb); 11 g Protein; 12 g total fat; 2 g saturated fat; 3 g monounsaturated fat; 6 g polyunsaturated fat; 5 g carb; 0 g fiber; 2 g sugar; 100 mg phosphorous; 16 mg calcium; 1 mg iron; 355 mg sodium; 224 mg potassium; 553 IU vitamin A; 8 mg ATE vitamin E; 28 mg vitamin C; 34 mg cholesterol

Glycemic Index: Low

Oven Fried Chicken

This is not the Colonel's fried chicken. Boneless breasts are dipped in pecan and cornmeal breading and then oven fried in hot oil for a delightfully crispy texture and a delicious taste.

2 pounds (900 g) boneless skinless chicken breast

¾ cup (175 ml) olive oil

3 tablespoons (33 g) Dijon mustard

¼ teaspoon black pepper

½ teaspoon paprika

1 cup (110 g) pecan, ground

½ cup (70 g) yellow cornmeal

Preheat the oven to 400°F (200°C, or gas mark 6). Pound the chicken breast halves to an even thickness. Pour ½ cup (120 ml) of the oil into a 9 x13-inch (23 x 33 cm) baking dish, and heat it in the hot oven for 10 minutes. Combine the remaining oil with the mustard, salt, pepper, and paprika in a shallow bowl and mix well. Combine the pecans and cornmeal on a sheet of wax paper. Dip the chicken pieces in the seasoned oil and then in the nut mixture. Remove the pan from the oven and place the chicken pieces in the pan. Bake for 10 minutes and then turn with tongs and bake for an additional 15 minutes. Drain on paper towels and serve immediately.

Yield: 6 servings

Each with: 121 g water; 586 calories (65% from fat, 26% from protein, 9% from carb); 38 g Protein; 43 g total fat; 5 g saturated fat; 28 g monounsaturated fat; 7 g polyunsaturated fat; 14 g carb; 3 g fiber; 1 g sugar; 370 mg phosphorous; 35 mg calcium; 2 mg iron; 185 mg sodium; 497 mg potassium; 177 IU vitamin A; 9 mg ATE vitamin E; 2 mg vitamin C; 88 mg cholesterol

Glycemic Index: Low

Cajun Beer Can Chicken

This recipe has been around a while. This version adds a Cajun flavor. It makes a nice tender, juicy bird, either on the grill or in the oven. For a nonalcoholic chicken, substitute ginger ale or use nonalcoholic beer. You should use the indirect method, which means that you set up your fire so that it is hottest away from the food. On a charcoal grill, arrange it in two piles at opposite sides of the grill. Place a foil drip pan in the center of the grill between the mounds of embers. On a gas grill, if it has two burners, light one side on high and cook the chicken on the other.

1 chicken, 4 to 6 pounds (1¾ to 2¾ kg)

3 tablespoons (12 g) Cajun seasoning

12 ounces (355 ml) beer

3 cloves garlic

Remove and discard the fat from inside the body cavities of the chicken. Remove the package of giblets and set aside for another use. Rinse the chicken, inside and out, under cold running water; then drain and blot dry, inside and out, with paper towels. Sprinkle 1 tablespoon (4 g) of the seasoning inside the body and neck cavities; then rub the rest all over the skin of the bird. If you wish, rub another ½-tablespoon of the seasoning between the flesh and the skin. Cover and refrigerate the chicken while you preheat the grill. Pop the tab on the beer can. Using a "church key" type of can opener, punch six or seven holes in the top of the can. Pour out the top inch (2½ cm) of beer; drop the peeled garlic cloves into the holes in the can. Holding the chicken upright (wings at top, legs at bottom), with the opening of the body cavity down, insert the beer can into the lower cavity. Oil the grill grate. Stand the chicken up in the center of the hot grate, over the drip pan. Spread out the legs to form a sort of tripod to support the bird. Cover the grill and cook the chicken until fall-off-the-bone tender, about an hour, depending on size. Use a thermometer to check for doneness. The internal temperature should be 180°F (82°C). Using tongs, lift the bird to a cutting board or platter, holding a metal spatula underneath the beer can for support.

Yield: 8 servings

Each with: 25 g water; 81 calories (66% from fat, 32% from protein, 2% from carb); 6 g protein; 6 g total fat; 2 g saturated fat; 2 g monounsaturated fat; 1 g polyunsaturated fat; 0 g carb; 0 g fiber; 0 g sugar; 6 mg calcium; 0 mg iron; 25 mg sodium; 76 mg potassium; 48 IU vitamin A; 0 mg vitamin C; 27 mg cholesterol

Glycemic Index: Low

Injector Chicken Breasts

Boneless chicken breast can be the basis for great meals that are low in sodium and fat as long as you make sure to find ones that don't have added broth and sodium. However, they also can tend to dry out on the grill without that extra liquid. Fortunately, you can find meat injectors in most stores that have a good selection of kitchen gadgets or grill accessories. And we can come up with a flavorful solution to inject that's a lot lower in sodium.

¼ cup (60 ml) low-sodium chicken broth

1 teaspoon Worcestershire sauce

1 tablespoon (15 ml) lemon juice

4 chicken breasts

Mix together broth, Worcestershire sauce, and lemon juice. Inject into chicken breasts. Grill over medium heat until done, about 15 minutes.

Yield: 4 servings

Each with: 71 g water; 81 calories (10% from fat, 87% from protein, 3% from carb); 17 g protein; 1 g total fat; 0 g saturated fat; 0 g monounsaturated fat; 0 g polyunsaturated fat; 1 g carb; 0 g fiber; 0 g sugar; 9 mg calcium; 1 mg iron; 59 mg sodium; 209 mg potassium; 16 IU vitamin A; 5 mg vitamin C; 41 mg cholesterol

Glycemic Index: Low

Chicken Kabobs

This is a little taste of the islands. It's mildly spicy and flavorful.

18 ounces (510 g) pineapple chunks

1 teaspoon cumin

1 teaspoon coriander

⅛ teaspoon garlic powder

(continued on page 162)

1 tablespoon (7 g) chili powder

1 teaspoon cilantro

2 tablespoons (30 g) plain yogurt

10 ounces (280 g) boneless skinless chicken breasts

1 red bell pepper

1 onion

8 cherry tomatoes

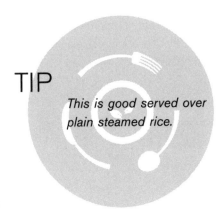

TIP

This is good served over plain steamed rice.

Drain pineapple, reserving juice. In a large bowl blend together spices and yogurt. Add juice from pineapple and stir to mix. Cut the chicken into cubes and add to the mixture. Cover and refrigerate for 1 to 1½ hours. Cut pepper and onion into cubes. Arrange chicken, pineapple, and vegetables on skewers. Grill over medium heat about 10 minutes, turning and basting with remaining marinade frequently.

Yield: 4 servings

Each with: 230 g water; 201 calories (15% from fat, 47% from protein, 38% from carb); 24 g protein; 3 g total fat; 1 g saturated fat; 1 g monounsaturated fat; 1 g polyunsaturated fat; 19 g carb; 3 g fiber; 13 g sugar; 67 mg calcium; 2 mg iron; 65 mg sodium; 613 mg potassium; 2,031 IU vitamin A; 91 mg vitamin C; 61 mg cholesterol

Glycemic Index: Low

Hawaiian Chicken Kabobs

Chicken kabobs with vegetables and fruit are a great start to any meal. You can also use shorter skewers to make appetizer-sized portions.

⅓ cup (80 ml) lime juice

1 tablespoon (15 ml) vegetable oil

1 tablespoon (21 g) honey

6 boneless skinless chicken breasts

12 pearl onions, peeled

1 green bell pepper, seeded, and cut into 2-inch (5 cm) pieces

1 papaya, peeled, seeded, and cut into 2-inch (5 cm) pieces

1½ cups (250 g) fresh pineapple chunks

Combine lime juice, vegetable oil, and honey in a shallow dish. Add chicken; toss gently. Cover and marinate in refrigerator 8 hours or overnight, stirring occasionally. Remove chicken from marinade. Alternate chicken, onion, pepper, papaya, and pineapple on 6 skewers. Coat grill rack with nonstick vegetable oil spray. Grill kabobs over medium-hot coals 15–20 minutes or until chicken is cooked through and vegetables are crisp-tender.

Yield: 6 servings

Each with: 264 g water; 161 calories (19% from fat, 44% from protein, 38% from carb); 18 g Protein; 3 g total fat; 1 g saturated fat; 1 g monounsaturated fat; 2 g polyunsaturated fat; 15 g carb; 2 g fiber; 11 g sugar; 184 mg phosphorous; 78 mg calcium; 1 mg iron; 515 mg sodium; 460 mg potassium; 138 IU vitamin A; 4 mg ATE vitamin E; 35 mg vitamin C; 41 mg cholesterol

Glycemic Index: Low

Chicken Fingers

Easy-to-make baked chicken fingers are not only healthier than the typical fried ones, but they actually taste better according to many people.

⅓ cup (10 g) cornflake crumbs

½ cup (55 g) pecans, finely chopped

1 tablespoon (1.3 g) parsley flakes

⅛ teaspoon garlic powder

12 ounces (340 g) boneless skinless chicken breast halves, cut into 1 x 3-inch (2½ x 7 ½ cm) strips

2 tablespoons (30 ml) skim milk

In a shallow dish, combine cornflake crumbs, pecans, parsley, and garlic powder. Dip chicken in milk and then roll in crumb mixture. Place in a 15 x 10 x 1-inch (38 x 25 x 2½ cm) baking pan. Bake in a 400°F (200°C, or gas mark 6). oven for 7–9 minutes or until chicken is tender and no longer pink.

Yield: 5 servings

(continued on page 164)

Each with: 47 g water; 213 calories (47% from fat, 46% from protein, 7% from carb); 24 g Protein; 11 g total fat; 2 g saturated fat; 6 g monounsaturated fat; 3 g polyunsaturated fat; 4 g carb; 1 g fiber; 1 g sugar; 207 mg phosphorous; 32 mg calcium; 1 mg iron; 59 mg sodium; 257 mg potassium; 67 IU vitamin A; 9 mg ATE vitamin E; 1 mg vitamin C; 62 mg cholesterol

Glycemic Index: Low

Chicken Scaloppini

This is the kind of recipe that you may be tempted to save for a special occasion. But it really isn't that difficult to make, so why not treat yourself more often?

4 tablespoons (55 g) unsalted butter, divided

4 cups (280 g) mushrooms, sliced

1½ pounds (680 g) boneless skinless chicken breasts, pounded flat

⅓ cup (34 g) green onions, thinly sliced

⅓ cup (80 ml) low-sodium chicken broth

¼ cup (60 ml) white wine

⅓ cup (80 ml) nonfat evaporated milk

Melt 2 tablespoons (28 g) of butter in large nonstick skillet. Sauté mushrooms until tender and any liquid has evaporated; remove from pan; set aside. Melt remaining 2 tablespoons (28 g) butter in same pan. Sauté chicken breasts on both sides until golden brown and cooked through. Remove from pan; set aside. Add onions to pan; sauté until tender. Add broth and wine to pan. Bring to boil. Cook and stir until mixture is reduced by half. Add milk to pan. Cook and stir until slightly thickened. Return mushrooms and chicken to sauce in pan. Reheat to serving temperature.

Yield: 6 servings

Each with: 167 g water; 226 calories (39% from fat, 54% from protein, 7% from carb); 29 g Protein; 9 g total fat; 5 g saturated fat; 2 g monounsaturated fat; 1 g polyunsaturated fat; 4 g carb; 1 g fiber; 3 g sugar; 300 mg phosphorous; 63 mg calcium; 1 mg iron; 99 mg sodium; 521 mg potassium; 372 IU vitamin A; 87 mg ATE vitamin E; 4 mg vitamin C; 87 mg cholesterol

Glycemic Index: Low

Chicken Breasts Stuffed with Cheese

Stuffed chicken breasts that are just oozing with cheese are bound to be a hit with kids and adults alike.

¾ cup (83 g) Swiss cheese, shredded

½ cup (125 g) ricotta cheese

1 tablespoon (4.3 g) thyme

⅛ teaspoon black pepper, coarse ground

6 boneless skinless chicken breasts

2 teaspoons (10 g) unsalted butter

In small bowl, fold together Swiss and ricotta cheeses, thyme, and cracked black pepper. Place a chicken breast on flat surface. Cut a 2½-inch (6 cm) horizontal slit into side of chicken breast to form a pocket. Repeat procedure with remaining breasts. Stuff each pocket with 2 tablespoons cheese mixture. Melt butter in skillet. Add chicken to skillet and cook 6 minutes. Turn; reduce heat to medium and cook 4–5 minutes until chicken is cooked through.

Yield: 6 servings

Each with: 75 g water; 181 calories (42% from fat, 53% from protein, 4% from carb); 23 g Protein; 8 g total fat; 5 g saturated fat; 2 g monounsaturated fat; 0 g polyunsaturated fat; 2 g carb; 0 g fiber; 0 g sugar; 278 mg phosphorous; 232 mg calcium; 1 mg iron; 75 mg sodium; 230 mg potassium; 287 IU vitamin A; 71 mg ATE vitamin E; 1 mg vitamin C; 66 mg cholesterol

Glycemic Index: Low

Curried Chicken and Apples

This is an easy and tasty curry recipe, with apples and raisins providing an extra amount of flavor.

2 boneless skinless chicken breasts

2 tablespoons (42 g) honey

2 teaspoons (4 g) curry powder

2 apples, peeled and chopped

3 tablespoons oil

½ cup (50 g) celery, sliced

¼ cup (35 g) raisins

3 tablespoons (12 g) fresh parsley

Cut chicken into cubes and place in bowl. Combine honey and curry and mix with chicken. Stir in apples. Heat oil in heavy skillet over high heat. Sauté celery for 1 minute. Add apple mixture and stir-fry 3–4 minutes, just until chicken is no longer pink. Add raisins and parsley, stir well, and serve over rice.

Yield: 4 servings

Each with: 100 g water; 229 calories (41% from fat, 15% from protein, 44% from carb); 9 g Protein; 11 g total fat; 1 g saturated fat; 3 g monounsaturated fat; 6 g polyunsaturated fat; 26 g carb; 2 g fiber; 22 g sugar; 96 mg phosphorous; 27 mg calcium; 1 mg iron; 37 mg sodium; 296 mg potassium; 336 IU vitamin A; 2 mg ATE vitamin E; 8 mg vitamin C; 21 mg cholesterol

Glycemic Index: Low

Chicken Breasts with Balsamic Sauce

Add a little extra flavor to your next meal of chicken breasts, with this balsamic sauce.

4 chicken breast halves

½ teaspoon salt

¼ teaspoon black pepper

2 tablespoons (28 g) butter, divided

1 tablespoon (15 ml) vegetable oil

1 tablespoon (10 g) shallots, finely chopped

3 tablespoons (45 ml) balsamic vinegar

1½ cups (355 ml) chicken broth

2 teaspoons (4 g) finely chopped fresh marjoram

Sprinkle chicken with pepper. Heat 1 tablespoon (14 g) butter and the oil in large, heavy frying pan over high heat. Add chicken, skin side down, and cook until skin is crisp. Reduce heat to medium-low; turn chicken breasts over and cook until chicken is no longer pink inside, about 12 minutes. Transfer chicken to heated platter and keep warm in oven. Pour off all but 1 tablespoon (15 ml) fat from frying pan. Add shallots and cook over medium-low heat for 3 minutes or until translucent, scraping up any browned bits. Add vinegar and bring to a boil. Boil for 3 minutes or until reduced to a glaze, stirring constantly. Add broth and boil until reduced to ½ cup (120 ml), stirring occasionally. Season to taste with salt and pepper. Remove sauce from heat and whisk in remaining butter and marjoram. Whisk in any juices from chicken. Spoon sauce over chicken and serve immediately.

Yield: 4 servings

Each with: 134 g water; 201 calories (55% from fat, 42% from protein, 3% from carb); 20 g protein; 12 g total fat; 5 g saturated fat; 4 g monounsaturated fat; 3 g polyunsaturated fat; 1 g carb; 0 g fiber; 0 g sugar; 180 mg phosphorus; 23 mg calcium; 1 mg iron; 964 mg sodium; 317 mg potassium; 241 IU vitamin A; 0 mg vitamin C; 60 mg cholesterol

Glycemic Index: Low

Spicy Grilled Chicken with Green Onions

Buy some carrot and celery sticks to dip into blue cheese dressing for a cool starter. Deli potato salad is good with the chicken, and classic southern ambrosia—sliced oranges with coconut—is a refreshing end.

(continued on page 168)

2 tablespoons (30 ml) vegetable oil

1 tablespoon (15 ml) Tabasco sauce

2 teaspoons honey

1 teaspoon paprika

7 green onions

2 chicken breasts, boned and skinned

Prepare the grill (medium-high heat). Whisk oil, Tabasco, honey, and paprika in a 9-inch (23 cm) glass pie dish to blend. Mince 1 green onion and mix into marinade. Transfer 2 tablespoons (30 ml) of the marinade to a small bowl and reserve. Add chicken to the pie dish marinade and turn to coat. Let stand 10 minutes, turning occasionally. Grill chicken and whole onions until chicken is cooked through and onions soften, turning occasionally, about 10 minutes. Transfer chicken and grilled onions to plates and drizzle with 1 tablespoon (15 ml) each of the reserved marinade.

Yield: 2 servings

Each with: 61 g water; 224 calories (59% from fat, 30% from protein, 12% from carb); 17 g protein; 15 g total fat; 2 g saturated fat; 4 g monounsaturated fat; 8 g polyunsaturated fat; 7 g carb; 0 g fiber; 6 g sugar; 145 mg phosphorus; 11 mg calcium; 1 mg iron; 91 mg sodium; 221 mg potassium; 737 IU vitamin A; 2 mg vitamin C; 41 mg cholesterol

Glycemic Index: Low

Chicken with Avocado and Tomato

When we first tried this recipe, I couldn't believe how much I liked it. The chicken is incredibly tender and flavorful. And the combination of avocados and tomatoes cooked with the chicken in a cheesy sauce is a real winner.

2 tablespoons (42 g) unsalted butter, melted

4 boneless skinless chicken breasts

2 avocados

1 cup (180 g) tomatoes, chopped

½ cup (115 g) sour cream

½ cup (58 g) Monterey jack cheese shredded

Slice chicken ½-inch (1 cm) thick. In large skillet, heat butter on medium-high. Add chicken slices and sauté 3–5 minutes, until they start to turn brown. Preheat oven to 350°F (180°C, or gas mark 4). Peel, pit, and thinly slice avocado. In medium casserole, layer chicken, avocado, and tomato. Top with sour cream. Sprinkle with cheese. Bake 30 minutes.

Yield: 2 servings

Each with: 339 g water; 705 calories (64% from fat, 26% from protein, 10% from carb); 46 g Protein; 52 g total fat; 21 g saturated fat; 22 g monounsaturated fat; 4 g polyunsaturated fat; 18 g carb; 10 g fiber; 1 g sugar; 577 mg phosphorous; 349 mg calcium; 2 mg iron; 313 mg sodium; 1323 mg potassium; 1527 IU vitamin A; 228 mg ATE vitamin E; 34 mg vitamin C; 166 mg cholesterol

Glycemic Index: Low

Orange Burgundy Chicken

My daughter made this one evening while I was busy taking advantage of a little sunshine to get some yard work done. It's definitely something we'll have again.

¼ cup (75 g) orange marmalade

½ teaspoon cornstarch

¼ cup (60 ml) burgundy wine

4 boneless chicken breasts

In a small saucepan, combine first 3 ingredients. Cook and stir until thickened and bubbly. Grill chicken breasts until done, about 15 minutes on a charcoal or gas grill. (It may also be baked in the oven.) Brush sauce over chicken during last 5 minutes of cooking. Serve remaining sauce over chicken.

Yield: 4 servings

(continued on page 170)

Each with: 54 g water; 147 calories (12% from fat, 47% from protein, 40% from carb); 16 g protein; 2 g total fat; 1 g saturated fat; 1 g monounsaturated fat; 0 g polyunsaturated fat; 14 g carb; 0 g fiber; 12 g sugar; 17 mg calcium; 1 mg iron; 50 mg sodium; 157 mg potassium; 23 IU vitamin A; 1 mg vitamin C; 44 mg cholesterol

Glycemic Index: Low

French Chicken

I don't know whether this is really a French way of cooking chicken or not, but somehow that was the first thing that came to mind thinking about the Dijon mustard and vermouth. Whatever you call it, it's good, and that is the main thing.

1 tablespoon (21 g) unsalted butter

1 tablespoon (15 ml) olive oil

2 boneless skinless chicken breasts

1 tablespoon (33 g) Dijon mustard

1 tablespoon (33 g) mustard, coarse grain

3 tablespoons (45 ml) vermouth

3 tablespoons (45 ml) water

2 tablespoons (30 ml) heavy cream

Melt the butter in a heavy-bottomed casserole. Add the oil. Brown the chicken on both sides, about 2 to 3 minutes each side. Carefully pour off any excess fat. Add the mustards, vermouth, and water. Bring the liquid to a simmer, scraping up the brown bits in the bottom of the pan. Cover and simmer for 10 minutes. Test the chicken to make sure it is done. Remove the meat to individual dishes and cover to keep warm. Add the cream and mix well. Serve the sauce over the chicken.

Yield: 2 servings

Each with: 106 g water; 245 calories (67% from fat, 31% from protein, 3% from carb); 17 g Protein; 17 g total fat; 7 g saturated fat; 8 g monounsaturated fat; 1 g polyunsaturated fat; 1 g carb; 0 g fiber; 0 g sugar; 157 mg phosphorous; 26 mg calcium; 1 mg iron; 137 mg sodium; 229 mg potassium; 313 IU vitamin A; 82 mg ATE vitamin E; 1 mg vitamin C; 67 mg cholesterol

Glycemic Index: Low

Chicken in Sour Cream Sauce

Chicken is cooked in a sherry flavored sour cream sauce for a delicious taste experience. Serve with sauce over rice or wild rice.

2 pounds (900 g) boneless skinless chicken breast

½ cup (112 g) unsalted butter

½ pint (230 g) fat-free sour cream

½ cup (120 ml) sherry

½ teaspoon rosemary

2 tablespoons (8 g) fresh parsley

½ teaspoon thyme

1 tablespoon (9 g) green pepper, finely chopped

Pepper to taste

½ cup (55 g) slivered almonds

Brown chicken in butter in skillet. Place in casserole. Add sour cream and sherry to chicken drippings. Add remaining ingredients and simmer 10 minutes. Pour mixture over chicken pieces. Bake 350°F (180°C, or gas mark 4) for 1 hour.

Yield: 4 servings

Each with: 248 g water; 686 calories (58% from fat, 36% from protein, 6% from carb); 58 g Protein; 42 g total fat; 21 g saturated fat; 15 g monounsaturated fat; 4 g polyunsaturated fat; 10 g carb; 2 g fiber; 3 g sugar; 598 mg phosphorous; 148 mg calcium; 3 mg iron; 179 mg sodium; 835 mg potassium; 1155 IU vitamin A; 265 mg ATE vitamin E; 8 mg vitamin C; 216 mg cholesterol

Glycemic Index: Low

Chicken Marsala

This is a traditional Italian recipe, and it's one that is definitely worth trying.

4 boneless skinless chicken breasts

4 tablespoons (55 g) butter, divided

4 shallots, finely chopped

½ pound (225 g) mushrooms, thinly sliced

¼ cup (60 ml) Marsala wine

½ cup (120 ml) heavy cream

1 teaspoon lemon juice

¼ teaspoon pepper

Using the flat (smooth) side of a meat mallet, pound the breasts to ¼ inch (½ cm) thickness. In a large frying pan, melt 2 teaspoons butter over medium heat. Add chicken and sauté, turning once, until lightly browned, about 2 minutes on each side. Remove and set aside. Melt remaining butter in pan. Add shallots and mushrooms. Cook until mushrooms are lightly browned, 3 to 5 minutes. Add Marsala and bring to a boil, scraping up any browned bits from bottom of pan. Add cream and lemon juice and return to a boil. Season with pepper to taste. Return chicken to pan and cook, turning in sauce, for about 3 minutes to reheat and finish cooking.

Yield: 4 servings

Each with: 128 g water; 268 calories (64% from fat, 29% from protein, 7% from carb); 19 g protein; 18 g total fat; 11 g saturated fat; 5 g monounsaturated fat; 1 g polyunsaturated fat; 5 g carb; 1 g fiber; 2 g sugar; 202 mg phosphorus; 25 mg calcium; 1 mg iron; 433 mg sodium; 393 mg potassium; 590 IU vitamin A; 3 mg vitamin C; 92 mg cholesterol

Glycemic Index: Low

Chicken Piccata

Here is another one of those classic recipes, updated to make it quicker and easier. Chicken is bathed in a lemon and vermouth sauce for an elegant flavor combination. Serve with rice or noodles.

4 boneless skinless chicken breasts

½ teaspoon black pepper, freshly ground

2 tablespoons (28 g) unsalted butter

1 teaspoon olive oil

½ cup (120 ml) low-sodium chicken broth

¼ cup (60 ml) vermouth

2 tablespoons (30 ml) fresh lemon juice

1 tablespoon (8.6 g) capers, drained, rinsed

Pat chicken dry. Season with pepper. Melt butter with oil in heavy large skillet over medium-high heat. Add chicken and cook until no longer pink, about 4 minutes per side. Remove from skillet; keep warm. Increase heat to high. Stir broth and vermouth into skillet. Boil until reduced by half, scraping up any browned bits. Remove from heat. Mix in lemon juice and capers. Place chicken on plates and pour sauce over. Garnish chicken with lemon slices, if desired.

Yield: 4 servings

Each with: 105 g water; 159 calories (49% from fat, 47% from protein, 5% from carb); 17 g Protein; 8 g total fat; 4 g saturated fat; 3 g monounsaturated fat; 1 g polyunsaturated fat; 2 g carb; 0 g fiber; 0 g sugar; 154 mg phosphorous; 15 mg calcium; 1 mg iron; 121 mg sodium; 233 mg potassium; 197 IU vitamin A; 52 mg ATE vitamin E; 5 mg vitamin C; 56 mg cholesterol

Glycemic Index: Low

Ranch Chicken Stir-Fry

This recipe pretty much defines "quick and tasty". You can probably do it start to finish in about 10 minutes, but the taste is exceptional, with the salad dressing mix taking it from plain to great.

1 tablespoon (15 ml) olive oil

½ pound (225 g) boneless skinless chicken breast, cut in strips

1 package ranch dressing mix

16 ounces (455 g) frozen winter vegetable mix, thawed

2 tablespoons (30 ml) water

(continued on page 174)

Heat vegetable oil in large skillet. Add chicken breast strips. Stir in Ranch Salad Dressing Mix to coat chicken. Add thawed vegetable medley and water. Stir-fry about 2 minutes.

Yield: 4 servings

Each with: 143 g water; 165 calories (25% from fat, 40% from protein, 36% from carb); 17 g Protein; 5 g total fat; 1 g saturated fat; 3 g monounsaturated fat; 1 g polyunsaturated fat; 15 g carb; 5 g fiber; 0 g sugar; 178 mg phosphorous; 35 mg calcium; 2 mg iron; 90 mg sodium; 385 mg potassium; 5770 IU vitamin A; 3 mg ATE vitamin E; 12 mg vitamin C; 33 mg cholesterol

Glycemic Index: Low

Hawaiian Chicken

This was kind of a throw-together one night when we didn't know what to have for dinner. We happened to have chicken thighs on hand, but you could use whatever pieces you prefer. The flavor is like a mild sweet-and-sour chicken.

8 ounces (225 g) pineapple chunks

¼ cup (85 g) honey

¼ cup (60 ml) red wine vinegar

4 chicken thighs

½ cup (75 g) chopped red bell pepper

½ cup (80 g) coarsely chopped onion

Drain pineapple, reserving juice. Combine juice, honey, and vinegar. Place chicken in an 8 × 12-inch (20 × 30 cm) baking pan. Sprinkle pineapple and vegetables over top. Pour juice mixture over. Bake at 350°F (180°C, gas mark 4) until chicken is done, about 45 minutes.

Yield: 4 servings

Each with: 126 g water; 144 calories (10% from fat, 23% from protein, 67% from carb); 9 g protein; 2 g total fat; 0 g saturated fat; 1 g monounsaturated fat; 0 g polyunsaturated fat; 26 g carb; 1 g fiber; 24 g sugar; 20 mg calcium; 1 mg iron; 38 mg sodium; 241 mg potassium; 337 IU vitamin A; 23 mg vitamin C; 34 mg cholesterol

Glycemic Index: Low

Slow Cooker Chicken in Tomato Cream Sauce

This meal in a pot does take a little work near the end, but it is well worth it. Your family will love the creamy taste of the sauce with the chicken and pasta.

2 chicken breasts halves

2 tablespoons (30 ml) olive oil

¼ cup (25 g) green onions, chopped

1 teaspoon garlic, minced

14½ ounces (410 g) canned tomatoes, drained and chopped

1 tablespoon (4.5 g) basil

1 cup (235 ml) fat-free evaporated milk

2 egg yolks

¾ cup (75 g) parmesan cheese, grated

8 ounces (225 g) fettuccine

1 cup (130 g) frozen peas, thawed

1½ cup (105 g) mushrooms, sliced

In skillet, brown chicken breasts in olive oil. Place chicken in slow cooker. Add green onions, garlic, tomatoes, and basil. Cover and cook on Low 7 to 9 hours. Remove chicken and cut into pieces. Return chicken pieces to pot. Stir in cream, egg yolks, and Parmesan cheese. Cover and cook on high 30 minutes to thicken. While sauce is thickening, cook fettuccine according to package directions; drain. Add fettuccine, peas, and mushrooms. Cover and cook on high 30 to 60 minutes.

Yield: 4 servings

Each with: 267 g water; 501 calories (33% from fat, 27% from protein, 40% from carb); 34 g Protein; 18 g total fat; 6 g saturated fat; 8 g monounsaturated fat; 2 g polyunsaturated fat; 51 g carb; 4 g fiber; 13 g sugar; 533 mg phosphorous; 479 mg calcium; 5 mg iron; 719 mg sodium; 807 mg potassium; 1607 IU vitamin A; 151 mg ATE vitamin E; 17 mg vitamin C; 188 mg cholesterol

Glycemic Index: Low

Chicken Breasts Baked In Creamy Herb Sauce

A creamy sauce made with yogurt and an assortment of herbs makes these chicken breasts special.

4 boneless skinless chicken breasts

1 cup (230 g) plain yogurt

¼ cup (60 g) sour cream

½ teaspoon lime peel, grated

½ teaspoon oregano

¼ teaspoon celery seed

¼ teaspoon garlic powder

¼ teaspoon coriander

¼ teaspoon parsley

¼ teaspoon thyme

3 tablespoons (45 ml) lime juice

Preheat oven to 375°F (190°C, or gas mark 5). Spray roasting pan with nonstick vegetable oil spray, place chicken breasts in it, and set aside. Combine all other ingredients. Baste chicken breasts with mixture and bake for 20 minutes. Remove from oven. Turn chicken breasts, baste with sauce, and bake 15 minutes longer until meat is tender. Turn off oven. Cover chicken with foil and let stand in oven 10 minutes. Remove aluminum foil, arrange chicken breasts on serving dish, and serve hot with any remaining sauce.

Yield: 4 servings

Each with: 122 g water; 164 calories (19% from fat, 48% from protein, 33% from carb); 19 g Protein; 3 g total fat; 2 g saturated fat; 1 g monounsaturated fat; 0 g polyunsaturated fat; 13 g carb; 0 g fiber; 12 g sugar; 224 mg phosphorous; 116 mg calcium; 1 mg iron; 85 mg sodium; 331 mg potassium; 122 IU vitamin A; 26 mg ATE vitamin E; 6 mg vitamin C; 50 mg cholesterol

Glycemic Index: Low

Quick Chicken and Mushroom Risotto

Although not really risotto, which requires a specific preparation and particular kind of rice to get the traditional creaminess and texture, this recipe still give you that same sort of impression while taking less time and effort.

2 tablespoons (28 g) unsalted butter, divided

¾ pound (340 g) boneless skinless chicken breasts, cut in cubes

½ cup (80 g) onion, finely chopped

½ cup (65 g) carrot, sliced

1 cup (185 g) long grain rice, uncooked

14½ ounces (410 g) low-sodium chicken broth

1 can (10¾ ounces or 305 g) cream of mushroom soup

⅛ teaspoon pepper

½ cup (65 g) frozen peas

In 3-quart saucepan over medium-high heat, in 1 tablespoon (14 g) melted butter, cook chicken until browned, stirring often. Remove; set aside. In same saucepan, add remaining butter. Reduce heat to medium; cook onion, carrot, and rice until rice is browned, stirring constantly. Stir in broth, soup, and pepper. Heat to boiling. Reduce heat to low. Cover; cook 15 minutes, stirring occasionally. Add peas and reserved chicken. Cover; cook 5 minutes or until chicken is no longer pink, rice is tender, and liquid is absorbed, stirring occasionally.

Yield: 4 servings

Each with: 326 g water; 425 calories (21% from fat, 27% from protein, 52% from carb); 28 g Protein; 10 g total fat; 5 g saturated fat; 3 g monounsaturated fat; 1 g polyunsaturated fat; 55 g carb; 3 g fiber; 5 g sugar; 346 mg phosphorous; 59 mg calcium; 4 mg iron; 646 mg sodium; 944 mg potassium; 3318 IU vitamin A; 55 mg ATE vitamin E; 6 mg vitamin C; 68 mg cholesterol

Glycemic Index: Low

Vidalia Onion Chicken Casserole

Make this in the spring when Vidalias are in season (or use another kind of sweet onion).

10 ounces (280 g) frozen broccoli

⅓ cup (53 g) chopped Vidalia onions

½ cup (35 g) sliced mushrooms

5 teaspoons (30 ml) olive oil, divided

1 cup (120 g) grated Cheddar cheese

2 large eggs, slightly beaten

½ cup (115 g) mayonnaise

1 cup (235 ml) water

1 cup (165 g) cooked rice

6 chicken breasts, boned and skinned

1 tablespoon (7 g) paprika

Cook broccoli according to directions. Drain and set aside. Sauté onions and mushrooms in 2 teaspoons olive oil until limp. Drain and combine with broccoli. Set aside. Combine cheese, eggs, mayonnaise, water, and rice. Set aside. Brown chicken breasts in remaining olive oil. To assemble, combine broccoli mixture with cheese mixture and pour into greased, shallow baking pan. Place chicken breasts on top and sprinkle with paprika. Bake uncovered in an oven heated to 350°F (180°C, gas mark 4) for 45 minutes.

Yield: 6 servings

Each with: 174 g water; 444 calories (58% from fat, 25% from protein, 17% from carb); 27 g protein; 29 g total fat; 8 g saturated fat; 8 g monounsaturated fat; 11 g polyunsaturated fat; 19 g carb; 2 g fiber; 2 g sugar; 355 mg phosphorus; 207 mg calcium; 3 mg iron; 337 mg sodium; 435 mg potassium; 1,716 IU vitamin A; 33 mg vitamin C; 150 mg cholesterol

Glycemic Index: Low

Chicken Alfredo

Kaye sent this recipe in. She comments that for the tomatoes, you could also use oven baked cherry tomatoes or sun-dried tomatoes.

2 boneless chicken breasts, cut in chunks

½ cup (90 g) chopped tomato

1 cup (70 g) sliced mushrooms

2 cloves garlic, minced

2 tablespoons (4 g) dried basil

1 slice low-sodium bacon, cooked and crumbled

8 ounces (225 g) no-salt-added tomato sauce

2 tablespoons (10 g) grated Parmesan cheese

4 ounces (120 ml) half-and-half

Sauté the chicken in olive oil until browned. Turn chicken and add tomato, mushrooms, and garlic and cook on medium heat until the mushrooms start to darken. Add basil, bacon, tomato sauce, and Parmesan. Heat on low for 15 minutes. Remove from heat. Add half-and-half to mixture. Mix well. Serve over pasta.

Yield: 4 servings

Each with: 135 g water; 133 calories (21% from fat, 49% from protein, 31% from carb); 13 g protein; 2 g total fat; 1 g saturated fat; 1 g monounsaturated fat; 0 g polyunsaturated fat; 8 g carb; 2 g fiber; 3 g sugar; 104 mg calcium; 1 mg iron; 107 mg sodium; 494 mg potassium; 572 IU vitamin A; 12 mg vitamin C; 36 mg cholesterol

Glycemic Index: Low

Pasta with Chicken and Broccoli

This is another meal in a pan. If you've longed for the days of Hamburger Helper, now is the time to cheer. This recipe is just as easy, and a boxed meal never tasted this good.

¼ cup (60 ml) olive oil

½ pound (225 g) boneless skinless chicken breasts, cut in ½-inch (1 cm) strips

½ pound (227 g) bow tie pasta, cooked

2 garlic cloves, minced

1½ cups (107 g) broccoli florets

1 teaspoon dried basil

¼ cup (60 ml) white wine

¾ cup (175 ml) low-sodium chicken broth

In a large skillet, heat oil over medium heat. Sauté garlic for about one minute, stirring constantly. Add the chicken and cook until well done. Add the broccoli and cook until crisp but tender. Add basil. Add pepper to taste, wine, and chicken broth. Cook for about 5 minutes. Add the cooked and drained pasta to the skillet and toss to combine. Heat for 1 to 2 minutes. Serve. Top with grated Parmesan cheese if desired.

Yield: 4 servings

Each with: 128 g water; 419 calories (34% from fat, 22% from protein, 44% from carb); 22 g Protein; 15 g total fat; 2 g saturated fat; 10 g monounsaturated fat; 2 g polyunsaturated fat; 45 g carb; 2 g fiber; 2 g sugar; 253 mg phosphorous; 38 mg calcium; 3 mg iron; 62 mg sodium; 413 mg potassium; 827 IU vitamin A; 3 mg ATE vitamin E; 26 mg vitamin C; 33 mg cholesterol

Glycemic Index: Low

Southwestern Skillet Supper

This southwestern flavored chicken and bean dish is good served over rice and sprinkled with a little cheddar cheese.

1 pound (455 g) boneless skinless chicken breasts

2 tablespoons (30 ml) olive oil

1 cup (160 g) onion, chopped

2 teaspoons (5.2 g) chili powder

½ teaspoon cumin

½ teaspoon oregano

½ cup (120 ml) chicken broth

1½ cups (355 ml) low-sodium V8 juice

19 ounces (532 g) kidney beans

Cut the chicken into ½-inch (1 cm) pieces. In hot oil, cook chicken, onion, chili powder, cumin, and oregano until the chicken turns white. Stir in broth and juice. Heat until boiling and then reduce heat to low. Simmer 10 minutes. Add beans, liquid and all, stir, cover, and simmer for another 10 minutes. Stir occasionally.

Yield: 4 servings

Each with: 324 g water; 395 calories (20% from fat, 41% from protein, 39% from carb); 40 g Protein; 9 g total fat; 1 g saturated fat; 5 g monounsaturated fat; 1 g polyunsaturated fat; 39 g carb; 14 g fiber; 5 g sugar; 448 mg phosphorous; 130 mg calcium; 6 mg iron; 242 mg sodium; 1143 mg potassium; 1825 IU vitamin A; 7 mg ATE vitamin E; 32 mg vitamin C; 66 mg cholesterol

Glycemic Index: Low

Easy Mexican Chicken and Rice

Ordinary chicken and rice gets a big flavor boost from the addition of salsa.

1 cup (185 g) rice, long cooking

1²/₃ cups (395 ml) low-sodium chicken broth

1 cup (160 g) onion, chopped

4 boneless skinless chicken breasts

1 cup (260 g) salsa

In a large pan, bring the broth to a boil. Add rice and onions, boil 10 minutes and then remove from the heat. Place into casserole dish, place chicken breasts on top, and pour salsa over the chicken breast and rice. Cover. Place into preheated 350°F (180°C, or gas mark 4) oven and bake for 1 hour.

Yield: 6 servings

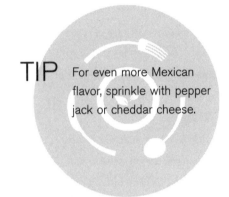

TIP For even more Mexican flavor, sprinkle with pepper jack or cheddar cheese.

Each with: 187 g water; 137 calories (22% from fat, 60% from protein, 18% from carb); 22 g Protein; 3 g total fat; 1 g saturated fat; 1 g monounsaturated fat; 1 g polyunsaturated fat; 7 g carb; 1 g fiber; 3 g sugar; 284 mg phosphorous; 34 mg calcium; 1 mg iron; 186 mg sodium; 428 mg potassium; 248 IU vitamin A; 36 mg ATE vitamin E; 9 mg vitamin C; 167 mg cholesterol

Glycemic Index: Low

Spanish Chicken

This is almost a soup. The spices give it a Spanish flavor. You can serve it as is or over rice the way we had it, but you'll need a bowl either way. I cut up a whole frying chicken, saving the back to make soup and skinning the rest before browning it.

2½ pounds (1 kg) chicken pieces

1 tablespoon (15 ml) oil

1 large onion, sliced

2 cloves garlic, minced

2 teaspoons thyme

¼ teaspoon black pepper

¼ teaspoon turmeric

2 cups (475 ml) low-sodium chicken broth

2 cups (480 g) no-salt-added canned tomatoes

2 green bell peppers, cut into strips

1 cup (130 g) no-salt-added frozen peas

In a large skillet, brown chicken pieces in oil on all sides. Place chicken in slow cooker. Add onion. Sprinkle with spices. Pour broth over. Cook on low for 6 to 8 hours or on high for4 to 5 hours. Add tomatoes, bell pepper, and peas in the last hour of cooking.

Yield: 6 servings

Each with: 161 g water; 356 calories (56% from fat, 30% from protein, 14% from carb); 27 g protein; 22 g total fat; 6 g saturated fat; 9 g monounsaturated fat; 6 g polyunsaturated fat; 12 g carb; 4 g fiber; 6 g sugar; 63 mg calcium; 3 mg iron; 121 mg sodium; 584 mg potassium; 1870 IU vitamin A; 59 mg vitamin C; 118 mg cholesterol

Glycemic Index: Low

Spanish Chicken Thighs

This recipe is from the card that came with my Turbocooker, a moment of weakness. It is designed to steam and cook at the same time, but you can get much the same effect from a skillet or Dutch oven with a tight-fitting lid. Don't be afraid of the amount of onion; it cooks down considerably. Besides, as we always have said in my family, you can never have too much onion.

1 teaspoon garlic powder

1 teaspoon paprika

1 teaspoon basil

1 teaspoon black pepper

(continued on page 184)

1 teaspoon parsley

4 chicken thighs

1 cup (160 g) chopped onion

1 can (8 ounces or 225 g) no-salt-added tomato sauce

¼ cup (60 ml) water

Combine spices in a plastic bag. Add chicken pieces and shake to coat evenly. Place chicken and onion in skillet with a lid. Add water. Cover and cook for 10 minutes. Turn and cook 10 minutes more. Pour tomato sauce over and continue cooking until done through, about 10 more minutes. Serve with pasta or rice. Spoon sauce and onion mixture over top.

Yield: 4 servings

Each with: 82 g water; 71 calories (22% from fat, 48% from protein, 30% from carb); 9 g protein; 2 g total fat; 0 g saturated fat; 1 g monounsaturated fat; 0 g polyunsaturated fat; 5 g carb; 1 g fiber; 2 g sugar; 21 mg calcium; 1 mg iron; 38 mg sodium; 188 mg potassium; 375 IU vitamin A; 4 mg vitamin C; 34 mg cholesterol

Glycemic Index: Low

Tequila Chicken

A little tequila never hurt any chicken, as you'll realize when you taste this.

4 chicken breast halves, boned and skinned

1 cup (235 ml) chicken stock

3 cloves garlic, minced

Olive oil

1 can (9 ounces or 255 g) tomatoes, undrained

½ cup (120 ml) tequila

¼ cup (60 ml) lime juice (2 limes)

¼ teaspoon cayenne pepper

1 teaspoon chili powder

1 teaspoon cumin

½ teaspoon coriander

Parmesan cheese

Fresh basil or parsley for garnish

Simmer the chicken breasts in the stock until tender. Remove and cube. Set aside, reserving stock. Sauté the garlic in olive oil. Add tomatoes (breaking up) and the remaining ingredients; simmer, covered, 30 minutes. Add chicken and reheat. Toss with cooked noodles. If sauce becomes too thick, add the chicken stock. Sprinkle with Parmesan cheese and garnish with fresh basil or parsley leaves.

Yield: 4 servings

Each with: 181 g water; 191 calories (23% from fat, 62% from protein, 16% from carb); 19 g protein; 3 g total fat; 1 g saturated fat; 1 g monounsaturated fat; 1 g polyunsaturated fat; 5 g carb; 1 g fiber; 2 g sugar; 170 mg phosphorus; 27 mg calcium; 1 mg iron; 538 mg sodium; 391 mg potassium; 793 IU vitamin A; 14 mg vitamin C; 47 mg cholesterol

Glycemic Index: Low

Greek Chicken

This chicken dish will make you think you are sitting at a little restaurant watching the sun going down on the Mediterranean. It's not difficult to make, but the flavor is excellent.

4 boneless skinless chicken breast halves

2 tablespoons (30 ml) olive oil

1 cup (160 g) onion, chopped

3 cloves garlic, minced

1 red bell pepper, cut in strips

1½ ounces (42 g) sun dried tomatoes

1½ cups (355 ml) dry white wine

⅓ cup (55 g) pitted ripe olives, sliced

1 lemon, sliced

1½ teaspoons cinnamon

1 teaspoon honey

(continued on page 186)

In large skillet over medium heat, sauté chicken breasts in oil about 5 minutes, turning once. Add onion, garlic, and red pepper. Sauté, stirring often, about 4 minutes until onion is limp. With kitchen shears, halve tomatoes; stir into skillet with remaining ingredients except parsley. Cover and simmer 15 minutes. Remove cover and cook 5 more minutes until chicken is tender and sauce is slightly reduced.

Yield: 4 servings

Each with: 206 g water; 303 calories (44% from fat, 31% from protein, 25% from carb); 19 g Protein; 12 g total fat; 2 g saturated fat; 8 g monounsaturated fat; 2 g polyunsaturated fat; 15 g carb; 3 g fiber; 6 g sugar; 183 mg phosphorous; 57 mg calcium; 2 mg iron; 175 mg sodium; 536 mg potassium; 1366 IU vitamin A; 4 mg ATE vitamin E; 69 mg vitamin C; 47 mg cholesterol

Glycemic Index: Low

Chicken Breasts with Crab Stuffing

This is not only a great tasting dish, but it looks like the kind of thing you can only get at a fancy restaurant. Don't let that discourage you. It really is easy to make.

1½ pounds (685 g) boneless skinless chicken breasts

½ cup (80 g) onion, chopped

½ cup (50 g) celery, chopped

5 tablespoons (70 g) unsalted butter, divided

3 tablespoons (45 ml) white wine, dry

7½ ounces (210 g) crabmeat, flaked

½ cup (54 g) stuffing mix

2 tablespoons (16 g) flour

½ teaspoon paprika

Pound chicken breasts to flatten. Cook onion and celery in 3 tablespoons (42 g) butter until tender. Remove from heat. Mix together the wine, the crab and stuffing mix and toss. Divide mixture among breasts. Roll up and secure with toothpicks. Combine flour and paprika. Coat chicken. Place in 11 x 7 x 2-inch (28 x 18 x 5 cm) baking dish, drizzle with 2 tablespoons (28 g) melted butter. Bake uncovered in 375°F (190°C, or gas mark 5) oven for 1 hour

Yield: 6 servings

Each with: 151 g water; 297 calories (41% from fat, 49% from protein, 10% from carb); 35 g Protein; 13 g total fat; 7 g saturated fat; 4 g monounsaturated fat; 1 g polyunsaturated fat; 7 g carb; 1 g fiber; 1 g sugar; 335 mg phosphorous; 64 mg calcium; 2 mg iron; 291 mg sodium; 491 mg potassium; 513 IU vitamin A; 105 mg ATE vitamin E; 4 mg vitamin C; 123 mg cholesterol

Glycemic Index: Low

Jellied Chicken Salad

This is chicken salad with a difference. It's molded into a gelatin base. This makes a great light dinner during warm weather and it is also good to take for workday lunches if you have a refrigerator available.

1 cup (235 ml) low-sodium chicken broth

1 package lemon flavor sugar free gelatin

¾ cup (175 ml) water, cold

1 tablespoon (15 ml) vinegar

¼ teaspoon black pepper

¼ cup (60 g) plain fat-free yogurt

2 tablespoons (30 g) fat-free sour cream

1 tablespoon (11 g) Dijon mustard

1 cup (140 g) cooked chicken breast finely chopped

1 cup (100 g) celery, finely chopped

½ cup (75 g) red bell pepper, finely chopped

Bring chicken broth to a boil in small saucepan. Completely dissolve gelatin in boiling broth. Add water, vinegar, and black pepper. Chill until slightly thickened. Stir in yogurt, sour cream, and mustard. Chill until slightly thickened. Stir in remaining ingredients. Spoon into 3 individual plastic containers or serving dishes. Chill until firm, about 2 hours.

Yield: 3 servings

(continued on page 188)

Each with: 256 g water; 136 calories (24% from fat, 54% from protein, 22% from carb); 19 g Protein; 4 g total fat; 1 g saturated fat; 1 g monounsaturated fat; 1 g polyunsaturated fat; 8 g carb; 1 g fiber; 3 g sugar; 220 mg phosphorous; 83 mg calcium; 1 mg iron; 184 mg sodium; 407 mg potassium; 982 IU vitamin A; 13 mg ATE vitamin E; 33 mg vitamin C; 44 mg cholesterol

Glycemic Index: Low

Barbecued Chicken Salad

This is a great way to use up grilled chicken leftovers. Serve it on a bed of greens.

2 cups (280 g) cubed cooked chicken

½ cup (50 g) chopped celery

½ cup (75 g) diced red bell pepper

½ cup (80 g) diced red onion

1 cup (130 g) frozen corn, cooked and drained

¼ cup (65 g) low-sodium barbecue sauce

2 tablespoons (28 g) mayonnaise

In a large bowl, toss together the chicken, celery, bell pepper, onion, and corn. In a small bowl, mix together the barbecue sauce and mayonnaise. Pour over the chicken and veggies. Stir and chill until ready to serve.

Yield: 4 servings

Each with: 132 g water; 239 calories (39% from fat, 32% from protein, 29% from carb); 19 g protein; 11 g total fat; 2 g saturated fat; 3 g monounsaturated fat; 4 g polyunsaturated fat; 17 g carb; 2 g fiber; 6 g sugar; 188 mg phosphorus; 24 mg calcium; 1 mg iron; 197 mg sodium; 409 mg potassium; 816 IU vitamin A; 29 mg vitamin C; 57 mg cholesterol

Glycemic Index: Low

Cumin Crusted Chicken Salad

I like the flavor of cumin, so this was a recipe that I just had to try. It turned out really well with the flavor on the chicken contrasting nicely with the vegetables.

¼ cup (45 g) tomato, chopped

3 tablespoons (25 g) cucumber, peeled and chopped

3 tablespoons (38 g) green pepper, chopped

1 tablespoon (10 g) red onion, chopped

1 small jalapeno pepper chopped

1 tablespoon (6.6 g) cumin

1 teaspoon pepper

4 boneless skinless chicken breasts

1 tablespoon (15 ml) red wine vinegar

Combine tomato, cucumber, green pepper, red onion, and jalapeno pepper in a small bowl and set aside. Combine cumin and pepper. Rub all sides of chicken breasts with this. Place a large cast iron skillet over medium high heat until hot. Add chicken and cook 6 minutes on each side or until tender. Remove from skillet, reserving drippings in skillet. Set chicken aside. Add vinegar to pan drippings and cook 2 minutes, stirring constantly. Pour over reserved vegetable mixture, tossing well. Thinly slice each chicken breast diagonally across grain and arrange on individual serving plates. Serve with reserved vegetable mixture.

Yield: 4 servings

Each with: 80 g water; 89 calories (13% from fat, 78% from protein, 8% from carb); 17 g Protein; 1 g total fat; 0 g saturated fat; 0 g monounsaturated fat; 0 g polyunsaturated fat; 2 g carb; 0 g fiber; 1 g sugar; 153 mg phosphorous; 25 mg calcium; 2 mg iron; 50 mg sodium; 256 mg potassium; 167 IU vitamin A; 4 mg ATE vitamin E; 9 mg vitamin C; 41 mg cholesterol

Glycemic Index: Low

Italian Chicken Pasta Salad

This is a nice variation on the usual pasta salad. The chicken makes it a complete meal.

2 quarts (1.1 L) water

½ cup (120 ml) dry white wine

4 boneless skinless chicken breasts

4 cloves garlic

3 tablespoons (7.5 g) fresh basil, thinly sliced

⅛ teaspoon pepper

2 tablespoons (30 ml) lemon juice

4 ounces (112 g) rigatoni

1 tablespoon (1.5 ml) olive oil

1 cup (150 g) red bell peppers, julienned

2 tablespoons (13 g) ripe olives, thinly sliced

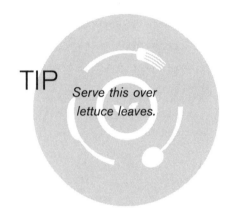

TIP

Serve this over lettuce leaves.

Bring water to a boil in medium sauce pan. Add wine, chicken, and garlic. Reduce heat and simmer 15 minutes. Or until chicken is done. Remove chicken and garlic from broth, reserving broth. Let chicken cool. Cut chicken into ½-inch (1 cm) pieces. Set aside. Crush garlic in a small bowl; add basil, pepper, and lemon juice. Mix well and set aside. Bring reserved broth to a boil. Add pasta. Cook 12 minutes or until al dente. Drain. Rinse under cold water. Drain. Toss pasta with olive oil. Combine reserved garlic-lemon mixture, chicken, pasta, bell peppers, and olives in a large bowl. Toss gently. Chill at least 1 hour.

Yield: 4 servings

Each with: 599 g water; 258 calories (20% from fat, 35% from protein, 44% from carb); 21 g Protein; 5 g total fat; 1 g saturated fat; 3 g monounsaturated fat; 1 g polyunsaturated fat; 26 g carb; 2 g fiber; 3 g sugar; 216 mg phosphorous; 71 mg calcium; 3 mg iron; 102 mg sodium; 413 mg potassium; 1350 IU vitamin A; 4 mg ATE vitamin E; 53 mg vitamin C; 41 mg cholesterol

Glycemic Index: Low

Injector Smoked Turkey Breast

This makes a nice hot-weather meal with a little potato salad and rolls.

3 pounds (1⅓ kg) turkey breast
½ cup (120 ml) apple juice

Inject the apple juice into the turkey breast. Smoke it until done, 6 to 8 hours. Fruit wood chips are preferred for smoking.

Yield: 12 servings

Each with: 93 g water; 131 calories (5% from fat, 91% from protein, 4% from carb); 28 g protein; 1 g total fat; 0 g saturated fat; 0 g monounsaturated fat; 0 g polyunsaturated fat; 1 g carb; 0 g fiber; 1 g sugar; 12 mg calcium; 1 mg iron; 56 mg sodium; 345 mg potassium; 0 IU vitamin A; 0 mg vitamin C; 70 mg cholesterol

Glycemic Index: Low

Turkey Vegetable Sauté

Here is a turkey and vegetable sauté with just a hint of Mexican flavor. I particularly like this one over whole wheat spaghetti, but it's also good over brown rice.

1 pound (455 g) ground turkey

1 cup (160 g) onion, cut in rings

15 black olives, halved

1 cup (130 g) sliced carrots

½ cup (50 g) sliced celery

½ cup (75 g) chunked green bell peppers

4 ounces (115 g) mushrooms, sliced

½ teaspoon cumin

½ teaspoon garlic salt

1 cup (180 g) chopped tomatoes

3 slices low-sodium bacon, cooked and broken into pieces (optional)

Brown meat. Add fresh vegetables, except tomatoes; add spices and cook over medium heat until vegetables are crisp-tender. Add remaining ingredients and heat through.

Yield: 6 servings

Each with: 161 g water; 197 calories (32% from fat, 52% from protein, 17% from carb); 25 g protein; 7 g total fat; 2 g saturated fat; 2 g monounsaturated fat; 1 g polyunsaturated fat; 8 g carb; 2 g fiber; 3 g sugar; 226 mg phosphorus; 50 mg calcium; 2 mg iron; 217 mg sodium; 521 mg potassium; 3,873 IU vitamin A; 20 mg vitamin C; 62 mg cholesterol

Glycemic Index: Low

Turkey Broccoli Casserole

This is a popular way to use leftover turkey around our house.

10 ounces (280 g) frozen broccoli

2 cups (350 g) turkey, cooked and diced

1 can (10 ounces or 280 g) cream of mushroom soup

½ cup (120 ml) skim milk

½ cup (60 g) grated Cheddar cheese

Preheat oven to 375°F (190°C, gas mark 5). Cook broccoli according to package directions. Layer the broccoli in 12 x 8-inch (30 x 20 cm) baking dish. Spread turkey evenly on top. Combine soup with milk, mix until smooth, and pour over turkey. Sprinkle grated cheese on top. Bake for 30 minutes. Let stand 5 minutes before serving.

Yield: 6 servings

Each with: 173 g water; 239 calories (50% from fat, 31% from protein, 19% from carb); 19 g protein; 14 g total fat; 5 g saturated fat; 4 g monounsaturated fat; 3 g polyunsaturated fat; 11 g carb; 3 g fiber; 2 g sugar; 243 mg phosphorus; 167 mg calcium; 2 mg iron; 458 mg sodium; 476 mg potassium; 1628 IU vitamin A; 62 mg vitamin C; 54 mg cholesterol

Glycemic Index: Low

White Bean and Smoked Turkey Casserole

This is a quick and tasty use for leftover smoked turkey. It's vaguely French in flavor.

1½ cups (375 g) dried great northern beans

3 tablespoons (45 ml) olive oil

1 onion, chopped

1½ cups (260 g) chopped smoked turkey

⅓ cup (80 ml) white wine

1 tablespoon (16 g) no-salt-added tomato paste

1 teaspoon thyme

1 bay leaf

½ teaspoon black pepper

½ teaspoon garlic powder

Cover beans with water. Bring to a boil and boil 1 minute. Remove from heat, cover, and let stand 1 hour. Return to heat and simmer 1 hour or until almost done. Drain, reserving 1 cup (235 ml) of the liquid. Heat oil in large frying pan or Dutch oven. Sauté onion until soft but not brown. Stir in turkey. Add wine and cook until liquid has evaporated. Add remaining ingredients and bean liquid. Simmer 20 minutes, adding water if needed. Discard bay leaf before serving.

Yield: 6 servings

Each with: 82 g water; 205 calories (38% from fat, 32% from protein, 31% from carb); 15 g protein; 8 g total fat; 1 g saturated fat; 2 g monounsaturated fat; 4 g polyunsaturated fat; 15 g carb; 3 g fiber; 1 g sugar; 172 mg phosphorus; 48 mg calcium; 2 mg iron; 29 mg sodium; 380 mg potassium; 48 IU vitamin A; 2 mg vitamin C; 24 mg cholesterol

Glycemic Index: Low

Turkey Meat Loaf

The glaze gives this a nice, sweet-tart taste without adding too many carbohydrates. The turkey is milder in flavor than beef, as well as being lower in fat.

1¼ pounds (570 g) ground turkey

½ cup (60 g) low-sodium bread crumbs

1 egg

1 tablespoon (4 g) parsley

½ teaspoon black pepper

½ teaspoon garlic powder

1 teaspoon onion powder

¼ cup (80 g) peach preserves

2 teaspoons Dijon mustard

Preheat oven to 350°F (180°C, gas mark 4). Combine first 8 ingredients in a large bowl and mix well. Shape mixture into a loaf on a baking sheet. Bake 45 minutes. Stir preserves and mustard together. Spread on top of loaf. Return to oven until internal temperature is 165°F (74°C), about 20 minutes.

Yield: 8 servings

Each with: 71 g water; 191 calories (23% from fat, 49% from protein, 28% from carb); 23 g protein; 5 g total fat; 1 g saturated fat; 1 g monounsaturated fat; 1 g polyunsaturated fat; 13 g carb; 1 g fiber; 6 g sugar; 42 mg calcium; 2 mg iron; 68 mg sodium; 293 mg potassium; 108 IU vitamin A; 4 mg vitamin C; 85 mg cholesterol

Glycemic Index: Low

Turkey Sausage and Pepper Patties

I happen to be one of the people who think that ground turkey tends to be pretty plain and lacking in real flavor. So I came up with this combination, which quite nicely solves the problem for me.

1 tablespoon (15 ml) olive oil

½ cup (75 g) green pepper, finely minced

½ cup (80 g) onion, finely minced

1¼ pounds (570 g) ground turkey

¼ teaspoon sage

¼ teaspoon thyme

¼ teaspoon marjoram

¼ teaspoon pepper

½ teaspoon fennel seeds

Heat oil in skillet; add peppers and onions and cook until tender, about 10 minutes. Cool. Combine peppers and onions with turkey and remaining ingredients, mixing well. Chill an hour or so to blend flavors. Form into 4 patties. Cook in nonstick skillet until lightly browned on both sides.

Yield: 4 servings

Each with: 127 g water; 284 calories (34% from fat, 61% from protein, 4% from carb); 42 g Protein; 11 g total fat; 3 g saturated fat; 4 g monounsaturated fat; 2 g polyunsaturated fat; 3 g carb; 1 g fiber; 1 g sugar; 313 mg phosphorous; 47 mg calcium; 3 mg iron; 101 mg sodium; 490 mg potassium; 83 IU vitamin A; 0 mg ATE vitamin E; 17 mg vitamin C; 108 mg cholesterol

Glycemic Index: Low

8

Main Dishes:
Beef

Despite what I said in the chicken chapter about eating less red meat, we still eat it on a regular basis. But that doesn't mean it needs to be unhealthy. This chapter contains recipes that not only taste great but are low in GI and saturated fat. We have recipes for the grill, meat loaves and meatballs, and soups and stews. And that's not to mention the good old-fashioned casseroles.

Steak Plus

Now I happen to be one of those people who usually feel a little pepper is the only thing a good steak needs. But I have to admit that a steak done up this way is maybe even better than a plain one. Give it a try and see if you agree.

1½ pounds (680 g) beefsteak

1 clove garlic, cut in half

2 teaspoons black peppercorns, crushed

¼ cup (55 g) unsalted butter

1 tablespoon (11 g) Dijon mustard

2 teaspoons Worcestershire sauce

½ teaspoon lime juice

Trim fat on beefsteaks to ¼-inch (½ cm) thickness. Rub garlic on beef. Press peppercorns into beef. Mix together the butter, mustard, Worcestershire sauce, and lime juice. Heat coals or gas grill. Apply sauce to steak; cover and grill beef 4 to 5 inches (10 to 13 cm) from medium heat. Turn steaks and apply sauce again; cook until desired doneness.

Yield: 4 servings

Each with: 115 g water; 437 calories (52% from fat, 46% from protein, 2% from carb); 50 g protein; 25 g total fat; 12 g saturated fat; 8 g monounsaturated fat; 1 g polyunsaturated fat; 2 g carb; 0 g fiber; 0 g sugar; 40 mg calcium; 4 mg iron; 114 mg sodium; 652 mg potassium; 366 IU vitamin A; 5 mg vitamin C; 161 mg cholesterol

Glycemic Index: Low

Texas Style Steak

This is similar to Swiss steak, except the flavor is definitely Southwestern United States. This is great with a side of baked beans and some coleslaw.

½ cup (63 g) flour

2½ teaspoons (6.5 g) chili powder, divided

1½ pounds (680 g) beef round steak

2 tablespoons (30 ml) vegetable oil

½ cup (75 g) green peppers, chopped

½ cup (80 g) onions, chopped

1 cup (235 ml) fat-free beef broth

½ cup (120 ml) tomato juice

¼ teaspoon garlic powder

¼ teaspoon ground cumin

Blend flour, salt, and 1½ teaspoons (4 g) chili powder well and place in pie pan. Dredge meat in the flour mixture. Place oil in a heavy frying pan and heat over moderate heat. Add meat and brown on both sides. Transfer steaks to a 1½ quart (1.5 L) casserole. Fry peppers and onions over moderate heat in the pan in which the meat was browned, stirring frequently. Remove vegetables with a slotted spoon and spread over meat. Pour out any remaining fat. Add beef broth to frying pan and cook and stir over moderate heat to absorb and brown particles remaining in the pan. Add remaining ingredients to broth. Mix well and pour over meat. Stir the meat and vegetables lightly with a fork to distribute the broth and vegetables. Cover tightly and bake at 325°F (170°C, or gas mark 3) for about 1–1½ hours or until the meat is tender.

Yield: 6 servings

Each with: 149 g water; 322 calories (31% from fat, 55% from protein, 14% from carb); 43 g Protein; 11 g total fat; 3 g saturated fat; 4 g monounsaturated fat; 3 g polyunsaturated fat; 11 g carb; 1 g fiber; 2 g sugar; 287 mg phosphorous; 19 mg calcium; 5 mg iron; 88 mg sodium; 522 mg potassium; 447 IU vitamin A; 0 mg ATE vitamin E; 15 mg vitamin C; 102 mg cholesterol

Glycemic Index: Low

Salsa Marinated Steak

A long time marinating in salsa and lime juice make what would ordinarily not be a very tender cut of beef tender and juicy. It also gives it a great flavor.

1¼ pounds (570 g) boneless beef chuck, cut 1-inch (2½ cm) thick

⅓ cup (87 g) salsa, prepared,

2 tablespoons (30 ml) lime juice, fresh

1 garlic clove, minced

1 teaspoon oregano leaves, dried

¼ teaspoon cumin, ground

Combine salsa, lime juice, garlic, oregano, and cumin; reserve 2 tablespoons (30 ml) marinade. Place beef steaks in plastic bag; add remaining marinade, turning to coat. Close bag securely and marinate in refrigerator 6 to 8 hours (or overnight, if desired), turning occasionally. Remove steaks from marinade and place on grill over medium coals. Grill 18 to 24 minutes for rare to medium, turning once. Brush with reserved marinade during last 5 minutes of cooking. Carve into thin slices.

Yield: 4 servings

Each with: 100 g water; 430 calories (58% from fat, 39% from protein, 2% from carb); 41 g Protein; 27 g total fat; 11 g saturated fat; 12 g monounsaturated fat; 1 g polyunsaturated fat; 2 g carb; 0 g fiber; 1 g sugar; 256 mg phosphorous; 35 mg calcium; 4 mg iron; 117 mg sodium; 407 mg potassium; 86 IU vitamin A; 0 mg ATE vitamin E; 3 mg vitamin C; 135 mg cholesterol

Glycemic Index: Low

Marinated London Broil

Flank steak is the traditional cut of meat to use for London broil. However, recently I've been seeing bottom round steak labeled as London broil. Either will work for this recipe. The secret to having tender meat is the marinating and slicing across the grain.

1½ pounds (680 g) flank steak or bottom round

¼ cup (40 g) onion, finely chopped

⅓ cup (80 ml) Worcestershire sauce

⅔ cup (30 ml) dry red wine

2 tablespoons olive oil

1 teaspoon thyme

With sharp knife, score steak on both sides. In shallow platter or plastic bag, combine onion, Worcestershire sauce, wine, oil, and thyme. Lay steak flat in marinade and turn to coat both sides thoroughly. Let stand for 30 minutes, turning occasionally. Prepare and heat grill. Grill about 5 minutes for first side and 4 minutes for second side, basting with marinade. To serve, cut crosswise in thin slanted slices. Heat remaining marinade to boiling and spoon over slices.

Yield: 6 servings

Each with: 105 g water; 296 calories (47% from fat, 48% from protein, 6% from carb); 32 g Protein; 14 g total fat; 5 g saturated fat; 7 g monounsaturated fat; 1 g polyunsaturated fat; 4 g carb; 0 g fiber; 0 g sugar; 262 mg phosphorous; 24 mg calcium; 3 mg iron; 196 mg sodium; 534 mg potassium; 21 IU vitamin A; 0 mg ATE vitamin E; 25 mg vitamin C; 62 mg cholesterol

Glycemic Index: Low

Texas Barbecued Steak

A quick sweet and spicy rub will make these steaks a favorite with children and adults alike.

4 sirloin steaks, 4 ounces (115 g) each

¼ cup (85 g) honey

4 garlic cloves minced

2 teaspoons (4 g) black pepper, fresh ground

2 teaspoons (6 g) dry mustard

2 teaspoons (5.2 g) chili powder

Rub each steak with 1 tablespoon (21 g) honey. Combine remaining ingredients and rub onto steaks. Let stand 20 to 30 minutes. Barbecue or broil to desired degree of doneness.

Yield: 4 servings

Each with: 82 g water; 457 calories (50% from fat, 33% from protein, 17% from carb); 38 g Protein; 25 g total fat; 10 g saturated fat; 10 g monounsaturated fat; 1 g polyunsaturated fat; 19 g carb; 1 g fiber; 17 g sugar; 282 mg phosphorous; 35 mg calcium; 3 mg iron; 87 mg sodium; 500 mg potassium; 376 IU vitamin A; 0 mg ATE vitamin E; 1 mg vitamin C; 131 mg cholesterol

Glycemic Index: Low

Soy and Ginger Flank Steak

Use the leftover marinade to season corn and red and yellow bell peppers. Add husked corn and halved and seeded bell peppers to the marinade after removing the steak and then cook on the grill, turning occasionally, until slightly browned.

1 flank steak (1¼ pounds or 570 g)

1 tablespoon (6 g) minced fresh ginger

2 teaspoons minced garlic

¼ cup (60 ml) Dick's Reduced-Sodium Soy Sauce (see chapter 2)

3 tablespoons (45 ml) dry red wine

1½ tablespoons (30 g) honey

Rinse the meat and pat dry. Place steak in a plastic freezer bag (1-gallon size) and add the remaining ingredients; seal bag and turn to coat. Lightly oil a barbecue grill and preheat to very hot. Remove the steak from the bag, reserving marinade for vegetables (see note). Cook steak, turning once until done as you like it (about 15 minutes total for medium-rare). To serve, slice diagonally across the grain into thin slices.

Yield: 4 servings

Each with: 115 g water; 320 calories (35% from fat, 53% from protein, 12% from carb); 40 g protein; 12 g total fat; 5 g saturated fat; 5 g monounsaturated fat; 0 g polyunsaturated fat; 9 g carb; 0 g fiber; 7 g sugar; 322 mg phosphorus; 28 mg calcium; 3 mg iron; 149 mg sodium; 538 mg potassium; 0 IU vitamin A; 1 mg vitamin C; 78 mg cholesterol

Glycemic Index: Low

Oriental-Style Flank Steak

I actually like to make this on the grill as well as in the oven. It has a great flavor, not quite barbecue and not quite Asian.

1½ pounds (680 g) flank steak

¼ cup (25 g) sliced green onion

2 tablespoons (16 g) sesame seeds, toasted

½ cup (125 g) barbecue sauce

1 clove garlic, minced

¼ cup (60 ml) Dick's Reduced-Sodium Soy Sauce (see chapter 2)

¼ teaspoon ground ginger

Score steak on both sides. Pour combined ingredients over steak. Cover; marinate in refrigerator several hours or overnight, turning once. Place steak on rack of broiler pan. Broil 15 to 20 minutes or until desired doneness, brushing frequently with barbecue sauce mixture and turning occasionally. To serve, carve steak across grain with slanted knife into thin slices.

Yield: 4 servings

(continued on page 204)

Each with: 134 g water; 395 calories (34% from fat, 50% from protein, 16% from carb); 48 g protein; 14 g total fat; 6 g saturated fat; 6 g monounsaturated fat; 1 g polyunsaturated fat; 16 g carb; 0 g fiber; 12 g sugar; 361 mg phosphorus; 30 mg calcium; 3 mg iron; 398 mg sodium; 594 mg potassium; 62 IU vitamin A; 1 mg vitamin C; 94 mg cholesterol

Glycemic Index: Low

Deviled Steak

This recipe is not spicy in a hot sort of way, just nicely flavored. This steak bakes until it is falling apart tender and is sure to be a hit.

2 pounds (900 g) beef round steak

2 tablespoons (30 ml) olive oil

3 tablespoons (30 g) minced onion

¾ cup (180 g) low-sodium catsup

¾ cup (175 ml) water

½ cup (120 ml) cider vinegar

1 tablespoon (15 g) brown sugar

1 tablespoon (11 g) prepared mustard

1 tablespoon (15 ml) Worcestershire sauce

Cut meat into serving pieces. In skillet, brown meat in oil over medium heat. Remove meat to Dutch oven. Add remaining ingredients to skillet. Simmer 5 minutes. Pour mixture over meat. Cover and bake 2 hours or until meat is tender.

Yield: 6 servings

Each with: 159 g water; 396 calories (29% from fat, 58% from protein, 13% from carb); 56 g Protein; 12 g total fat; 3 g saturated fat; 6 g monounsaturated fat; 1 g polyunsaturated fat; 13 g carb; 0 g fiber; 10 g sugar; 364 mg phosphorous; 24 mg calcium; 6 mg iron; 102 mg sodium; 708 mg potassium; 285 IU vitamin A; 0 mg ATE vitamin E; 11 mg vitamin C; 136 mg cholesterol

Glycemic Index: Low

Bourbon Barbecue-Sauced Beef Ribs

This is not a particularly simple meal, but it's well worth the effort. This recipe came about because I found quite by accident a bag of wood chips for the grill that are made from Jack Daniel's whiskey barrels. The sauce is a variation of a recipe on the back of the bag.

3 pounds (1⅓ kg) beef ribs

½ cup (120 ml) Jack Daniel's whiskey

¼ cup (60 g) brown sugar

½ cup (120 g) low-sodium ketchup

1 teaspoon Worcestershire sauce

1 tablespoon (15 ml) vinegar

2 teaspoons lemon juice

½ teaspoon garlic powder

½ teaspoon dry mustard

Precook ribs 1 hour in oven heated to 350°F (180°C, gas mark 4). Meanwhile, preheat grill. Combine sauce ingredients. Transfer ribs to grill. Brush with sauce. Baste and turn until done and crisp on the outside, about 30 minutes.

Yield: 6 servings

Each with: 187 g water; 466 calories (42% from fat, 44% from protein, 14% from carb); 45 g protein; 19 g total fat; 8 g saturated fat; 8 g monounsaturated fat; 1 g polyunsaturated fat; 14 g carb; 0 g fiber; 13 g sugar; 445 mg phosphorus; 30 mg calcium; 5 mg iron; 163 mg sodium; 923 mg potassium; 188 IU vitamin A; 5 mg vitamin C; 134 mg cholesterol

Glycemic Index: Low

Braised Short Ribs

Beef short ribs are browned and then given a long, slow braising in the slow cooker, resulting in falling off the bone tenderness.

4 pounds (1.8 kg) beef short ribs

½ cup (63 g) flour

1½ teaspoons paprika

½ teaspoon dry mustard

1½ cups (240 g) onion, sliced and separated into rings

1 clove garlic, chopped

1 cup (235 ml) beer or beef broth

Place short ribs in skillet and brown to remove fat; drain well. Combine flour with the paprika and dry mustard; toss with short ribs. Place in slow cooker. Place remaining ingredients over beef. Cook on low for 8–10 hours.

Yield: 6 servings

Each with: 283 g water; 596 calories (49% from fat, 42% from protein, 9% from carb); 59 g Protein; 31 g total fat; 13 g saturated fat; 13 g monounsaturated fat; 1 g polyunsaturated fat; 13 g carb; 1 g fiber; 2 g sugar; 605 mg phosphorous; 38 mg calcium; 7 mg iron; 200 mg sodium; 1174 mg potassium; 304 IU vitamin A; 0 mg ATE vitamin E; 3 mg vitamin C; 178 mg cholesterol

Glycemic Index: Low

Spinach and Mushroom-Stuffed Tenderloin

This looks fancy and tastes great, but it's not really that hard to make.

Mushroom Stuffing

4 tablespoons (55 g) butter (or margarine)

1 pound (455 g) mushrooms, coarsely chopped

2 tablespoons (30 ml) dry vermouth

10 ounces (280 g) frozen chopped spinach, thawed and squeezed dry

2 tablespoons (10 g) grated Parmesan cheese

2 tablespoons (14 g) plain bread crumbs

1 teaspoon thyme

¼ teaspoon black pepper

¼ teaspoon salt

Tenderloin

2 teaspoons (2.8 g) thyme

1 teaspoon salt

1 teaspoon black pepper

4½ pounds (2 kg) whole beef tenderloin

3 tablespoons (42 g) butter (or margarine)

¼ cup (30 g) bread crumbs

2 tablespoons (30 ml) vermouth

1 can (13 ounces or 364 g) chicken broth

½ pound (225 g) mushrooms, sliced

2 tablespoons (16 g) flour

Thyme sprigs for garnish (optional)

For the stuffing (prepare it first and set it aside): In a 12-inch (30 cm) skillet, heat butter over medium-high heat and add mushrooms. Cook until golden and liquid evaporates, 12 to 15 minutes. Stir in vermouth and cook another minute. Remove skillet from heat and stir in the spinach, cheese, bread crumbs, and spices. For the tenderloin: Preheat oven to 425°F (220°C, gas mark 7). In a cup, mix the thyme, salt, and pepper and rub evenly over the tenderloin. With a sharp knife, cut a 1½-inch-deep (3½ cm deep) slit in the tenderloin 2 inches (5 cm) from each end. Spoon the stuffing mixture into the slit and tie the tenderloin closed using cooking twine at 2-inch (5-cm) intervals. Roast for 30 minutes. Meanwhile in a small saucepan, melt 1 tablespoon (14 g) butter over low heat and then remove pan from heat and stir in the bread crumbs. Sprinkle the bread crumb mixture over the tenderloin and roast 10 to 15 minutes longer or until internal temperature reaches 145°F (63°C) for medium-rare. Transfer to a platter and let rest. While resting, prepare the mushroom gravy. Add vermouth and ½ cup (120 ml) chicken broth to the roasting pan and stir over low heat until the browned bits are loosened. Skim off the fat and add

(continued on page 208)

the remaining chicken broth. In a separate pan, heat remaining butter over medium-high heat, add mushrooms, and cook until golden and liquid evaporates, about 12 minutes. Stir in flour. Gradually stir in the meat juice mixture and cook, stirring constantly, until the gravy boils and thickens slightly. To serve: Remove cooking twine, cut tenderloin into slices, and garnish with thyme sprigs (optional). Serve with mushroom gravy.

Yield: 10 servings

Each with: 231 g water; 808 calories (70% from fat, 27% from protein, 3% from carb); 54 g protein; 62 g total fat; 26 g saturated fat; 24 g monounsaturated fat; 3 g polyunsaturated fat; 7 g carb; 2 g fiber; 2 g sugar; 522 mg phosphorus; 93 mg calcium; 8 mg iron; 784 mg sodium; 1,054 mg potassium; 3685 IU vitamin A; 2 mg vitamin C; 198 mg cholesterol

Glycemic Index: Low

Barbecue Meat Loaf

Catsup and liquid smoke give this meat loaf a barbecue flavor, even though it is cooked in the oven.

¼ cup (40 g) onion, finely chopped

¼ cup (25 g) celery, finely chopped

¼ cup (60 g) low-sodium catsup

1 egg

¼ cup (30 g) dry bread crumbs

1 teaspoon (5 ml) liquid smoke

Dash black pepper

1½ pounds (680 g) lean ground beef

Place all ingredients except beef in mixing bowl and mix well. Add beef to catsup mixture and mix until blended. Shape into a loaf about 3½ x 7-inch (9 x 18 cm). Place in a pan that has been sprayed with nonstick vegetable oil spray or lined with aluminum foil. Bake at 325°F (170°C, or gas mark 3) about 1 hour or until browned and firm. Pour off any fat and drippings and let set for 10 minutes before cutting into 6 equal slices.

Yield: 6 servings

Each with: 94 g water; 311 calories (61% from fat, 30% from protein, 9% from carb); 23 g Protein; 21 g total fat; 8 g saturated fat; 9 g monounsaturated fat; 1 g polyunsaturated fat; 7 g carb; 0 g fiber; 3 g sugar; 189 mg phosphorous; 26 mg calcium; 3 mg iron; 96 mg sodium; 401 mg potassium; 168 IU vitamin A; 15 mg ATE vitamin E; 2 mg vitamin C; 113 mg cholesterol

Glycemic Index: Low

Home-Style Meat Loaf

An iron-rich food like meat loaf can help keep you warm on winter nights. When researchers at the U.S. Department of Agriculture deprived a group of women of iron, they became chilled more quickly when exposed to lower temperatures. Besides, it tastes good.

¾ cup (180 g) ketchup, divided

½ cup (40 g) quick-cooking oats

¼ cup (40 g) minced onion

2 tablespoons (8 g) chopped parsley

1 tablespoon (15 g) brown sugar

¼ teaspoon black pepper

2 large egg whites, lightly beaten

1½ pounds (680 g) ground round

Preheat oven to 350°F (180°C, gas mark 4). Combine ½ cup (120 g) ketchup, oats, and next 6 ingredients (oats through egg whites) in a large bowl. Add meat; stir just until blended. Shape meat mixture into an 8 × 4-inch (20 × 10 cm) loaf on a broiler pan coated with nonstick vegetable oil spray. Brush remaining ketchup over meat loaf. Bake 1½ hours or until done.

Yield: 6 servings

Each with: 110 g water; 363 calories (51% from fat, 28% from protein, 21% from carb); 25 g protein; 20 g total fat; 8 g saturated fat; 9 g monounsaturated fat; 1 g polyunsaturated fat; 19 g carb; 2 g fiber; 9 g sugar; 243 mg phosphorus; 27 mg calcium; 3 mg iron; 528 mg sodium; 536 mg potassium; 386 IU vitamin A; 7 mg vitamin C; 78 mg cholesterol

Glycemic Index: Low

German Meatballs

These German-flavored meatballs would traditionally be served over spaetzle, but they are also good with noodles, rice, or mashed potatoes.

1 egg

¼ cup (60 ml) skim milk

¼ cup (30 g) bread crumbs

¼ teaspoon poultry seasoning

1 pound (455 g) extra-lean ground beef

2 cups (475 ml) low-sodium beef broth

½ cup (35 g) sliced mushrooms

½ cup (80 g) chopped onion

1 cup (230 g) fat-free sour cream

1 tablespoon (8 g) flour

1 teaspoon caraway seed

Combine egg and milk. Stir in crumbs and seasoning. Add meat and mix well. Form into 24 meatballs, about 1½ inches (3½ cm). Brown meatballs in skillet. Drain. Add broth, mushrooms, and onion. Cover and simmer for 30 minutes. Stir together sour cream, flour, and caraway seed. Stir into skillet. Cook and stir until thickened.

Yield: 6 servings

Each with: 194 g water; 281 calories (32% from fat, 47% from protein, 21% from carb); 19 g protein; 6 g total fat; 2 g saturated fat; 2 g monounsaturated fat; 1 g polyunsaturated fat; 8 g carb; 1 g fiber; 1 g sugar; 199 mg phosphorus; 87 mg calcium; 2 mg iron; 172 mg sodium; 417 mg potassium; 212 IU vitamin A; 2 mg vitamin C; 68 mg cholesterol

Glycemic Index: Low

Meatballs with Barbecue Sauce

These barbecue flavored meatballs are great for a main dish served over noodles or rice, but they also are a great appetizer or party food that will keep guests coming back for one more.

1 pound (455 g) ground beef

¼ cup (30 g) bread crumbs

¼ cup (40 g) onions, chopped

⅓ cup (80 ml) milk

1 egg, slightly beaten

1 cup (240 g) low-sodium catsup

¾ cup (210 g) chili sauce (see chapter 2)

2 tablespoons (22 g) prepared mustard

2 tablespoons (30 g) brown sugar

2 cloves garlic, chopped

1 tablespoon (6.5 g) celery seed

2 tablespoons (30 ml) Worcestershire sauce

1½ cups (355 ml) water

1 dash Tabasco

Mix first 5 ingredients. Form into balls. Place in baking dish. Mix together remaining ingredients. Pour sauce over meatballs. Bake (foil covered) at 350°F (180°C, or gas mark 4) for 45 minutes.

Yield: 4 servings

Each with: 281 g water; 449 calories (45% from fat, 24% from protein, 31% from carb); 27 g Protein; 23 g total fat; 8 g saturated fat; 9 g monounsaturated fat; 1 g polyunsaturated fat; 35 g carb; 1 g fiber; 25 g sugar; 257 mg phosphorous; 118 mg calcium; 5 mg iron; 237 mg sodium; 749 mg potassium; 1453 IU vitamin A; 35 mg ATE vitamin E; 32 mg vitamin C; 131 mg cholesterol

Glycemic Index: Low

Sweet and Sour Meatballs

These tasty meatballs have a fairly traditional sweet and sour flavor and are great served over rice.

1½ pounds (680 g) lean ground beef

⅔ cup (86 g) cracker crumbs

⅓ cup (60 g) onion, minced

1 egg

¼ teaspoon ginger

¼ cup (60 ml) milk

1 tablespoon (15 ml) olive oil

2 tablespoons (16 g) cornstarch

13 ounces (365 g) pineapple tidbits, drained (reserve syrup)

½ cup (8 g) brown sugar substitute, such as Splenda

⅓ cup (80 ml) cider vinegar

⅓ cup (50 g) green bell pepper, chopped

Mix thoroughly beef, crumbs, onion, egg, ginger, and milk. Shape mixture by rounded teaspoonfuls into balls. Heat oil in large skillet; brown and cook meatballs. Remove meatballs; keep warm. Pour fat from skillet. Mix cornstarch and sugar. Stir in reserved pineapple syrup and vinegar. Pour into skillet; cook over medium heat, stirring constantly until mixture thickens and boils. Add meatballs, pineapple tidbits, and bell pepper; heat through.

Yield: 6 servings

Each with: 172 g water; 402 calories (53% from fat, 25% from protein, 22% from carb); 25 g Protein; 24 g total fat; 9 g saturated fat; 11 g monounsaturated fat; 2 g polyunsaturated fat; 22 g carb; 1 g fiber; 10 g sugar; 214 mg phosphorous; 60 mg calcium; 3 mg iron; 97 mg sodium; 489 mg potassium; 131 IU vitamin A; 21 mg ATE vitamin E; 12 mg vitamin C; 113 mg cholesterol

Glycemic Index: Low

Swiss Steak

Swiss steak was one of those recipes that we hadn't made in years, when suddenly it occurred to me to wonder why. I did a little research, came up with this recipe, and now we have it frequently.

2 pounds (900 g) round steak

¼ cup (32 g) flour

⅛ teaspoon black pepper

3 tablespoons (45 ml) olive oil

1 onion, sliced

½ teaspoon oregano

¼ teaspoon garlic powder

½ cup (50 g) chopped celery

½ cup (75 g) chopped green bell pepper

2 cups (480 g) canned no-salt-added tomatoes, mashed

¼ cup (60 ml) water

TIP

This may be served with mashed potatoes or over rice or noodles.

Pound meat with meat mallet to tenderize; set aside. In a pie plate, combine flour and pepper. Dredge meat in flour mixture. Reserve flour mixture. Brown both sides of meat in oil in a 4-quart (4 L) casserole dish. Add onion; cook until transparent. Stir in reserved flour mixture, oregano, garlic powder, celery, bell pepper, tomatoes with liquid, and water. Be sure meat is covered with liquid. Cover and cook at 350°F (180°C, gas mark 4) for 45 to 55 minutes or until meat is tender, stirring every 15 minutes.

Yield: 6 servings

Each with: 212 g water; 411 calories (40% from fat, 49% from protein, 10% from carb); 49 g protein; 18 g total fat; 6 g saturated fat; 8 g monounsaturated fat; 2 g polyunsaturated fat; 11 g carb; 2 g fiber; 4 g sugar; 44 mg calcium; 6 mg iron; 94 mg sodium; 733 mg potassium; 202 IU vitamin A; 23 mg vitamin C; 145 mg cholesterol

Glycemic Index: Low

Coca-Cola Pot Roast

I know it sounds funny, but it works.

3 pounds (1 ⅓ kg) beef

2 tablespoons (30 ml) olive oil

1 can (14½ ounces or 410 g) no-salt-added tomatoes

1 cup (235 ml) Coca-Cola

1 onion, chopped

1 package spaghetti sauce mix

1½ teaspoons salt

½ teaspoon garlic salt

Brown meat in oil for 10 minutes on each side; remove to slow cooker. Drain fat. Break up tomatoes in their juice; add remaining ingredients, stirring until spaghetti sauce mix is dissolved. Pour over meat. Cover; simmer until meat is tender. Thicken gravy; serve over sliced meat.

Yield: 8 servings

Each with: 179 g water; 621 calories (64% from fat, 29% from protein, 7% from carb); 45 g protein; 44 g total fat; 17 g saturated fat; 18 g monounsaturated fat; 3 g polyunsaturated fat; 10 g carb; 1 g fiber; 5 g sugar; 368 mg phosphorus; 35 mg calcium; 5 mg iron; 997 mg sodium; 784 mg potassium; 414 IU vitamin A; 8 mg vitamin C; 141 mg cholesterol

Glycemic Index: Low

Slow Cooker Pot Roast

Powdered dressing mixes add great flavor to this pot roast.

2 tablespoons (30 ml) olive oil

3 pounds (1⅓ kg) beef chuck roast

1½ tablespoons (11 g) dry Italian salad dressing mix

2 tablespoons (14 g) dry ranch-style dressing mix

2 tablespoons (12 g) low-sodium beef bouillon

1 can (14½ ounces or 410 g) low-sodium beef broth

1 large onion, diced

Heat oil in a large skillet. Brown the roast on all sides in the hot oil. Place roast in slow cooker. In a small cup or bowl, mix together the Italian salad dressing mix, ranch dressing mix, and bouillon. Sprinkle them evenly over the roast. Pour in the beef broth and add the chopped onion. Cover and cook on high 4 to 5 hours or low 8 to 10 hours. You can use the juices as is or thicken with flour or cornstarch to make gravy.

Yield: 9 servings

Each with: 88 g water; 345 calories (40% from fat, 60% from protein, 0% from carb); 50 g protein; 15 g total fat; 5 g saturated fat; 6 g monounsaturated fat; 2 g polyunsaturated fat; 0 g carb; 0 g fiber; 0 g sugar; 406 mg phosphorus; 14 mg calcium; 6 mg iron; 119 mg sodium; 437 mg potassium; 0 IU vitamin A; 0 mg vitamin C; 153 mg cholesterol

Glycemic Index: Low

Beef Bourguignon

This slow cooked beef is tender and wonderfully seasoned with its red wine sauce.

2½ pounds (1 kg) lean beef, cubed

1 cup (235 ml) red wine

⅓ cup (80 ml) olive oil

1 teaspoon thyme

1 teaspoon black pepper

4 slices bacon, diced

2 cloves garlic, crushed

1 cup (160 g) onion, diced

1 pound (454 g) mushrooms, sliced

⅓ cup (42 g) flour

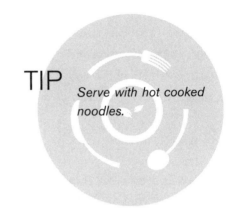

TIP

Serve with hot cooked noodles.

Marinate beef in wine, oil, thyme, and pepper 4 hours at room temp or overnight in the refrigerator. In large pan, cook bacon until soft. Add garlic and onion, sautéing until soft. Add mushrooms and cook until slightly softened. Drain beef, reserving liquid. Place beef in slow cooker. Sprinkle flour over the beef stirring until well coated. Add mushroom mixture on top. Pour reserved marinade over all. Cook on low 8–9 hours.

Yield: 8 servings

Each with: 175 g water; 537 calories (59% from fat, 34% from protein, 7% from carb); 43 g Protein; 34 g total fat; 11 g saturated fat; 17 g monounsaturated fat; 2 g polyunsaturated fat; 9 g carb; 1 g fiber; 2 g sugar; 390 mg phosphorous; 26 mg calcium; 5 mg iron; 187 mg sodium; 740 mg potassium; 7 IU vitamin A; 0 mg ATE vitamin E; 3 mg vitamin C; 126 mg cholesterol

Glycemic Index: Low

Beef Burgundy

This is a great beef and noodles dish, and it's so easy to prepare in your slow cooker. The beef gets very tender from the long cooking process.

4 slices low-sodium bacon

2 pounds (900 g) beef stew meat

1 cup (130 g) carrots, cut into chunks

1 onion, sliced

½ cup (64 g) all-purpose flour

½ teaspoon marjoram

¼ teaspoon garlic powder

¼ teaspoon black pepper

1 cup (235 ml) low-sodium beef broth

½ cup (120 ml) burgundy wine

1 tablespoon (15 ml) Worcestershire sauce

3 cups (210 g) sliced mushrooms

8 ounces (225 g) uncooked egg noodles

2 tablespoons (8 g) fresh parsley (optional)

Cook bacon until crisp; drain and crumble. Place beef, bacon, carrots, and onions in the bottom of the slow cooker. Whisk together flour, marjoram, garlic powder, and pepper with broth, wine, and Worcestershire sauce. Pour mixture into slow cooker. Cook on high for 1 hour. Reduce to low and cook for 5 to 6 hours. Add mushrooms to slow cooker. Cook on high for 30 minutes or until mushrooms are tender. While mushrooms are cooking, prepare noodles according to package directions. Serve beef over noodles and garnished with parsley, if desired.

Yield: 8 servings

Each with: 195 g water; 476 calories (43% from fat, 35% from protein, 22% from carb); 40 g protein; 22 g total fat; 8 g saturated fat; 9 g monounsaturated fat; 1 g polyunsaturated fat; 15 g carb; 1 g fiber; 2 g sugar; 32 mg calcium; 5 mg iron; 140 mg sodium; 563 mg potassium; 2,023 IU vitamin A; 7 mg vitamin C; 137 mg cholesterol

Glycemic Index: Low

Braised Sirloin Tips

These tips are very tender and flavorful.

2 pounds (900 g) sirloin tips

1 tablespoon (15 ml) olive oil

⅓ cup (80 ml) cranberry juice

1 can (10½ ounces or 295 g) beef consommé

3 tablespoons (45 ml) Dick's Reduced-Sodium Soy Sauce (see chapter 2)

⅛ teaspoon garlic powder

⅛ teaspoon ginger

Cornstarch

Cut sirloin tips into bite-size pieces; brown on all sides in oil in skillet; add juice, consommé, soy sauce, garlic, and ginger. Simmer for 1½ hours or until tender. Blend small amount of cornstarch with water (use cold so it won't lump). Stir into beef until thickened, stirring constantly.

Yield: 4 servings

Each with: 234 g water; 542 calories (45% from fat, 53% from protein, 3% from carb); 69 g protein; 26 g total fat; 9 g saturated fat; 10 g monounsaturated fat; 3 g polyunsaturated fat; 4 g carb; 0 g fiber; 0 g sugar; 535 mg phosphorus; 53 mg calcium; 5 mg iron; 1386 mg sodium; 865 mg potassium; 2 IU vitamin A; 2 mg vitamin C; 166 mg cholesterol

Glycemic Index: Low

Roast Beef with Root Vegetables

This makes a lot of food, but it's just as good left over. Or you can add fewer vegetables and use the extra beef in other meals.

3 pounds (1⅓ kg) beef rump roast

1 can (14½ ounces or 405 g) low-sodium beef broth

4 turnips, cubed

1 pound (455 g) parsnips, sliced

1 pound (455 g) carrots, sliced

½ pound (225 g) mushrooms

1 onion, quartered

Place beef roast in large roasting pan. Pour broth over top. Slice vegetables into large pieces. Place around meat. Cover and roast at 325°F (170°C, gas mark 3) until vegetables are tender and meat is desired doneness.

Yield: 10 servings

Each with: 293 g water; 360 calories (42% from fat, 36% from protein, 22% from carb); 32 g protein; 17 g total fat; 7 g saturated fat; 7 g monounsaturated fat; 20 g carb; 5 g fiber; 8 g sugar; 81 mg calcium; 3 mg iron; 176 mg sodium; 1,015 mg potassium; 5,460 IU vitamin A; 27 mg vitamin C; 83 mg cholesterol

Glycemic Index: Low

Beef and Barley Casserole

This quick casserole has a great flavor from a unique combination of ingredients.

⅓ cup (67 g) pearl barley

1 pound (455 g) ground beef, browned

1 cup (160 g) onion, cut up

1 cup (130 g) carrot, sliced

2 tablespoons (40 g) molasses

2 tablespoons (30 ml) Dick's Reduced-Sodium Soy Sauce (see chapter 2)

In a 2-quart (2 L) casserole, mix barley, browned beef, onion, carrots, and molasses; mix well. Add enough water to cover. Bake at 350°F (180°C, or gas mark 4) for 1 hour covered. Before serving, stir in soy sauce. Mix. You may have to add more water during baking.

Yield: 4 servings

(continued on page 220)

Each with: 145 g water; 384 calories (47% from fat, 25% from protein, 28% from carb); 24 g Protein; 20 g total fat; 8 g saturated fat; 8 g monounsaturated fat; 1 g polyunsaturated fat; 27 g carb; 4 g fiber; 9 g sugar; 235 mg phosphorous; 56 mg calcium; 4 mg iron; 107 mg sodium; 721 mg potassium; 5384 IU vitamin A; 0 mg ATE vitamin E; 5 mg vitamin C; 78 mg cholesterol

Glycemic Index: Low

Skillet Beef and Peppers

This is a variation of Salisbury steak with peppers and onions and a tomato-based sauce. It's great with just about any starch, from rice to noodles to pasta.

2 pounds (900 g) lean ground beef

⅛ teaspoon pepper

1 tablespoon (15 ml) olive oil

1 cup (160 g) onion, sliced

1½ cups (225 g) green bell peppers, chopped

16 ounces (245 g) no-salt-added tomato sauce

½ teaspoon ginger

2 tablespoons (30 ml) Dick's Reduced-Sodium Soy Sauce (see chapter 2)

Sprinkle beef with pepper, shape into 6 oval steaks. In large skillet lightly brown steak in oil. Drain off excess fat. Add onion and peppers. Pour in tomato sauce. Blend in ginger and soy sauce. Cover and simmer 15 to 25 minutes or until desired doneness.

Yield: 6 servings

Each with: 225 g water; 423 calories (61% from fat, 29% from protein, 10% from carb); 30 g Protein; 28 g total fat; 11 g saturated fat; 13 g monounsaturated fat; 1 g polyunsaturated fat; 10 g carb; 2 g fiber; 5 g sugar; 259 mg phosphorous; 32 mg calcium; 4 mg iron; 112 mg sodium; 826 mg potassium; 403 IU vitamin A; 0 mg ATE vitamin E; 42 mg vitamin C; 104 mg cholesterol

Glycemic Index: Low

Beef and Tomato Pie

Here is an easy main-dish pie.

1 pound (455 g) ground beef, cooked

1 cup (160 g) chopped onion

1 cup (100 g) chopped celery

3 tomatoes, chopped

1½ cups (173 g) shredded Swiss cheese

2 cups (475 ml) skim milk

¼ cup (56 g) unsalted butter, melted

3 eggs

1 cup (120 g) baking mix, such as Bisquick

½ teaspoon garlic powder

Preheat oven to 350°F (180°C, gas mark 4). Grease a 13 × 9 × 2-inch (33 × 23 × 5 cm) baking dish. Layer beef, onion, celery, tomatoes, and cheese in dish. Beat remaining ingredients until smooth. Pour into dish. Bake 40 to 50 minutes.

Yield: 8 servings

Each with: 136 g water; 319 calories (62% from fat, 29% from protein, 9% from carb); 23 g protein; 22 g total fat; 12 g saturated fat; 7 g monounsaturated fat; 1 g polyunsaturated fat; 7 g carb; 1 g fiber; 2 g sugar; 329 mg phosphorus; 309 mg calcium; 2 mg iron; 155 mg sodium; 358 mg potassium; 667 IU vitamin A; 3 mg vitamin C; 163 mg cholesterol

Glycemic Index: Low

Beef and Beer Stew with Root Vegetables

This flavorful stew cooks well in a cast iron Dutch oven, but any large heavy pan will do. The flavor of the dark beer and root vegetables combine for a real taste treat.

2 pounds (900 g) beef stew meat

2 bay leaves

1 tablespoon (4.3 g) dry thyme

1 tablespoon (3.3 g) rosemary

¼ cup (60 ml) olive oil

2 tablespoons (28 g) unsalted butter

1 cup (160 g) onion, peeled and diced

¼ cup (31 g) flour

12 ounces (355 ml) dark beer

1 quart (950 ml) low-sodium beef broth

½ cup crushed tomatoes

2 teaspoons (4 g) black pepper, fresh ground

¼ cup (35 g) carrots, peeled and diced

½ cup (50 g) celery, diced

1 cup (150 g) rutabaga, peeled and diced,

1 cup (225 g) parsnips, peeled and diced

Season the beef with pepper. Tie the bay leaves, thyme and rosemary into cheesecloth. In a large skillet, combine the oil and butter and heat until the butter bubbles. Add the beef in one flat and not too tightly-packed layer and brown the beef well on all sides. Remove the beef, set aside, and add the onions and cook to a golden-caramelized color. Sprinkle the onions with the flour and stir to combine well. Return the beef to the pan; add the beer, broth, herbs, tomatoes, and pepper. Bring to a boil and reduce the heat to a slow simmer. Cover and cook for ¾ hour. Add the carrots, celery, rutabaga, and parsnips and continue to cook for 1 additional hour.

Yield: 6 servings

Each with: 409 g water; 425 calories (47% from fat, 37% from protein, 17% from carb); 37 g Protein; 21 g total fat; 7 g saturated fat; 11 g monounsaturated fat; 2 g polyunsaturated fat; 17 g carb; 3 g fiber; 4 g sugar; 388 mg phosphorous; 82 mg calcium; 5 mg iron; 289 mg sodium; 902 mg potassium; 981 IU vitamin A; 32 mg ATE vitamin E; 15 mg vitamin C; 92 mg cholesterol

Glycemic Index: Low

Curried Beef

Beef is not a traditional ingredient for curried dishes, but once you try this you'll wonder why.

½ pound (225 g) lean ground beef

½ cup (80 g) onion, chopped

1 clove garlic, minced

¾ cup (94 g) apple, chopped, unpeeled

¼ cup (15 g) fresh parsley, chopped

1½ teaspoons curry powder

½ teaspoon cumin

⅛ teaspoon cayenne

¼ cup (60 ml) apple juice, unsweetened

16 ounces (455 g) no-salt-added tomatoes undrained

TIP

Serve this over rice or whole wheat pasta.

Cook ground beef, onion and garlic in 10-inch (25 cm) nonstick skillet over medium heat, stirring frequently, until no longer pink; drain. Stir in remaining ingredients; break up tomatoes. Heat to boiling; reduce heat. Simmer uncovered about 5 minutes or until apple is tender, stirring occasionally.

Yield: 4 servings

Each with: 195 g water; 182 calories (49% from fat, 26% from protein, 25% from carb); 12 g Protein; 10 g total fat; 4 g saturated fat; 4 g monounsaturated fat; 1 g polyunsaturated fat; 12 g carb; 2 g fiber; 7 g sugar; 117 mg phosphorous; 57 mg calcium; 3 mg iron; 57 mg sodium; 479 mg potassium; 491 IU vitamin A; 0 mg ATE vitamin E; 18 mg vitamin C; 39 mg cholesterol

Glycemic Index: Low

Beef and Tomato Curry

Beef, tomatoes, and other vegetables are simmered in a mild curry sauce to make this tasty dish. Serve over noodles or rice.

½ pound (225 g) round steak

½ cup (120 ml) low-sodium beef broth

1½ cups (270 g) tomatoes, coarsely chopped

1 cup (150 g) green bell pepper cut in 1-inch (2½ cm) pieces

1½ cups (240 g) onion, coarsely chopped

1 teaspoon curry powder

1 tablespoon (8 g) cornstarch

1 tablespoon (15 ml) water

Cut meat into 1 x 2-inch (2½ x 5 cm) strips. Spray skillet with nonstick vegetable oil spray. Cook meat in broth until tender. Add tomatoes, peeled and cut up, green peppers, onion, and curry powder and heat to boiling. Cover and cook on medium for 3 to 5 minutes. Mix cornstarch and water. Stir into mixture and cook until thick and boiling.

Yield: 4 servings

Each with: 212 g water; 146 calories (18% from fat, 49% from protein, 33% from carb); 18 g Protein; 3 g total fat; 1 g saturated fat; 1 g monounsaturated fat; 0 g polyunsaturated fat; 12 g carb; 2 g fiber; 3 g sugar; 147 mg phosphorous; 28 mg calcium; 2 mg iron; 48 mg sodium; 435 mg potassium; 492 IU vitamin A; 0 mg ATE vitamin E; 49 mg vitamin C; 33 mg cholesterol

Glycemic Index: Low

Stuffed Red Bell Peppers

The original recipe called for green bell peppers, but I modified it because I like the taste of red peppers better (at least they're ripe).

6 red bell peppers

½ cup (60 g) bread crumbs

1 cup (235 ml) cream

¾ cup (120 g) chopped onion

2 tablespoons (30 ml) olive oil

2 pounds (900 g) hamburger

¼ cup (25 g) scallions

2 cups (475 ml) water

Blanch peppers, cut off tops, and finely chop as much of the tops as possible. Combine bread crumbs and cream and let soak. Cook onion in oil until tender. Combine all ingredients and stuff peppers. Place in a dish, add water, and cook at 375°F (190°C, gas mark 5) for 1 hour.

Yield: 6 servings

Each with: 267 g water; 616 calories (77% from fat, 17% from protein, 6% from carb); 27 g protein; 52 g total fat; 22 g saturated fat; 23 g monounsaturated fat; 3 g polyunsaturated fat; 9 g carb; 2 g fiber; 4 g sugar; 239 mg phosphorus; 46 mg calcium; 3 mg iron; 143 mg sodium; 562 mg potassium; 2,667 IU vitamin A; 98 mg vitamin C; 156 mg cholesterol

Glycemic Index: Low

Bulgogi

I spent some time in Korea when I was in the Army. My favorite Korean food was bulgogi, beef skewers marinated in a spicy ginger, red pepper, and soy-based sauce. At that time, Korean food wasn't well known in the United States, but now there are a number of Korean restaurants serving bulgogi and other dishes. You can also make a good bulgogi at home, and if your family is like mine, they'll be glad you did.

2 pound (900 g) flank steak

1½ tablespoons (12 g) gingerroot, grated

2 tablespoons (30 ml) olive oil

1 teaspoon sesame oil

2 teaspoons (5.4 g) sesame seeds

⅔ cups Dick's Reduce-Sodium Teriyaki Sauce (see chapter 2)

(continued on page 226)

2 garlic cloves, minced

½ teaspoon red pepper flakes

Lightly freeze steak and slice into thin slices. Mix all but sesame seeds together and marinate meat at least 3 hours. Skewer and broil or barbecue. Sprinkle with sesame seeds.

Yield: 6 servings

Each with: 120 g water; 374 calories (45% from fat, 48% from protein, 6% from carb); 44 g Protein; 18 g total fat; 6 g saturated fat; 9 g monounsaturated fat; 2 g polyunsaturated fat; 6 g carb; 0 g fiber; 4 g sugar; 376 mg phosphorous; 41 mg calcium; 4 mg iron; 97 mg sodium; 597 mg potassium; 61 IU vitamin A; 0 mg ATE vitamin E; 0 mg vitamin C; 83 mg cholesterol

Glycemic Index: Low

Easy Cheeseburger Pie

This is a variation of the Bisquick impossible pie recipe with most of the sodium removed. The nice part about this is you can quickly mix it up and put it in the oven without worrying about making pie crust.

1 pound (455 g) lean ground beef

1 onion, chopped

¼ teaspoon black pepper

½ cup (64 g) flour

¾ teaspoon sodium-free baking powder

2 tablespoons (28 g) unsalted butter

1 cup (235 ml) skim milk

1 egg

1 tomato, sliced

4 ounces (115 g) Swiss cheese, shredded

Cook beef and onion until beef is brown and onion soft. Stir in pepper. Place in bottom of a greased 9-inch (23 cm) pie plate. Stir together dry ingredients. Cut in butter. Stir in milk and egg. Pour over beef mixture. Bake at 400°F (200°C, gas mark 6) for 25 minutes. Top with tomato slices and cheese. Cook an additional 5 to 8 minutes until cheese melts and knife inserted in center comes out clean.

Yield: 6 servings

Each with: 120 g water; 261 calories (50% from fat, 29% from protein, 21% from carb); 19 g protein; 14 g total fat; 6 g saturated fat; 5 g monounsaturated fat; 1 g polyunsaturated fat; 14 g carb; 1 g fiber; 2 g sugar; 105 mg calcium; 2 mg iron; 81 mg sodium; 429 mg potassium; 456 IU vitamin A; 5 mg vitamin C; 98 mg cholesterol

Glycemic Index: Low

Blue Cheese Burgers

A creamy blue cheese and mustard sauce lifts these hamburger patties out of the ordinary and into that category of special meals that get repeated regularly.

2 tablespoons (30 g) plain yogurt

2 tablespoons (16 g) blue cheese, crumbled

1 tablespoon (14 g) mayonnaise

1 teaspoon Dijon mustard

1½ pounds (680 g) lean ground beef

⅛ teaspoon pepper

For sauce, stir together yogurt, blue cheese, mayonnaise, and mustard; cover and chill up to 2 4 hours. Crumble ground beef into a large bowl. Shape ground beef into 6 patties ¾-inch (2 cm) thick. Sprinkle with pepper. Grill patties on an uncovered grill 14 to 18 minutes or to desired doneness, turning patties once halfway through grilling time. Serve patties in rolls, topped with sauce.

Yield: 6 servings

Each with: 79 g water; 304 calories (68% from fat, 30% from protein, 2% from carb); 22 g Protein; 23 g total fat; 9 g saturated fat; 9 g monounsaturated fat; 2 g polyunsaturated fat; 1 g carb; 0 g fiber; 1 g sugar; 185 mg phosphorous; 41 mg calcium; 2 mg iron; 166 mg sodium; 345 mg potassium; 47 IU vitamin A; 12 mg ATE vitamin E; 0 mg vitamin C; 83 mg cholesterol

Glycemic Index: Low

Inside Out Bacon Cheeseburgers

Bacon, cheese, and other good things are cooked right into these great tasting burgers. They are good on a bun but are equally good just on a plate with veggies for a lower carbohydrate option.

4 slices bacon

¼ cup (38 g) onions, chopped

4 ounces (115 g) mushroom, diced

1 pound (455 g) lean ground beef

1 pound (455 g) sausage

¼ cup (25 g) parmesan, grated

½ teaspoon pepper

½ teaspoon garlic powder

2 tablespoons (30 g) steak sauce

Cook bacon until crisp. Drain all but 2 tablespoons (30 ml) drippings and sauté onions and mushrooms in drippings. Crumble bacon and add to skillet. Set aside. Combine beef, pork, cheese, pepper, garlic powder, and steak sauce in a large bowl. Shape into 16 patties. Divide bacon mixture and place over eight of the patties. Place remaining patties on top and press edges tightly to seal. Grill over medium coals until well done.

Yield: 8 servings

Each with: 85 g water; 376 calories (71% from fat, 25% from protein, 4% from carb); 23 g Protein; 30 g total fat; 11 g saturated fat; 14 g monounsaturated fat; 3 g polyunsaturated fat; 4 g carb; 0 g fiber; 2 g sugar; 228 mg phosphorous; 50 mg calcium; 2 mg iron; 691 mg sodium; 377 mg potassium; 21 IU vitamin A; 4 mg ATE vitamin E; 1 mg vitamin C; 90 mg cholesterol

Glycemic Index: Low

Slow Cooker Beef for Sandwiches

A beef rump roast is turned tender and delicious by long, slow cooking. Yes, that says to cook it 16 hours on low. Put it in before you go to bed for tomorrow night's dinner. You won't be disappointed.

3 pounds (1.5 kg) beef rump roast

3 tablespoons (24 g) flour

16 ounces (450 g) tomato sauce

½ cup (75 g) onion, chopped

2 tablespoons (30 g) brown sugar, packed

2 tablespoons (30 ml) lemon juice

1½ tablespoons (11.3 g) chili powder

1 clove garlic, chopped fine

1 teaspoon dry mustard

Rub flour into roast. Place in bottom of slow cooker and add remaining ingredients. Cook on low for about 14–16 hours. Slice thinly to serve.

Yield: 10 servings

Each with: 140 g water; 294 calories (36% from fat, 52% from protein, 12% from carb); 38 g Protein; 12 g total fat; 4 g saturated fat; 5 g monounsaturated fat; 1 g polyunsaturated fat; 9 g carb; 1 g fiber; 5 g sugar; 247 mg phosphorous; 22 mg calcium; 4 mg iron; 298 mg sodium; 495 mg potassium; 493 IU vitamin A; 0 mg ATE vitamin E; 6 mg vitamin C; 127 mg cholesterol

Glycemic Index: Low

Mediterranean Stew

This is a Greek-style stew adapted for the slow cooker. The spices give it the characteristic Mediterranean flavor. The eggplant will be very soft.

2 eggplants, cut in 1-inch (2½ cm) cubes

2 pounds (900 g) stew beef, cut in 1½-inch (3½ cm) chunks

2 medium onions, sliced thin

2 cloves garlic, minced

¼ cup (60 ml) olive oil

1 cup (235 ml) low-sodium beef broth

8 ounces (225 g) no-salt-added tomato sauce

1 tablespoon (15 ml) red wine vinegar

¾ teaspoon sugar

½ teaspoon cinnamon

⅛ teaspoon allspice

⅛ teaspoon ground cloves

¼ cup (15 g) minced parsley

TIP

This is terrific served over thick pasta, like penne or rigatoni.

Wash the eggplant, peel, and cut into 1-inch (2½ cm) cubes. In large skillet, brown the beef, onion, garlic, and eggplant in olive oil until dark golden-brown; drain. Place in slow cooker. Combine the beef broth with the tomato sauce, vinegar, sugar, and spices and stir it into the meat. Cover and cook on low heat for 8 to 10 hours. If serving with pasta, prepare pasta, pour onto a large serving platter, and cover with meat, eggplant, and sauce. Sprinkle minced parsley over top.

Yield: 8 servings

Each with: 247 g water; 467 calories (57% from fat, 31% from protein, 11% from carb); 37 g protein; 30 g total fat; 10 g saturated fat; 15 g monounsaturated fat; 2 g polyunsaturated fat; 13 g carb; 5 g fiber; 6 g sugar; 48 mg calcium; 4 mg iron; 75 mg sodium; 728 mg potassium; 289 IU vitamin A; 11 mg vitamin C; 93 mg cholesterol

Glycemic Index: Low

Southwestern Beef Stew

Salsa helps to give this stew its southwestern flavor. I particularly like this as a meal to serve when we have people over, not just because it tastes great, but it makes a great presentation with the pieces of fresh corn mixed in.

2 tablespoons (30 ml) olive oil

1½ pounds (680 g) beef stew meat

2 cups (320 g) onion, quartered

2 cloves garlic, minced

28 ounces no-salt-added tomatoes

2 cups (475 ml) low-sodium beef broth

1 cup (235 ml) water

¾ teaspoon thyme

¾ teaspoon marjoram

2 cups (240 g) celery, cut in 1-inch (2½ cm) pieces

2 cups (260 g) carrot, sliced

½ cup (75 g) red bell peppers, diced

½ cup (30 g) fresh parsley, chopped

¼ cup (65 g) salsa

½ cup (50 g) elbow macaroni

3 ears of corn, husked and cut into 1½-inch (3½ cm) pieces

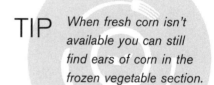

TIP *When fresh corn isn't available you can still find ears of corn in the frozen vegetable section.*

Brown meat in oil in 5 or 6 quart pot. Add onions and garlic; stir until limp. Add tomatoes, break up with spoon. Add liquids and spices. Bring to a boil. Cover and simmer until meat is very tender, approximately 2 hours. Stir in vegetables and continue to simmer for 15 minutes. Stir in salsa, macaroni, and corn. Cook until carrots and macaroni are tender, about 10 minutes.

Yield: 6 servings

Each with: 497 g water; 341 calories (29% from fat, 35% from protein, 36% from carb); 31 g Protein; 11 g total fat; 3 g saturated fat; 6 g monounsaturated fat; 1 g polyunsaturated fat; 31 g carb; 6 g fiber; 10 g sugar; 350 mg phosphorous; 122 mg calcium; 5 mg iron; 239 mg sodium; 1134 mg potassium; 8333 IU vitamin A; 0 mg ATE vitamin E; 44 mg vitamin C; 61 mg cholesterol

Glycemic Index: Low

Mexican Beef Soup

This is one of those throw-together meals that turned out to be a keeper. It's quick and easy and has a lot of flavor.

½ pound (225 g) extra-lean ground beef, 93 percent lean

½ cup (80 g) chopped onion

1 cup (70 g) shredded cabbage

1 cup (240 g) no-salt-added canned tomatoes

2 cups (500 g) Mexican-flavored beans

1 cup (235 ml) water

TIP *For variety, replace the cabbage with packaged coleslaw or broccoli slaw mix.*

Brown beef and onion in a large saucepan. Drain. Add cabbage and continue cooking until cabbage is soft, about 5 minutes. Add tomatoes, beans, and water. Bring to boil and simmer 10 minutes to blend the flavors.

Yield: 5 servings

Each with: 199 g water; 213 calories (16% from fat, 37% from protein, 47% from carb); 16 g protein; 3 g total fat; 1 g saturated fat; 1 g monounsaturated fat; 0 g polyunsaturated fat; 20 g carb; 8 g fiber; 2 g sugar; 179 mg phosphorus; 77 mg calcium; 4 mg iron; 44 mg sodium; 570 mg potassium; 76 IU vitamin A; 13 mg vitamin C; 31 mg cholesterol

Glycemic Index: Low

Mexican Steak Salad

If you have leftover London broil or other beef, this salad is a great tasting, healthy way to use it.

½ cup (115 g) sour cream

½ cup (130 g) salsa

2 tablespoons (2 g) fresh cilantro, divided

1 cup (256 g) kidney beans, rinsed and drained

½ cup (58 g) Monterey jack cheese

¼ cup (25 g) green onions, sliced

8 ounces (225 g) beef round steak, cooked and sliced (about 2 cups)

1 small head iceberg lettuce, shredded

5 radishes, thinly sliced

1 avocado, peeled and sliced

30 tortilla chips (about 2 ounces)

In small bowl, combine sour cream, salsa, and 1 tablespoon (1 g) cilantro; set aside. In medium bowl combine beans, cheese, green onions, and remaining 1 tablespoon (1 g) cilantro. To serve, on four individual plates arrange bean mixture, beef, lettuce, radishes, avocado, olives, and tortilla chips. Serve with dressing.

Yield: 4 servings

Each with: 225 g water; 2325 calories (31% from fat, 12% from protein, 57% from carb); 68 g Protein; 82 g total fat; 19 g saturated fat; 34 g monounsaturated fat; 23 g polyunsaturated fat; 331 g carb; 32 g fiber; 5 g sugar; 1688 mg phosphorous; 894 mg calcium; 11 mg iron; 4483 mg sodium; 1983 mg potassium; 1165 IU vitamin A; 62 mg ATE vitamin E; 10 mg vitamin C; 90 mg cholesterol

Glycemic Index: Low

9

Main Dishes:
Pork and Lamb

Pork, like beef, can contain a lot of saturated fats, which we all should be trying to avoid. This chapter features a number of recipes using low-fat pork chops, as well as some grilling recipes for ribs and some great, low-GI pork stews. There also are a couple of tasty, low-GI lamb recipes.

Memphis Spareribs

These ribs are done in the traditional way, cooked most of the way with just a spice rub and then "mopped" with sauce near the end. This helps to keep the meat from getting too dried out. I personally prefer to smoke the ribs until they are nearly done and then move them to the grill for the last 20 minutes or so to sear the sauce into them.

2 pounds (900 g) pork spareribs

¼ cup (60 ml) cider vinegar

Rub

½ cup (115 g) brown sugar

1½ teaspoons black pepper

1 teaspoon cayenne pepper

Sauce

8 ounces (225 g) no-salt-added tomato sauce

½ cup (120 ml) cider vinegar

¼ cup (85 g) honey

1 teaspoon onion powder

1 teaspoon dry mustard

1 teaspoon garlic powder

½ teaspoon cayenne pepper

Brush ribs with vinegar. Mix rub ingredients together and rub into ribs. Smoke or grill until done. While ribs are cooking, combine sauce ingredients. Brush with sauce during the last 30 minutes of cooking.

Yield: 4 servings

Each with: 162 g water; 529 calories (45% from fat, 15% from protein, 39% from carb); 21 g protein; 27 g total fat; 10 g saturated fat; 12 g monounsaturated fat; 3 g polyunsaturated fat; 53 g carb; 1 g fiber; 49 g sugar; 78 mg calcium; 3 mg iron; 106 mg sodium; 694 mg potassium; 487 IU vitamin A; 8 mg vitamin C; 88 mg cholesterol

Glycemic Index: Low

Pineapple-Stuffed Pork Chops

Do you feel like you need a trip to the islands? Let these pineapple-stuffed chops ferry you away.

4 pork loin chops, 1-inch (2½ cm) thick

8 ounces (225 g) pineapple slices

¼ cup (60 g) low-sodium ketchup

1 tablespoon (6 g) chopped green onion

½ teaspoon dry mustard

Cut a pocket in each chop to make room for pineapple. Drain pineapple, reserving liquid. Cut two slices in half; cut up remaining pineapple and set aside. Place a half pineapple slice in the pocket of each chop. Heat grill to medium and grill about 20 minutes, turning once. Meanwhile, in a small saucepan combine ketchup, green onion, mustard, and the reserved pineapple juice and pieces. Heat to boiling, reduce heat, and simmer 10 minutes. Grill chops 5 minutes more, brushing with sauce and turning several times.

Yield: 4 servings

Each with: 131 g water; 189 calories (21% from fat, 46% from protein, 33% from carb); 22 g protein; 4 g total fat; 1 g saturated fat; 2 g monounsaturated fat; 0 g polyunsaturated fat; 15 g carb; 1 g fiber; 13 g sugar; 230 mg phosphorus; 25 mg calcium; 1 mg iron; 55 mg sodium; 495 mg potassium; 171 IU vitamin A; 8 mg vitamin C; 64 mg cholesterol

Glycemic Index: Low

Sweet and Sour Skillet Pork Chops

This is a low GI version of an old favorite. Pork chops are skillet cooked in a sweet and sour sauce for great taste, but the traditional breading of sweet and sour dishes is eliminated, lowering the carbohydrate count.

6 pork chops

6 pineapple rings, juice packed

½ cup (120 ml) pineapple juice

2 tablespoons (30 ml) cider vinegar

¼ tablespoon brown sugar substitute, such as Splenda

¼ teaspoon cinnamon

Dash rosemary

1 cup (100 g) celery, cut into strips

1 cup (150 g) green bell pepper, cut into strips

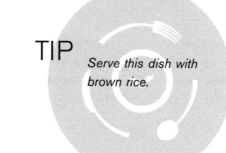

TIP

Serve this dish with brown rice.

Trim all fat from chops. Brown meat on both sides in skillet sprayed with nonstick vegetable oil spray. Remove chops. In skillet, mix pineapple juice, vinegar, and sugar substitute. Add cinnamon and rosemary. Put chops in pan. Add celery and cover. Simmer about 30 minutes. Add green pepper strips. Place pineapple rings on each chop. Cover and cook about 10 minutes longer. Arrange chops on serving platter. Place pineapple and pepper strips on top. Spoon juice over top.

Yield: 6 servings

Each with: 98 g water; 274 calories (50% from fat, 35% from protein, 15% from carb); 24 g Protein; 15 g total fat; 5 g saturated fat; 7 g monounsaturated fat; 2 g polyunsaturated fat; 10 g carb; 1 g fiber; 8 g sugar; 14 mg phosphorous; 40 mg calcium; 1 mg iron; 15 mg sodium; 579 mg potassium; 193 IU vitamin A; 0 mg ATE vitamin E; 26 mg vitamin C; 74 mg cholesterol

Glycemic Index: Low

Oriental Barbecued Pork Chops

An Oriental flavored barbecue sauce is used first to marinate, then as a topping for these flavorful chops. If you prefer, you can also pan fry or broil the chop instead of grilling.

4 pork loin chops

6 tablespoons (90 ml) Dick's Reduced-Sodium Soy Sauce (see chapter 2)

½ teaspoon garlic powder

2 teaspoons (10 ml) sherry

½ cup (60 g) no-salt-added tomato sauce

¼ cup (60 ml) water

(continued on page 238)

Trim fat away. Mix soy sauce, garlic, sherry, and tomato sauce. Pour over meat in flat pan. Let stand, covered, in refrigerator for 3 hours. Drain off marinade and pour into small pan. Add water and heat to boiling. Reduce heat and simmer 5 minutes. Grill over medium heat until done, turning once. Serve hot sauce with meat.

Yield: 4 servings

Each with: 135 g water; 158 calories (26% from fat, 61% from protein, 13% from carb); 23 g Protein; 4 g total fat; 1 g saturated fat; 2 g monounsaturated fat; 0 g polyunsaturated fat; 5 g carb; 1 g fiber; 2 g sugar; 258 mg phosphorous; 22 mg calcium; 2 mg iron; 65 mg sodium; 536 mg potassium; 113 IU vitamin A; 2 mg ATE vitamin E; 5 mg vitamin C; 64 mg cholesterol

Glycemic Index: Low

Slow Cooker Pork Chops

Do you feel like some barbecue but don't want to fire up the grill? These chops are a perfect alternative. They're cooked with minimum effort in the slow cooker.

4 pork loin chops

1 cup (160 g) onion, sliced

1 tablespoon (15 g) brown sugar

¼ cup (60 g) low-sodium catsup

1 tablespoon (15 ml) lemon juice

¼ cup (60 ml) water

Cut fat from chops. In a slow cooker, layer pork chops, onion, brown sugar, catsup and lemon juice. Pour water over all. Cook on low 8–10 hours.

Yield: 4 servings

Each with: 139 g water; 174 calories (23% from fat, 51% from protein, 26% from carb); 22 g Protein; 4 g total fat; 1 g saturated fat; 2 g monounsaturated fat; 0 g polyunsaturated fat; 11 g carb; 1 g fiber; 9 g sugar; 238 mg phosphorous; 29 mg calcium; 1 mg iron; 58 mg sodium; 506 mg potassium; 149 IU vitamin A; 2 mg ATE vitamin E; 8 mg vitamin C; 64 mg cholesterol

Glycemic Index: Low

Zucchini Stuffed Pork Chops

Boneless pork chops are stuffed with a flavorful vegetable mixture, giving maximum flavor and a very low GI.

1½ cup (188 g) zucchini, shredded

1 clove garlic, crushed

2 tablespoons (10 g) parmesan cheese, grated

¼ teaspoon black pepper

4 boneless pork loin chops

1 teaspoon (5 ml) olive oil

½ cup (120 ml) dry white wine or chicken broth

1 tablespoon (11 g) Dijon mustard

TIP *If you prefer, you could also cut a pocket in each chop to hold the mixture rather than pounding and rolling them.*

Squeeze zucchini with paper towels to remove moisture. Spray 10-inch (25 cm) nonstick skillet with nonstick cooking spray. Cook zucchini and garlic in skillet over medium heat about 3 minutes or until tender. Stir in cheese and pepper. Remove zucchini mixture from skillet; cool. Trim fat from pork chops. Flatten each pork chop to ¼-inch (5 mm) thickness between waxed paper or plastic wrap. Spread one-fourth of the zucchini mixture over each piece of pork. Roll up; secure with wooden picks. Add oil and pork rolls to skillet. Cover and cook over medium heat 15 to 20 minutes, turning once, until done. Remove wooden picks. Remove pork rolls from skillet; keep warm. Add wine to skillet. Cook over high heat 2 to 3 minutes or until reduced by half. Stir in mustard. Pour sauce over pork rolls.

Yield: 4 servings

Each with: 148 g water; 187 calories (36% from fat, 57% from protein, 7% from carb); 23 g Protein; 7 g total fat; 2 g saturated fat; 3 g monounsaturated fat; 1 g polyunsaturated fat; 3 g carb; 1 g fiber; 1 g sugar; 270 mg phosphorous; 60 mg calcium; 1 g iron; 148 mg sodium; 527 mg potassium; 117 IU vitamin A; 6 mg ATE vitamin E; 9 mg vitamin C; 66 mg cholesterol

Glycemic Index: Low

Pork Chops in Onion Sauce

Savory pork chops and onions are simmered in beer and beef broth for added flavor. Serve this over noodles or brown rice.

4 pork loin chops

¼ teaspoon pepper

1½ tablespoons (12 g) flour

1½ tablespoons (25 ml) olive oil

4 small onions, thinly sliced

½ cup (120 ml) beer

½ cup (120 ml) low-sodium beef broth

1 teaspoon cornstarch

Season pork chops with pepper; coat with flour. Heat oil in a heavy skillet. Add pork chops; fry for 3 minutes on each side. Add onions; cook for another 5 minutes, turning chops once. Pour in beer and beef broth; cover and simmer 15 minutes. Remove pork shops to a preheated platter. Blend cornstarch with a small amount of cold water. Stir into sauce and cook until thick and bubbly. Pour over pork chops.

Yield: 4 servings

Each with: 238 g water; 250 calories (36% from fat, 39% from protein, 25% from carb); 23 g Protein; 10 g total fat; 2 g saturated fat; 6 g monounsaturated fat; 1 g polyunsaturated fat; 15 g carb; 2 g fiber; 5 g sugar; 266 mg phosphorous; 44 mg calcium; 1 mg iron; 75 mg sodium; 577 mg potassium; 16 IU vitamin A; 2 mg ATE vitamin E; 10 mg vitamin C; 64 mg cholesterol

Glycemic Index: Low

Barbecued Pork

This recipe for pulled pork is done in the oven, but it could also be cooked on a smoker or with indirect heat on a grill.

3 pounds (1⅓ kg) pork loin roast

1 cup (160 g) sliced onion

1 teaspoon red pepper flakes

1 teaspoon black pepper

1 cup (235 ml) apple cider

1 cup (235 ml) apple cider vinegar

½ teaspoon minced garlic

Preheat the oven to 300°F (150°C, gas mark 2). Coat a large baking pan with nonstick vegetable oil spray. Rub the pork shoulder with the pepper flakes and pepper and place in the baking pan. Pour the cider and vinegar over and around the pork. Scatter the onion and garlic over and around the pork. Cover with aluminum foil. Roast for 3 hours. Uncover and continue to roast until an instant-read thermometer inserted into the thickest part of the pork registers 180°F (82°C), about 1 hour. Remove the pork from the oven and transfer to a plate. Let stand for 1 hour. Using 2 forks, shred the pork by steadying the meat with 1 fork and pulling it away with the other, discarding any fat.

Yield: 12 servings

Each with: 132 g water; 165 calories (28% from fat, 62% from protein, 10% from carb); 24 g protein; 5 g total fat; 2 g saturated fat; 2 g monounsaturated fat; 1 g polyunsaturated fat; 4 g carb; 0 g fiber; 3 g sugar; 255 mg phosphorus; 22 mg calcium; 1 mg iron; 60 mg sodium; 484 mg potassium; 70 IU vitamin A; 2 mg vitamin C; 71 mg cholesterol

Glycemic Index: Low

Dijon Pork Chops

It's a little hard to categorize the marinade for these chops. The soy sauce and spices say Asian, but the mustard gives it a really unique flavor.

1 pound (455 g) boneless pork loin chops

1 tablespoon (11 g) Dijon mustard

3 tablespoons (45 ml) Dick's Reduced-Sodium Soy Sauce (see chapter 2)

⅛ teaspoon garlic powder

(continued on page 242)

¼ cup (60 ml) dry white wine

2 teaspoons (10 ml) vegetable oil

2 teaspoons (10 ml) sherry extract

Combine marinade ingredients and pour over chops. Marinate several hours or overnight. Broil or grill, turning occasionally and basting until done.

Yield: 4 Servings

Each with: 108 g water; 187 calories (38% from fat, 58% from protein, 4% from carb); 25 g Protein; 7 g total fat; 2 g saturated fat; 3 g monounsaturated fat; 2 g polyunsaturated fat; 2 g carb; 0 g fiber; 0 g sugar; 267 mg phosphorous; 20 mg calcium; 1 mg iron; 106 mg sodium; 458 mg potassium; 11 IU vitamin A; 2 mg ATE vitamin E; 1 mg vitamin C; 71 mg cholesterol

Glycemic Index: Low

Ginger-Orange Pork Chops

These are good either as an Asian-style meal with stir-fried vegetables and rice or with more American-type side dishes like pasta or potatoes.

4 boneless pork chops

1 tablespoon (15 ml) oil

¼ teaspoon black pepper

1 teaspoon ground ginger

¼ cup (60 ml) orange juice

Brown chops in oil on both sides. Sprinkle with spices and pour orange juice over top. Cover and cook until done, 10 to 15 minutes.

Yield: 4 servings

Each with: 77 g water; 173 calories (49% from fat, 46% from protein, 5% from carb); 19 g protein; 9 g total fat; 2 g saturated fat; 3 g monounsaturated fat; 3 g polyunsaturated fat; 2 g carb; 0 g fiber; 0 g sugar; 7 mg calcium; 1 mg iron; 40 mg sodium; 408 mg potassium; 19 IU vitamin A; 5 mg vitamin C; 48 mg cholesterol

Glycemic Index: Low

Onion-Pork Sauté

My daughter found this recipe one night when she decided to get dinner ready before the rest of the family got home. It is a simple but wonderfully flavorful dish. Serve the sauce over some mashed potatoes or noodles.

6 pork chops

1 onion, peeled and sliced

1 teaspoon sodium-free beef bouillon

¼ cup (60 ml) water

½ cup (120 ml) skim milk

Brown the chops on both sides in a large skillet. Top each with a slice of onion. Dissolve bouillon in water. Pour over chops. Cover and simmer 40 minutes or until chops are tender. Remove chops. Stir milk into drippings in pan. Heat, stirring constantly, until bubbly. Spoon sauce over chops.

Yield: 6 servings

Each with: 278 calories (68% from fat, 27% from protein, 5% from carb); 18 g protein; 20 g total fat; 7 g saturated fat; 9 g monounsaturated fat; 3 g carb; 0 g fiber; 27 mg calcium; 1 mg iron; 64 mg sodium; 305 mg potassium; 6 IU vitamin A; 2 mg vitamin C; 69 mg cholesterol

Glycemic Index: Low

Grilled Pork Chops with Bourbon-Mustard Glaze

Corn muffins, coleslaw, and boiled green beans round out the main course.

⅓ cup (92 g) chili sauce

¼ cup (60 ml) bourbon

1½ tablespoons (17 g) Dijon mustard

(continued on page 244)

1½ tablespoons (25 ml) Dick's Reduced-Sodium Soy Sauce (see chapter 2)

4 pork rib chops (3 ounces or 85 g each), ¼ to ⅓ inch (½ cm) thick

Prepare grill (medium-high heat). Combine chili sauce, bourbon, mustard, and soy sauce in a saucepan and simmer over medium heat until it's reduced enough to coat a spoon, whisking occasionally, about 4 minutes. Sprinkle both sides of chops with salt and pepper. Brush 1 side of chops generously with sauce and place sauce side down on the grill. Brush tops generously with remaining sauce. Grill until cooked through and glazed, about 3 minutes per side.

Yield: 2 servings

Each with: 167 g water; 569 calories (61% from fat, 36% from protein, 4% from carb); 44 g protein; 33 g total fat; 9 g saturated fat; 16 g monounsaturated fat; 4 g polyunsaturated fat; 4 g carb; 0 g fiber; 3 g sugar; 288 mg phosphorus; 52 mg calcium; 3 mg iron; 431 mg sodium; 577 mg potassium; 681 IU vitamin A; 9 mg vitamin C; 141 mg cholesterol

Glycemic Index: Low

Pork and Squash Packets

Pork and acorn squash wrapped in foil bake in the oven for an easy meal and exceptional tenderness.

2 boneless pork loin chops, 1-inch (2½ cm) thick

1 dash black pepper

6 slices acorn squash, ½-inch (1 cm) thick

2 tablespoons (28 g) unsalted butter

2 tablespoons (30 g) brown sugar

Cut two 18 x 12-inch (45 x 30 cm) pieces of heavy foil; place pork chop in center of lower half of each piece of foil. Sprinkle with pepper. Lay squash slices on top of chops. Dot butter in center of each slice. Sprinkle with brown sugar. Fold upper edge of foil over ingredients to meet bottom edge. Turn foil edges to form a ½-inch (1 cm) fold. Smooth fold. Double over again; press very tightly to seal, allowing room for expansion and heat circulation. Repeat folding and sealing at each end. Place packet on a baking sheet; bake in a 425°F (220°C, or gas mark 7) oven, 25–30 minutes or until chops and squash are tender.

Each with: 266 g water; 369 calories (38% from fat, 24% from protein, 38% from carb); 23 g Protein; 16 g total fat; 9 g saturated fat; 5 g monounsaturated fat; 1 g polyunsaturated fat; 36 g carb; 3 g fiber; 13 g sugar; 304 mg phosphorous; 99 mg calcium; 3 mg iron; 65 mg sodium; 1172 mg potassium; 1153 IU vitamin A; 97 mg ATE vitamin E; 25 mg vitamin C; 94 mg cholesterol

Glycemic Index: Low

Pork Chop Sweet Potato Bake

Pork chops, sweet potatoes, and apples, baked in apple juice, make a great meal without the need for anything else.

4 pork loin chops

2 sweet potatoes, peeled and sliced

¼ cup (4 g) brown sugar substitute, such as Splenda

2 apples, peeled and sliced

1 cup (235 ml) apple juice

Brown pork chops in skillet sprayed with nonstick vegetable oil spray. Place in 8 x 8-inch (20 x 20 cm) baking pan. Slice sweet potatoes over top. Sprinkle with brown sugar substitute. Slice apples over top. Pour apple juice over all. Bake 1½ hours at 350°F (180°C, or gas mark 4).

Yield: 4 servings

Each with: 243 g water; 255 calories (16% from fat, 35% from protein, 49% from carb); 23 g Protein; 5 g total fat; 2 g saturated fat; 2 g monounsaturated fat; 1 g polyunsaturated fat; 31 g carb; 3 g fiber; 20 g sugar; 256 mg phosphorous; 40 mg calcium; 2 mg iron; 76 mg sodium; 680 mg potassium; 11915 IU vitamin A; 2 mg ATE vitamin E; 13 mg vitamin C; 64 mg cholesterol

Glycemic Index: Low

Schnitzel

This is properly called wienerschnitzel if you use veal chops and schweineschnitzel if you use pork, which I do. Some people serve this with a fried egg placed on top of the schnitzel.

2 tablespoons (30 ml) olive oil

4 pork loin chops, boneless

2 eggs

½ cup (60 g) low-sodium fine bread crumbs

¼ teaspoon pepper

2 lemons

Heat the oil in a large skillet at medium-high heat. Place each chop between 2 sheets of plastic and pound with the smooth side of a meat tenderizer until thin (¼ inch to ½ inch or ½ to 1 cm thick). Beat the 2 eggs in a bowl that is wide enough to dip the meat into. Spread the bread crumbs onto a plate or flat surface. Take each cutlet, season with pepper, and dip both sides of meat into eggs to coat. Then coat the entire cutlet with the bread crumbs. Place in hot oil and cook on both sides until golden brown. It only takes about 1 to 2 minutes per side. Serve each cutlet with half a lemon on the side. Some people go ahead and squeeze the lemon onto the schnitzel before serving.

Yield: 4 servings

Each with: 112 g water; 372 calories (54% from fat, 29% from protein, 17% from carb); 28 g protein; 23 g total fat; 7 g saturated fat; 12 g monounsaturated fat; 2 g polyunsaturated fat; 16 g carb; 3 g fiber; 1 g sugar; 274 mg phosphorus; 96 mg calcium; 2 mg iron; 109 mg sodium; 465 mg potassium; 159 IU vitamin A; 42 mg vitamin C; 184 mg cholesterol

Glycemic Index: Low

Roast Pork Tenderloin and Vegetables

This is a great pork tenderloin meal in a pan, with roasted carrots and new potatoes surrounding it.

1 ½ pounds (680 g) pork tenderloin

1 pound (455 g) carrots, peeled and cut 2-inch (5 cm) slices

2 pounds (900 g) new potatoes, halved

1 cup (160 g) onion, cut wedges

1 tablespoon (15 ml) olive oil

2 teaspoons (2.4 g) dried rosemary, crushed

1 teaspoon dried sage, crushed

¼ teaspoon pepper

Preheat oven 450°F (230°C, or gas mark 8). Generously spray roasting pan with nonstick cooking spray. Place tenderloin in pan. Place vegetables around. Drizzle oil evenly over all. Sprinkle spices over. Bake uncovered 30–40 minutes or until thermometer inserted in thickest part reads 165°F (74°C) and vegetables are tender. Stir vegetables occasionally.

Yield: 8 Servings

Each with: 217 g water; 254 calories (17% from fat, 34% from protein, 49% from carb); 21 g Protein; 5 g total fat; 1 g saturated fat; 3 g monounsaturated fat; 1 g polyunsaturated fat; 31 g carb; 4 g fiber; 5 g sugar; 297 mg phosphorous; 46 mg calcium; 3 mg iron; 94 mg sodium; 1131 mg potassium; 9561 IU vitamin A; 2 mg ATE vitamin E; 17 mg vitamin C; 55 mg cholesterol

Glycemic Index: Low

Cinnamon Apple Pork Tenderloin

Pork tenderloins cook quickly and provide a great low fat meat to build your meal around. This one is baked in under an hour surrounded by apples for even more flavor.

1 pound (455 g) pork tenderloin

2 tablespoons (16 g) cornstarch

1 teaspoon ground cinnamon

2 apples, peeled, cored, sliced

2 tablespoons (18 g) raisins

(continued on page 248)

Preheat the oven to 400°F (200°C, or gas mark 6). Place the pork tenderloin in a roasting pan or casserole dish with a lid. Combine the remaining ingredients in a bowl and stir. Spoon the apple mixture around the pork tenderloin. Cover and bake 40 minutes. Remove the lid and spoon the apple mixture over the tenderloin. Return to the oven and bake 15–20 minutes longer until tenderloin is browned and cooked through.

Yield: 4 servings

Each with: 142 g water; 199 calories (18% from fat, 49% from protein, 33% from carb); 24 g Protein; 4 g total fat; 1 g saturated fat; 2 g monounsaturated fat; 0 g polyunsaturated fat; 16 g carb; 1 g fiber; 10 g sugar; 269 mg phosphorous; 18 mg calcium; 2 mg iron; 58 mg sodium; 514 mg potassium; 33 IU vitamin A; 2 mg ATE vitamin E; 4 mg vitamin C; 74 mg cholesterol

Glycemic Index: Low

Pork Loin Roast

This pork roast has a sort of Latin flavor.

3 pounds (1⅓ kg) pork loin roast

1 tablespoon (7 g) chili powder

½ cup (120 ml) lime juice

1 teaspoon ground cumin

1 teaspoon oregano

½ teaspoon black pepper

½ teaspoon minced garlic

6 ounces (213 g) orange juice concentrate, thawed, divided

¼ cup (60 ml) dry white wine

½ cup (115 g) fat-free sour cream

Place pork roast in a shallow glass dish. Mix ground chili powder, lime juice, cumin, oregano, pepper, garlic, and ¼ cup (60 ml) of orange juice concentrate and brush mixture onto the pork roast. Cover and refrigerate at least 8 hours. Heat oven to 325°F (170°C, gas mark 3). Place pork on a rack in a shallow roasting pan. Roast uncovered until thermometer registers 170°F (77°C),

1½ to 2 hours. Remove pork and rack from the pan. Strain the drippings from the pan and set aside. Add enough water to remaining orange juice concentrate to measure ¾ cup (175 ml); stir juice and wine into the drippings. Stir in sour cream. Serve with the pork roast.

Yield: 9 servings

Each with: 151 g water; 255 calories (26% from fat, 57% from protein, 17% from carb); 33 g protein; 7 g total fat; 2 g saturated fat; 3 g monounsaturated fat; 1 g polyunsaturated fat; 10 g carb; 1 g fiber; 7 g sugar; 361 mg phosphorus; 49 mg calcium; 2 mg iron; 93 mg sodium; 748 mg potassium; 397 IU vitamin A; 32 mg vitamin C; 100 mg cholesterol

Glycemic Index: Low

Greek Pork Loin

A Mediterranean style sauce makes these thin pork slices a little different meal. Serve with couscous or a small pastalike orzo.

12 ounces (340 g) pork loin, cut into ¼-inch (5 mm) thick slices

⅛ teaspoon black pepper

2 teaspoons (10 ml) olive oil

1½ cups (240 g) onion, cut into thin wedges

1 cup (150 g) green bell pepper, cut into thin bite-size strips

½ cup (35 g) mushroom, sliced

2 cloves garlic, minced

½ teaspoon oregano

⅓ cup (34 g) pimento stuffed olives, sliced

Spray a large skillet with nonstick vegetable oil spray. Heat over medium-high heat. Season pork with pepper. Cook half of the pork slices at a time in skillet for 2 to 3 minutes or until meat is browned and no longer pink in center, turning once. Remove from heat; keep warm. Add olive oil to skillet. Heat over medium-high heat. Cook onions, peppers, mushrooms, garlic, and oregano in skillet about 4 minutes or until crisp-tender. Stir in olives; heat through. Serve vegetable mixture with pork slices.

(continued on page 250)

Yield: 4 servings

Each with: 159 g water; 163 calories (33% from fat, 47% from protein, 19% from carb); 19 g Protein; 6 g total fat; 2 g saturated fat; 3 g monounsaturated fat; 1 g polyunsaturated fat; 8 g carb; 2 g fiber; 4 g sugar; 218 mg phosphorous; 31 mg calcium; 1 mg iron; 47 mg sodium; 498 mg potassium; 154 IU vitamin A; 2 mg ATE vitamin E; 35 mg vitamin C; 54 mg cholesterol

Glycemic Index: Low

Cranberry Pork Roast

A spicy cranberry orange sauce makes this a great choice for a holiday meal. But you don't have to wait for a holiday; the slow cooker makes it easy to cook even on a workday.

3 pounds (1⅓ kg) pork loin roast

1 cup (110 g) cranberries, finely chopped

¼ cup (85 g) honey

1 teaspoon orange peel, grated

⅛ teaspoon cloves

⅛ teaspoon nutmeg

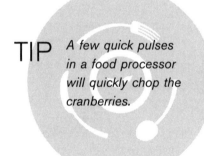

TIP *A few quick pulses in a food processor will quickly chop the cranberries.*

Place roast in slow cooker. Combine remaining ingredients. Pour over roast. Cover. Cook on low for 8 to 10 hours.

Yield: 8 servings

Each with: 139 g water; 257 calories (26% from fat, 57% from protein, 17% from carb); 36 g Protein; 7 g total fat; 2 g saturated fat; 3 g monounsaturated fat; 1 g polyunsaturated fat; 11 g carb; 1 g fiber; 9 g sugar; 373 mg phosphorous; 25 mg calcium; 2 mg iron; 88 mg sodium; 648 mg potassium; 21 IU vitamin A; 3 mg ATE vitamin E; 4 mg vitamin C; 107 mg cholesterol

Glycemic Index: Low

Smoked Pork Shoulder

This recipe uses a pork shoulder roast and makes a lot of smoked pork. This makes it great for a get-together, or you can freeze some of the leftovers for quick meals later. We found that you can easily shred the pork for pulled pork sandwiches when it's hot, but that it slices easily after it's been refrigerated.

6 pounds (2¾ kg) pork shoulder roast

Rub

¼ cup (28 g) paprika

1 tablespoon freshly ground black pepper

¼ cup (60 g) brown sugar

1 tablespoon (7 g) chili powder

1 tablespoon (7 g) onion powder

1 tablespoon (9 g) garlic powder

Sauce

2 cups (475 ml) cider vinegar

3 tablespoons (18 g) black pepper, freshly ground

1 tablespoon (15 ml) Worcestershire sauce

1 tablespoon (7 g) paprika

1 teaspoon cayenne pepper

The night before you plan to barbecue, massage the rub into the roast, place in a plastic bag, and refrigerate. Remove from refrigerator and allow to come to room temperature while the grill or smoker heats. Bring the temperature of the grill or smoker to about 250°F (120°C, gas mark ½). Add wood chips as appropriate for your type of cooker. Place the roast in the cooker and cook over indirect heat for about 6 hours. Combine sauce ingredients and baste roast with the sauce about once an hour. At the end of the 6 hours, remove from cooker and place on a sheet of heavy-duty aluminum foil. Pour the remaining sauce over the roast. Return to cooker and cook an additional 3 hours. Remove from cooker and allow to stand 10 minutes before cutting and serving.

Yield: 18 servings

(continued on page 252)

Each with: 122 g water; 365 calories (68% from fat, 29% from protein, 3% from carb); 26 g protein; 27 g total fat; 9 g saturated fat; 12 g monounsaturated fat; 3 g polyunsaturated fat; 3 g carb; 0 g fiber; 2 g sugar; 30 mg calcium; 2 mg iron; 107 mg sodium; 514 mg potassium; 258 IU vitamin A; 3 mg vitamin C; 107 mg cholesterol

Glycemic Index: Low

Glazed Pork Roast

I actually grill this when it's warm enough. If you want to do that, it's best to grill with indirect heat. Place a pan of water under the roast and mound the charcoal around it. Close the grill to hold in the heat and smoke. This makes excellent sandwiches when it's cold and sliced thinly.

2 pounds (900 g) pork tenderloin

¼ cup (85 g) honey

1 tablespoon (9 g) dry mustard

¼ cup (60 ml) white wine vinegar

1 teaspoon chili powder

Mix together last 4 ingredients. Trim excess fat from pork roast. Brush with glaze. Roast at 350°F (180°C, gas mark 4) until done, 1 to 1½ hours, occasionally brushing with remaining glaze.

Yield: 8 servings

Each with: 94 g water; 173 calories (22% from fat, 57% from protein, 21% from carb); 24 g protein; 4 g total fat; 1 g saturated fat; 2 g monounsaturated fat; 0 g polyunsaturated fat; 9 g carb; 0 g fiber; 9 g sugar; 258 mg phosphorus; 9 mg calcium; 2 mg iron; 61 mg sodium; 436 mg potassium; 101 IU vitamin A; 1 mg vitamin C; 74 mg cholesterol

Glycemic Index: Low

Apple Pork Roast

A pork loin roast, cooked with apples and onions, makes a great looking as well as great tasting meal. This recipe makes enough for a large get together, but if you have a smaller family the leftovers are also good.

4 pounds (1.8 kg) pork loin roast

¾ teaspoon pepper

8 apples, cored

8 small onions, peeled but left whole

2 tablespoons (16 g) flour

2½ cups (570 ml) apple cider

Sprinkle pepper over pork roast and place in roasting pan. Roast at 325°F (170°C, or gas mark 3) for 1½ hours. Pour off fat. Place onions and apples in alternate positions around roast. Add 1½ cups cider and roast an additional 1½ hours, basting often. Skim off fat when done. Add flour and remaining cider to pan liquid. Cook mixture until smooth and thickened, stirring frequently. Place roast on platter and pour sauce over to serve.

Yield: 8 servings

Each with: 418 g water; 427 calories (21% from fat, 46% from protein, 32% from carb); 49 g Protein; 10 g total fat; 3 g saturated fat; 4 g monounsaturated fat; 1 g polyunsaturated fat; 34 g carb; 3 g fiber; 25 g sugar; 539 mg phosphorous; 60 mg calcium; 3 mg iron; 121 mg sodium; 1166 mg potassium; 76 IU vitamin A; 5 mg ATE vitamin E; 14 mg vitamin C; 143 mg cholesterol

Glycemic Index: Low

Sour Cream Pork Chop Bake

In this recipe, German-style pork chops are cooked in white wine and sour cream.

6 pork loin chops

1 garlic clove, minced

1 teaspoon caraway seeds, crushed

(continued on page 254)

2 teaspoons (5 g) paprika, mild

¼ teaspoon pepper

1 cup (235 ml) white wine, dry

1 cup (230 g) sour cream

TIP *Use Hungarian mild paprika. It is available at many larger stores and at specialty shops.*

Place the pork chops in a 9 x 13-inch (23 x 33 cm) ovenproof casserole. Mix the remaining ingredients, except sour cream, and pour over the chops. Marinate the chops 2 to 3 hours in the refrigerator. Bake the chops, uncovered, in the marinade in a preheated 325°F (170°C, or gas mark 3). oven for 1 hour or until tender. Add more wine if necessary. Stir sour cream into pan juices and heat through but DO NOT boil. Serve chops with sour cream gravy.

Yield: 6 servings

Each with: 141 g water; 220 calories (44% from fat, 48% from protein, 7% from carb); 23 g Protein; 9 g total fat; 5 g saturated fat; 3 g monounsaturated fat; 1 g polyunsaturated fat; 3 g carb; 0 g fiber; 1 g sugar; 270 mg phosphorous; 63 mg calcium; 1 mg iron; 70 mg sodium; 477 mg potassium; 567 IU vitamin A; 42 mg ATE vitamin E; 2 mg vitamin C; 79 mg cholesterol

Glycemic Index: Low

Pork and Green Bean Skillet

An updated version of the old favorite green bean casserole adds pork chops and easy skillet preparation for a great weeknight dinner.

2 tablespoons (10 g) unsalted butter

4 boneless pork loin chops ¾-inch (2 cm) thick

1½ cups (105 g) mushrooms, sliced

½ teaspoon rosemary, crushed

1 can (10¾ ounces or 305 g) cream of mushroom soup

2 tablespoons (30 ml) water

½ pound (225 g) fresh green beans, cut into 2-inch (5 cm) pieces

In skillet, in 1 tablespoon (5 g) melted butter, cook chops 10 minutes or until browned on both sides. Remove. In remaining butter, cook mushrooms with rosemary until tender and liquid is evaporated, stirring often. Add soup, water, and green beans. Heat to boiling. Return chops to skillet. Cover; cook over low heat 10 minutes or until chops are no longer pink and green beans are tender, stirring occasionally.

Yield: 4 servings

Each with: 220 g water; 240 calories (42% from fat, 40% from protein, 18% from carb); 24 g Protein; 11 g total fat; 6 g saturated fat; 4 g monounsaturated fat; 1 g polyunsaturated fat; 11 g carb; 3 g fiber; 3 g sugar; 302 mg phosphorous; 46 mg calcium; 2 mg iron; 329 mg sodium; 843 mg potassium; 583 IU vitamin A; 51 mg ATE vitamin E; 11 mg vitamin C; 81 mg cholesterol

Glycemic Index: Low

Pork Chop and Potato Bake

This recipe makes a great one pan casserole meal. Canned soup and onions and frozen hash brown potatoes make this dish an easy one.

6 pork loin chops

1 can (10¾ ounces or 304 g) cream of celery soup

½ cup skim milk

½ cup sour cream

¼ teaspoon black pepper

12 ounces (340 g) frozen hash brown potatoes

1 cup (115 g) cheddar cheese, shredded, divided

1 can (2.8 ounces or 79 g) French fried onions, divided

Brown pork chops in skillet sprayed with nonstick vegetable oil spray. Combine soup, milk, sour cream, and pepper. Stir in potatoes, ½ cup (5.8 g) cheese, and ½ can fried onions. Spoon mixture into 9 x 13-inch (23 x 33 cm) baking dish. Arrange pork chops over potatoes. Bake, covered, at 350°F (180°C, or gas mark 4) for 40 minutes. Top with remaining cheese and onions and bake uncovered 5 minutes longer.

Yield: 6 servings

(continued on page 256)

Each with: 242 g water; 426 calories (49% from fat, 29% from protein, 22% from carb); 31 g Protein; 23 g total fat; 11 g saturated fat; 8 g monounsaturated fat; 3 g polyunsaturated fat; 23 g carb; 2 g fiber; 1 g sugar; 433 mg phosphorous; 249 mg calcium; 2 mg iron; 624 mg sodium; 765 mg potassium; 469 IU vitamin A; 111 mg ATE vitamin E; 5 mg vitamin C; 101 mg cholesterol

Glycemic Index: Low

Stuffed Acorn Squash

This acorn squash stuffed with a ground pork mixture is a favorite around our house. For variety you can also use ground turkey.

1 acorn squash, about 1 pound (455 g)

¼ cup (25 g) celery, chopped

¼ teaspoon cinnamon

1 slice whole wheat bread, cubed

6 ounces (170 g) ground pork

¼ cup (40 g) chopped onion

¼ teaspoon curry powder

½ cup (125 g) applesauce, unsweetened

Spray a 10 x 6 x 2-inch (25 x 15 x 5 cm) baking dish with nonstick cooking spray. Halve squash; discard seeds. Place squash, cut side down, in baking dish. Bake, uncovered, in 350°F (180°C, or gas mark 4) oven 50 minutes. While that is roasting, prepare the stuffing. In a skillet, cook pork, celery, and onion until meat is no longer pink and vegetables are tender. Drain fat. Stir in curry powder and cinnamon; cook 1 minute more. Stir in applesauce and bread cubes. Turn squash cut side up in dish. Place stuffing in squash halves. Bake uncovered, 20 minutes more.

Yield: 2 servings

Each with: 322 g water; 410 calories (40% from fat, 24% from protein, 36% from carb); 25 g Protein; 18 g total fat; 7 g saturated fat; 8 g monounsaturated fat; 2 g polyunsaturated fat; 38 g carb; 5 g fiber; 8 g sugar; 303 mg phosphorous; 124 mg calcium; 3 mg iron; 146 mg sodium; 1192 mg potassium; 875 IU vitamin A; 2 mg ATE vitamin E; 27 mg vitamin C; 80 mg cholesterol

Glycemic Index: Low

Pork Turnovers

The preparation of these turnovers is similar to many Latin American meat turnovers, but the flavor is American, with mustard providing a little zip. If you like them spicier, add a small amount of red pepper flakes to the meat mixture.

8 teaspoons (112 g) unsalted butter

¾ cup (94 g) flour

3 tablespoons (45 ml) water

4 ounces (120 g) ground pork, cooked and crumbled

2 ounces (60 g) Monterey jack cheese shredded

1 teaspoon prepared mustard

1 egg, separated

1 tablespoon (15 ml) skim milk

In small bowl, with pastry blender or 2 knives, cut margarine into flour until mixture resembles cornmeal; sprinkle with ice water and use fork to mix until it forms soft dough. Roll dough between 2 sheets of wax paper to form a rectangle about ¼ inch (5 mm) thick; remove paper and use 2-inch (5 cm) diameter cookie cutter to cut dough into rounds. Roll scraps of dough and continue cutting until all dough has been used (should yield 24 rounds). Combine pork, cheese, and mustard in small bowl and set aside. Preheat oven to 375°F (190°C, or gas mark 5). Beat egg white lightly and brush an equal amount onto each pastry round. Spoon an equal amount of the meat mixture (about ½ rounded teaspoon) onto center of each round; fold pastry over, turnover-fashion, to enclose filling. Press edges of dough together to seal. Transfer turnovers to nonstick cookie sheet. Add milk to egg yolk and beat lightly; brush an equal amount of mixture over each turnover. Bake until turnovers are golden brown, 15 to 20 minutes.

Yield: 8 servings

Each with: 24 g water; 158 calories (57% from fat, 19% from protein, 23% from carb); 8 g Protein; 10 g total fat; 5 g saturated fat; 3 g monounsaturated fat; 1 g polyunsaturated fat; 9 g carb; 0 g fiber; 0 g sugar; 91 mg phosphorous; 66 mg calcium; 1 mg iron; 62 mg sodium; 84 mg potassium; 220 IU vitamin A; 58 mg ATE vitamin E; 0 mg vitamin C; 56 mg cholesterol

Glycemic Index: Low

Barbecued Pork Chops

A nice sweet and sour sort of barbecue sauce gives these chops great flavor.

4 loin pork chops, 1 inch (2½ cm) thick

1 cup (160 g) finely chopped onion

2 tablespoons (30 ml) vinegar

1 tablespoon (15 ml) canola oil

½ teaspoon dry mustard

1 tablespoon (15 ml) Worcestershire sauce

1 teaspoon black pepper

1 tablespoon (13 g) sugar

½ teaspoon paprika

Score edges of chops to prevent curling. Place into a large baking pan and set aside. Combine remaining ingredients and mix well. Pour over chops to coat well. Cover and chill for 2 to 4 hours. Grill chops to desired doneness, basting often.

Yield: 4 servings

Each with: 118 g water; 196 calories (37% from fat, 46% from protein, 17% from carb); 22 g protein; 8 g total fat; 2 g saturated fat; 4 g monounsaturated fat; 2 g polyunsaturated fat; 8 g carb; 1 g fiber; 5 g sugar; 238 mg phosphorus; 26 mg calcium; 1 mg iron; 91 mg sodium; 482 mg potassium; 166 IU vitamin A; 11 mg vitamin C; 64 mg cholesterol

Glycemic Index: Low

Slow-Cooker Barbecued Pork

This is an easy way to make pork barbecue, even if it's not quite the traditional slow-smoked kind.

½ cup (120 ml) cider vinegar

¼ cup (40 g) chopped onion

1 teaspoon Worcestershire sauce

1 teaspoon hot pepper sauce

3 pounds (1⅓ kg) pork shoulder roast boneless, trimmed, tied

½ tablespoon liquid smoke

1 tablespoon (13 g) sugar

1 teaspoon paprika

¼ teaspoon black pepper

2 tablespoons (30 g) low-sodium ketchup

In a large bowl, combine cider vinegar, onion, Worcestershire sauce, and hot pepper sauce. Add the pork roast, cover, and marinate in refrigerator for 6 to 10 hours. Turn occasionally to keep roast coated with marinade. Remove the pork from the marinade, scraping the onion back into the marinade. Lightly pat the roast dry with paper towels. Pour the marinade into a slow cooker and add the liquid smoke. Place a slow cooker meat rack or ring of foil in the slow cooker. Combine the sugar, paprika, and pepper in a cup. Rub the pork roast with the sugar and spice mixture and place on the rack in slow cooker. Cover and cook on low for 7 to 9 hours or until very tender. Transfer the pork to a cutting board; cover with foil to keep warm. Skim the fat from the surface of the cooking liquid. Stir in the ketchup; pour into a bowl. Using 2 forks, pull the pork apart into shreds or chop the pork into small pieces. Serve the pork on buns. Serve the sauce separately.

Yield: 8 servings

Each with: 145 g water; 268 calories (42% from fat, 51% from protein, 7% from carb); 33 g protein; 12 g total fat; 4 g saturated fat; 6 g monounsaturated fat; 1 g polyunsaturated fat; 4 g carb; 0 g fiber; 4 g sugar; 27 mg calcium; 2 mg iron; 137 mg sodium; 634 mg potassium; 211 IU vitamin A; 4 mg vitamin C; 114 mg cholesterol

Glycemic Index: Low

Crushed Herb Lamb

For carving, select a leg of lamb with an exposed bone shank. It makes a great handle. Slice the meat parallel to the bone. The outside slices will be well done and the center rare. Serve with oven-roasted new potatoes.

(continued on page 260)

1 leg of lamb (5½ pounds or 2½ kg)

6 cloves garlic

2 shallots

2 tablespoons (9 g) dried thyme

2 tablespoons (6 g) dried rosemary

2 tablespoons (12 g) pepper, freshly ground

¼ cup (60 ml) olive oil

Trim and discard fat and any transparent membrane from the surface of the lamb. Peel garlic and shallots and cut into ¼-inch-thick (½ cm thick) slivers. Pierce lamb all over with the tip of a small knife and insert garlic and shallots into cuts (lamb will look like a porcupine). Mix thyme, rosemary, pepper, and olive oil and pat the mixture all over the lamb. Roast at 350°F (180°C, gas mark 4) or grill over indirect heat until internal temperature reaches 125°F (52°C) for rare or 135°F (57°C) for medium rare, about 1 hour and 10 minutes to 1 hour and 30 minutes.

Yield: 8 servings

Each with: 180 g water; 871 calories (62% from fat, 38% from protein, 1% from carb); 80 g protein; 58 g total fat; 22 g saturated fat; 27 g monounsaturated fat; 4 g polyunsaturated fat; 2 g carb; 1 g fiber; 0 g sugar; 600 mg phosphorus; 57 mg calcium; 8 mg iron; 797 mg sodium; 1,005 mg potassium; 46 IU vitamin A; 1 mg vitamin C; 290 mg cholesterol

Glycemic Index: Low

Lamb Stew

We don't eat lamb very often, but this stew is one recipe that has proved popular when lamb is on sale.

1 tablespoon (15 ml) olive oil

2 cups (320 g) onion, thinly sliced

1 tablespoon (10 g) garlic, minced

¼ cup (60 ml) red wine vinegar

2 pounds (900 g) lamb shoulder, trimmed and cut into 1-inch (2½ cm) cubes

14 ounces (400 g) no-salt-added tomatoes

2 tablespoons (32 g) no-salt-added tomato paste

1 teaspoon basil

1 teaspoon oregano

2 bay leaves

¼ teaspoon black pepper

1 cup (150 g) red bell pepper, sliced

1 cup (150 g) green bell pepper, sliced

⅓ cup (20 g) fresh parsley, finely minced

In Dutch oven, heat oil. Sauté onions and garlic until onions are soft, about 2 minutes. Stir in vinegar and cook for 1 to 2 minutes over medium heat, scraping any browned bits from the bottom. Add lamb, tomatoes, tomato paste, basil, oregano, bay leaves, salt and pepper to taste. Stir well to blend. Bring to boil, reduce heat, cover, and cook until lamb is fork tender, about 1 to 1½ hours. Remove bay leaves; stir in the red and green peppers. Cover and simmer over medium heat until peppers are crisp-tender, another 5 to 8 minutes. Remove the bay leaves and stir in the parsley just before serving.

Yield: 4 servings

Each with: 404 g water; 534 calories (35% from fat, 51% from protein, 14% from carb); 67 g Protein; 21 g total fat; 7 g saturated fat; 9 g monounsaturated fat; 2 g polyunsaturated fat; 18 g carb; 5 g fiber; 9 g sugar; 583 mg phosphorous; 108 mg calcium; 8 mg iron; 204 mg sodium; 1344 mg potassium; 2002 IU vitamin A; 0 mg ATE vitamin E; 102 mg vitamin C; 204 mg cholesterol

Glycemic Index: Low

10

Soups, Stews, and Chilies

Soups and stews traditionally offer great taste and nutrition. And if you are careful about the ingredients, they can also be a great choice for filling meals that are very low on the GI scale. And that's not even to mention chili, with its healthy beans and high-energy flavor. We usually have stew or soup at least once a week, more often in colder weather, and these recipes are some of our favorites.

Amish Chicken Soup

When I was growing up along the Maryland-Pennsylvania border, Amish chicken corn soup was always one of the highlights of volunteer fire company carnivals and suppers. This soup has a similar flavor.

4 cups (950 ml) low-sodium chicken broth

2 cups (280 g) chicken, cooked and chopped

½ cup (50 g) chopped celery

½ cup (65 g) sliced carrot

½ cup (80 g) chopped onion

1 tablespoon (4 g) parsley

¼ teaspoon garlic powder

2 cups (475 ml) water

12 ounces (340 g) egg noodles

Place all ingredients in a large kettle and simmer until noodles are tender.

Yield: 8 servings

Each with: 248 g water; 148 calories (22% from fat, 37% from protein, 41% from carb); 14 g protein; 4 g total fat; 1 g saturated fat; 1 g monounsaturated fat; 1 g polyunsaturated fat; 15 g carb; 3 g fiber; 1 g sugar; 144 mg phosphorus; 20 mg calcium; 1 mg iron; 49 mg sodium; 262 mg potassium; 1,456 IU vitamin A; 2 mg vitamin C; 31 mg cholesterol

Glycemic Index: Low

Italian Turkey Soup

I was looking for something a little different from the usual turkey noodle soup to make with the turkey carcass one year, and this was the result.

4 cups (950 ml) low-sodium chicken or turkey broth

1 can (14½ ounces or 410 g) no-salt-added tomatoes

(continued on page 264)

1 cup (160 g) coarsely chopped onion

1 cup (130 g) sliced carrot

½ teaspoon garlic powder

1 teaspoon Italian seasoning

1 tablespoon (4 g) parsley

2 cups (350 g) cooked turkey

6 ounces (128 g) whole wheat pasta, any shape desired

Combine all ingredients except pasta in a large Dutch oven. Bring to a boil. Stir in pasta, lower heat, and simmer until pasta is cooked and veggies are tender.

Yield: 8 servings

Each with: 57 g water; 148 calories (12% from fat, 36% from protein, 52% from carb); 14 g protein; 2 g total fat; 1 g saturated fat; 0 g monounsaturated fat; 1 g polyunsaturated fat; 20 g carb; 3 g fiber; 2 g sugar; 142 mg phosphorus; 30 mg calcium; 2 mg iron; 40 mg sodium; 238 mg potassium; 2,738 IU vitamin A; 3 mg vitamin C; 27 mg cholesterol

Glycemic Index: Low

Turkey Barley Soup

This is little different soup to make with leftover turkey. We've found it to be more popular than turkey noodle.

6 cups (1.4 L) low-sodium chicken broth

1 cup (140 g) cooked turkey, diced

1 cup (200 g) pearl barley

1 cup (160 g) onion, chopped

1 cup (100 g) celery, chopped

¾ cup (83 g) carrot, sliced

1 bay leaf

1 teaspoon dried thyme

¼ teaspoon dried marjoram

¼ teaspoon black pepper

2 tablespoons (2.6 g) dried parsley

Combine all the ingredients in soup pot or slow cooker. Cook over low heat in the slow cooker for 6 hours or simmer on the stove for 1 hour until the carrots are tender and the barley is soft. Remove bay leaf before serving.

Yield: 6 servings

Each with: 304 g water; 203 calories (12% from fat, 31% from protein, 57% from carb); 16 g Protein; 3 g total fat; 1 g saturated fat; 1 g monounsaturated fat; 1 g polyunsaturated fat; 30 g carb; 7 g fiber; 3 g sugar; 220 mg phosphorous; 48 mg calcium; 3 mg iron; 118 mg sodium; 550 mg potassium; 2887 IU vitamin A; 0 mg ATE vitamin E; 5 mg vitamin C; 23 mg cholesterol

Glycemic Index: Low

Cabbage Beef Soup

The combination may seem a little strange, but I really like it.

½ pound (225 g) lean ground beef

½ onion, chopped

1 cup (70 g) coleslaw mix or shredded cabbage

1 can (14½ ounces or 406 g) no-salt-added tomatoes

2 cups (500 g) Mexican beans

Break beef up into fine pieces and brown with the chopped onion and slaw mix or cabbage until the vegetables become clear and not scorched. Add canned tomatoes, beans, and 1 cup (235 ml) water. Bring to a boil and simmer 10 minutes to blend the flavors.

Yield: 5 servings

Each with: 145 g water; 212 calories (32% from fat, 34% from protein, 34% from carb); 18 g protein; 8 g total fat; 3 g saturated fat; 3 g monounsaturated fat; 0 g polyunsaturated fat; 18 g carb; 7 g fiber; 1 g sugar; 60 mg calcium; 3 mg iron; 38 mg sodium; 490 mg potassium; 20 IU vitamin A; 9 mg vitamin C; 37 mg cholesterol

Glycemic Index: Low

Beef Barley Skillet

This is an easy one pan meal that will please everyone. Don't tell them that it's also good for them.

¼ pound (110 g) lean ground beef

4 tablespoons (40 g) onion, chopped

2 tablespoons (13 g) celery, chopped

2 tablespoons (19 g) green pepper, chopped

⅛ teaspoon thyme

½ teaspoon (30 g) Worcestershire

1½ tablespoons (30 g) chili sauce, see recipe in chapter 2

⅔ cup (120 g) no-salt-added tomatoes

½ cup (120 ml) water

¼ cup (50 g) pearl barley

Sauté beef, onion, celery, and green pepper until meat is done. Pour off fat and stir in rest of the ingredients. Bring to a boil and then turn down heat and simmer until barley is cooked.

Yield: 4 servings

Each with: 108 g water; 122 calories (38% from fat, 24% from protein, 38% from carb); 7 g Protein; 5 g total fat; 2 g saturated fat; 2 g monounsaturated fat; 0 g polyunsaturated fat; 12 g carb; 3 g fiber; 2 g sugar; 83 mg phosphorous; 25 mg calcium; 1 mg iron; 74 mg sodium; 244 mg potassium; 177 IU vitamin A; 0 mg ATE vitamin E; 10 mg vitamin C; 20 mg cholesterol

Glycemic Index: Low

Beef and Black Bean Stew

This is not quite a chili, but it has definite southwestern flavor. This one is always a big hit at our house.

2 pounds (900 g) extra-lean ground beef

½ teaspoon minced garlic

1 cup (160 g) chopped onion

2 cups (480 g) no-salt-added canned tomatoes

1 cup (260 g) salsa

1 teaspoon ground cumin

½ teaspoon freshly ground black pepper

6 ounces (130 g) frozen corn

1½ cups (150 g) black beans, drained and rinsed

1 tablespoon (1 g) chopped fresh cilantro

TIP *To make a meal, top with grated cheese, guacamole, or sour cream and serve with tortilla chips or cornbread.*

In a large skillet, brown ground beef with garlic and onion. Drain and transfer to a slow cooker. Add tomatoes, salsa, cumin, pepper, corn, and black beans. Cook on low 6 to 8 hours or on high for 3 to 4 hours. Add cilantro during the last hour of cooking.

Yield: 8 servings

Each with: 213 g water; 355 calories (50% from fat, 29% from protein, 20% from carb); 26 g protein; 20 g total fat; 8 g saturated fat; 9 g monounsaturated fat; 1 g polyunsaturated fat; 18 g carb; 5 g fiber; 4 g sugar; 253 mg phosphorus; 52 mg calcium; 4 mg iron; 163 mg sodium; 741 mg potassium; 237 IU vitamin A; 9 mg vitamin C; 78 mg cholesterol

Glycemic Index: Low

Oven Beef Stew

This stew is easy to make, but full of flavor, and it will definitely satisfy the meat lovers in your family.

2 pound (900 g) beef round steak, cut in 1-inch (2½ cm) cubes

4 cups (520 g) carrot, sliced

2 cups (200 g) celery, sliced

2 cups (320 g) onion, sliced

8 ounces (227 g) mushroom, sliced

¼ cup (31 g) flour

32 ounces (909 g) no-salt-added tomatoes

2 cups (475 ml) burgundy wine

(continued on page 268)

In roasting pan or Dutch oven, mix meat, carrots, celery, onions, and mushrooms. Add flour. Stir in tomatoes and Burgundy wine. Cover and bake 4 hours.

Yield: 6 servings

Each with: 490 g water; 482 calories (18% from fat, 56% from protein, 26% from carb); 59 g Protein; 8 g total fat; 3 g saturated fat; 3 g monounsaturated fat; 1 g polyunsaturated fat; 27 g carb; 6 g fiber; 12 g sugar; 480 mg phosphorous; 115 mg calcium; 8 mg iron; 181 mg sodium; 1453 mg potassium; 14675 IU vitamin A; 0 mg ATE vitamin E; 25 mg vitamin C; 136 mg cholesterol

Sausage and Lentil Soup

This soup doesn't have a lot of spices and other seasonings added. Instead it lets the flavor of the ham bone, lentils, and veggies shine through. But I don't think you'll get any complaints, because it would be hard to imagine a soup with more flavor.

2 cups (384 g) dried lentils

2 quarts (1.9 L) water

1 ham hock

1 cup (130 g) carrot, chopped

1 cup (160 g) onion, chopped

¾ cup (75 g) celery, chopped

1 bay leaf

2 garlic cloves, peeled and quartered

¼ teaspoon pepper, fresh ground

½ pound (225 g) kielbasa sausage, diced

1 tablespoon (15 ml) olive oil

Wash lentils and pick over. Drain. Put in large kettle with remaining ingredients except sausage. Bring soup to a boil, reduce heat, and simmer for 1½ hours. Meanwhile, during last 10 minutes of cooking hour, dice sausage and sauté in skillet in oil until golden brown on all sides. Remove ham bone and bay leaf from soup. Garnish each serving with diced cooked sausage.

Yield: 8 servings

Each with: 329 g water; 183 calories (49% from fat, 20% from protein, 31% from carb); 9 g Protein; 10 g total fat; 3 g saturated fat; 5 g monounsaturated fat; 1 g polyunsaturated fat; 14 g carb; 5 g fiber; 3 g sugar; 149 mg phosphorous; 43 mg calcium; 2 mg iron; 365 mg sodium; 375 mg potassium; 2740 IU vitamin A; 0 mg ATE vitamin E; 4 mg vitamin C; 21 mg cholesterol

Glycemic Index: Low

Vegetable and Chickpea Stew

This is vegetarian stew with a great assortment of veggies and a wonderful flavor.

2 tablespoons (30 ml) olive oil

2 garlic cloves, minced

1 cup (160 g) onion, chopped

½ cup (50 g) celery, chopped

¾ cup (98 g) carrot, cut into discs

2 parsnips, cut into discs

1 large potato, cubed

3 cups (705 ml) low-sodium vegetable juice

5 cups (1.2 L) water

½ cup (30 g) fresh parsley, chopped

1 teaspoon marjoram

15 ounces (420 g) chickpeas, drained

2 cups (140 g) cabbage, shredded

Heat the oil in a large pan and toss the onion, garlic, celery, carrots, parsnips and potato in it over a low heat. Add the juice and water and marjoram. Increase the heat and simmer for 20 minutes. Add the drained chickpeas and the cabbage and cook for another 10 minutes.

Yield: 6 servings

Each with: 511 g water; 289 calories (20% from fat, 13% from protein, 66% from carb); 10 g Protein; 7 g total fat; 1 g saturated fat; 4 g monounsaturated fat; 1 g polyunsaturated fat; 50 g carb; 11 g fiber; 14 g sugar; 239 mg phosphorous; 114 mg calcium; 4 mg iron; 245 mg sodium; 1101 mg potassium; 5095 IU vitamin A; 0 mg ATE vitamin E; 68 mg vitamin C; 0 mg cholesterol

Glycemic Index: Low

Mushroom Barley Soup with Short Ribs

Here's a hearty soup with beef ribs, barley, and lots of mushrooms. This is the sort of warm filling meal we start looking for when the weather gets cooler.

2 pounds (900 g) beef short ribs

1 cup (160 g) onion, diced

2 tablespoons (20 g) minced garlic

1 cup (100 g) celery, finely sliced

6 cups (1.4 L) low-sodium chicken broth

2/3 cup (133 g) pearl barley

1 tablespoon (3 g) dried dill weed

Pepper to taste

2 pounds (900 g) mushrooms

Place ribs, onion, garlic, and celery in a soup pot. Add the liquid, cover, bring to a boil, and simmer over low heat for 1 hour. Add the barley, dill, and pepper and cook another 50 minutes. Add the mushrooms and cook another 10 minutes. Serve hot.

Yield: 8 servings

Each with: 389 g water; 318 calories (37% from fat, 38% from protein, 25% from carb); 31 g Protein; 13 g total fat; 5 g saturated fat; 6 g monounsaturated fat; 1 g polyunsaturated fat; 20 g carb; 4 g fiber; 3 g sugar; 422 mg phosphorous; 45 mg calcium; 4 mg iron; 147 mg sodium; 1073 mg potassium; 83 IU vitamin A; 0 mg ATE vitamin E; 5 mg vitamin C; 67 mg cholesterol

Glycemic Index: Low

Potato Corn Chowder

This may be simple vegetable soup, but it's one with lots of flavor. This is the kind of soup that makes a great meal with just a slice of fresh baked bread.

1 cup (160 g) onion, chopped

3 medium potatoes, diced

1 cup (130 g) carrot, sliced

½ cup (50 g) celery, chopped

2 bay leaves

2 tablespoons (30 ml) olive oil

3 cups (492 g) frozen corn

14 ounces (400 g) no-salt-added tomatoes, chopped

1½ teaspoons coriander

1 teaspoon savory

½ teaspoon thyme

1 cup (235 ml) water

Place onions, potatoes, carrots, celery, bay leaves and oil in large soup pot. Add just enough water to cover. Bring to a boil and simmer over low heat for 10 minutes. Add the corn and tomatoes with their liquid and simmer for 10 minutes. Add the seasonings and simmer for another 10 minutes. Remove ¾ cup of potatoes and mash well. Return to the pot with the 1 cup (235ml) of water. Stir well. Simmer for another 5 minutes. Remove bay leaves before serving.

Yield: 8 servings

Each with: 247 g water; 203 calories (17% from fat, 10% from protein, 74% from carb); 5 g Protein; 4 g total fat; 1 g saturated fat; 3 g monounsaturated fat; 1 g polyunsaturated fat; 40 g carb; 5 g fiber; 6 g sugar; 139 mg phosphorous; 44 mg calcium; 2 mg iron; 41 mg sodium; 897 mg potassium; 2799 IU vitamin A; 0 mg ATE vitamin E; 24 mg vitamin C; 0 mg cholesterol

Glycemic Index: Low

Potato Leek Soup

This simple soup of potatoes and leeks is the kind of thing you need on a cold winter night. Something about it just says "comfort food" and makes everything seem a little warmer.

(continued on page 272)

3 cups (312 g) chopped leeks

1 cup (100 g) celery, peeled, diced

3 large potatoes, peeled and cubed

6 cups (1.4 L) water

¼ teaspoon pepper

1 teaspoon white wine vinegar

In a 4-quart (4 L) soup pot over medium heat, sauté leeks, celery, and potatoes in a little water for 5 to 7 minutes. Add more water as needed to prevent sticking. Add the 6 cups (1.4 L) of water and pepper. Bring to a boil, lower heat, and simmer potatoes are very soft, about 15 minutes. Add vinegar. Puree soup 2 to 3 cups at a time in a blender or food processor until very smooth. Return to soup pot and rewarm if needed.

Yield: 6 servings

Each with: 440 g water; 159 calories (2% from fat, 10% from protein, 87% from carb); 4 g Protein; 0 g total fat; 0 g saturated fat; 0 g monounsaturated fat; 0 g polyunsaturated fat; 36 g carb; 4 g fiber; 4 g sugar; 132 mg phosphorous; 59 mg calcium; 2 mg iron; 41 mg sodium; 967 mg potassium; 835 IU vitamin A; 0 mg ATE vitamin E; 22 mg vitamin C; 0 mg cholesterol

Glycemic Index: Low

Broccoli Soup

This broccoli soup looks great, but that isn't the real point. It also tastes great, which is of course even more important.

1 cup (160 g) onion, chopped

1 clove garlic, crushed

1 tablespoon (15 ml) olive oil

1 bay leaf

1 pound (455 g) broccoli, chopped

2 cups (475 ml) low-sodium vegetable broth

2 tablespoons (30 ml) lemon juice

Sauté onion and garlic in oil with the bay leaf for 3 to 4 minutes. Remove 4 ounces (114 g) of broccoli florets. Add the rest of the broccoli and stock. Bring to a boil and simmer gently, covered for 10 minutes. The broccoli should be tender but still bright green. Remove the bay leaf and cool slightly. Blend the soup until it is completely smooth. Add the lemon juice. Reheat gently in a clean pot. Meanwhile, steam the reserved florets till tender, 8 minutes or so. Scatter them over the soup, stir, and serve.

Yield: 4 servings

Each with: 261 g water; 106 calories (36% from fat, 21% from protein, 43% from carb); 6 g Protein; 5 g total fat; 1 g saturated fat; 3 g monounsaturated fat; 1 g polyunsaturated fat; 12 g carb; 4 g fiber; 4 g sugar; 124 mg phosphorous; 100 mg calcium; 1 mg iron; 109 mg sodium; 531 mg potassium; 714 IU vitamin A; 1 mg ATE vitamin E; 108 mg vitamin C; 0 mg cholesterol

Glycemic Index: Low

Broccoli Cheese Soup

This creamy soup makes an excellent first course for a larger dinner or a simple dinner by itself. It goes together quickly, so it's a good answer when you have no idea what to fix.

2 cup (475 ml) milk

3 tablespoons (42 g) unsalted butter

2 tablespoons (20 g) onion, finely chopped

3 tablespoons (24 g) flour

½ teaspoon salt

⅛ teaspoon white pepper

½ teaspoon thyme

½ teaspoon garlic powder

1½ cup (355 ml) low-sodium chicken broth

2 cups (225 g) cheddar cheese, shredded

1 cup (71 g) broccoli, cooked and finely chopped

Cook onions in butter until tender. Blend in flour and seasonings and cook 3 to 4 minutes, stirring

(continued on page 274)

constantly. Add chicken broth and cook slowly until thick. Stir in the milk until smooth. Add the cheese and broccoli and heat through.

Yield: 6 servings

Each with: 166 g water; 287 calories (65% from fat, 22% from protein, 14% from carb); 16 g Protein; 21 g total fat; 13 g saturated fat; 6 g monounsaturated fat; 1 g polyunsaturated fat; 10 g carb; 1 g fiber; 5 g sugar; 344 mg phosphorous; 434 mg calcium; 1 mg iron; 528 mg sodium; 284 mg potassium; 882 IU vitamin A; 211 mg ATE vitamin E; 14 mg vitamin C; 63 mg cholesterol

Glycemic Index: Low

Squash Soup

This is really a simple soup, with butternut squash the only "real" ingredient. But it flavored with a long list of ingredients, giving it a complex depth of tastes.

½ cup (80 g) chopped onions

2 tablespoons (20 g) minced garlic

1 tablespoon (6 g) gingerroot, minced

⅓ cup (120 ml) dry sherry

1 tablespoon (15 ml) olive oil

2 cups (475 g) low-sodium vegetable broth

4 cups (560 g) butternut squash, peeled, seeded, cubed

1 tablespoon (15 ml) lemon juice

½ teaspoon coriander

½ teaspoon nutmeg

½ teaspoon cumin

½ teaspoon cinnamon

1 tablespoon (6 g) lemon peel

In a large pot, sauté onions, garlic, and ginger in oil and sherry for 10 minutes. Stir frequently. If the vegetables stick, add a little broth. Add remaining ingredients and simmer until squash is tender. Process in a blender until smooth.

Yield: 5 servings

Each with: 223 g water; 132 calories (26% from fat, 12% from protein, 62% from carb); 4 g Protein; 4 g total fat; 1 g saturated fat; 2 g monounsaturated fat; 1 g polyunsaturated fat; 19 g carb; 3 g fiber; 5 g sugar; 80 mg phosphorous; 102 mg calcium; 1 mg iron; 64 mg sodium; 549 mg potassium; 11918 IU vitamin A; 1 mg ATE vitamin E; 29 mg vitamin C; 0 mg cholesterol

Glycemic Index: Low

Indian Vegetable Soup

This makes a great vegetarian meal. The amount of ginger gives it a sneaky sort of spiciness. I prefer the mild curry powder, but if you want something even hotter, you could use the hot curry.

1 eggplant, peeled and cubed

1 pound (455 g) potatoes, cubed

2 cups (480 g) no-salt-added canned tomatoes

1½ cups (246 g) precooked chickpeas

1 cup (160 g) coarsely chopped onion

1½ teaspoons curry powder

1½ teaspoons ground ginger

1 teaspoon coriander

¼ teaspoon black pepper

4 cups (950 ml) low-sodium vegetable broth

In a slow cooker, combine the vegetables. Sprinkle spices over top. Pour broth over all. Cover and cook on low for 8 to 10 hours or on high for 4 to 5 hours.

Yield: 6 servings

Each with: 426 g water; 196 calories (9% from fat, 18% from protein, 73% from carb); 9 g protein; 2 g total fat; 0 g saturated fat; 1 g monounsaturated fat; 1 g polyunsaturated fat; 38 g carb; 8 g fiber; 6 g sugar; 193 mg phosphorus; 76 mg calcium; 3 mg iron; 246 mg sodium; 969 mg potassium; 146 IU vitamin A; 21 mg vitamin C; 0 mg cholesterol

Glycemic Index: Low

Moroccan Stew

This spicy stew of vegetables and dried fruit is sure to be a hit. Serve with toasted pita bread triangles.

1 tablespoon (15 ml) olive oil

1½ cup (270 g) onion, chopped

2 garlic cloves, minced

1 teaspoon cinnamon, ground

½ teaspoon ginger, ground

½ teaspoon turmeric, ground

¼ teaspoon nutmeg, ground

¼ teaspoon red pepper, ground

2 cups (475 ml) water

3 cloves, whole

2 cups (260 g) carrot, sliced

2 cups (280 g) butternut squash, cubed

2 cups (480 g) chickpeas, cooked or canned, drained and rinsed

1½ cups (165 g) sweet potatoes, cubed

½ cup (75 g) raisins

⅓ cup (43 g) dried apricots, diced

3 tablespoons (3 g) brown sugar substitute, such as Splenda

In a 4-quart (4 L) saucepan, heat the oil over medium-high heat. Add the onion and garlic and cook, stirring, until softened. Add the cinnamon, ginger, turmeric, nutmeg, and red pepper, stirring until absorbed. Add the water and cloves; bring to a boil. Add the carrot, squash, chickpeas, sweet potato, raisins, apricots, and brown sugar and return to a boil. Reduce the heat and simmer uncovered, stirring occasionally, 40 to 45 minutes or until the sweet potato is tender.

Yield: 4 servings

Each with: 458 g water; 422 calories (12% from fat, 11% from protein, 77% from carb); 12 g Protein; 6 g total fat; 1 g saturated fat; 3 g monounsaturated fat; 2 g polyunsaturated fat; 86 g carb; 15 g fiber; 34 g sugar; 267 mg phosphorous; 166 mg calcium; 5 mg iron; 95 mg sodium; 1264 mg potassium; 37936 IU vitamin A; 0 mg ATE vitamin E; 42 mg vitamin C; 0 mg cholesterol

Glycemic Index: Low

Mediterranean Vegetable Stew

It's half casserole and half stew, but this dish is good tasting no matter what you call it.

2 cups (240 g) zucchini, sliced

1 eggplant, sliced and peeled

1 cup (160 g) onion, sliced

½ pound (225 g) okra, stemmed

1 cup (100 g) fresh green beans, halved

1 large potato, thinly sliced

4 medium tomatoes, peeled and sliced

¼ cup (60 ml) olive oil

2 tablespoons (5 g) fresh basil

2 garlic cloves, minced

¼ teaspoon pepper

Preheat oven to 350 °F (180 °C, or gas mark 4). In a deep casserole, make a layer of each vegetable. Dribble a little oil over each layer and sprinkle lightly with garlic, basil, and pepper. Layer in any order but have potatoes in the middle and end with tomatoes. Bake covered for 1½ hours, basting once or twice.

Yield: 4 servings

Each with: 473 g water; 299 calories (41% from fat, 9% from protein, 50% from carb); 7 g Protein; 15 g total fat; 2 g saturated fat; 10 g monounsaturated fat; 2 g polyunsaturated fat; 40 g carb; 11 g fiber; 8 g sugar; 205 mg phosphorous; 121 mg calcium; 3 mg iron; 39 mg sodium; 1488 mg potassium; 1598 IU vitamin A; 0 mg ATE vitamin E; 82 mg vitamin C; 0 mg cholesterol

Glycemic Index: Low

African Chicken and Groundnut Stew

This chicken stew is moderately spicy and flavored with peanut butter in a style similar to the traditional stews of West Africa.

2 boneless skinless chicken breasts, cut into ½-inch (1 cm) pieces

1 tablespoon (15 ml) olive oil

1 cup (160 g) onion, chopped

1 garlic clove, minced

28 ounces (795 g) no-salt-added tomatoes, undrained, cut up

15½ ounces (440 g) great northern beans, undrained

10 ounces (280 g) frozen corn

1 large sweet potato, peeled and chopped

¾ cup (175 ml) water

¼ cup (65 g) peanut butter

1 tablespoon (16 g) no-salt-added tomato paste

1 teaspoon chili powder

½ teaspoon ginger

½ teaspoon cayenne

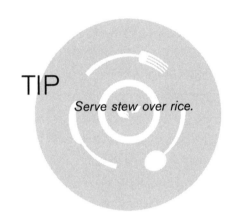

TIP

Serve stew over rice.

In a 4 quart (4 L) Dutch oven over medium-high heat, cook chicken in oil until chicken is lightly browned and no longer pink, stirring frequently. Add onion and garlic; cook and stir 3 to 4 minutes or until onion is tender. Add remaining ingredients; mix well. Bring to a boil. Reduce heat to medium-low; cover and cook 30 minutes or until sweet potato is tender, stirring occasionally. If stew becomes too thick, add additional water.

Yield: 8 servings

Each with: 263 g water; 248 calories (23% from fat, 20% from protein, 57% from carb); 13 g Protein; 7 g total fat; 1 g saturated fat; 3 g monounsaturated fat; 2 g polyunsaturated fat; 38 g carb; 7 g fiber; 9 g sugar; 203 mg phosphorous; 91 mg calcium; 3 mg iron; 53 mg sodium; 738 mg potassium; 9971 IU vitamin A; 1 mg ATE vitamin E; 21 mg vitamin C; 10 mg cholesterol

Glycemic Index: Low

Black Bean Soup

Here's a flavorful Latin-style soup that's low in fat.

1½ cups (375 g) dried black beans

4 cups (950 ml) water

1 cup (160 g) finely chopped onion

½ cup (75 g) finely chopped green bell pepper

½ teaspoon minced garlic

½ cup (65 g) finely chopped carrot

½ cup (50 g) finely chopped celery

1 tablespoon (15 ml) olive oil

1 teaspoon cumin

¼ teaspoon cayenne pepper

1 tablespoon (15 ml) lime juice

¼ cup (65 g) salsa

Soak beans in water overnight. In a large Dutch oven, sauté onion, bell pepper, garlic, carrot, and celery in oil until almost soft. Add spices and sauté a few minutes more. Add beans, water, lime juice, and salsa and simmer until beans are beginning to fall apart, 1½ to 2 hours.

Yield: 6 servings

Each with: 251 g water; 101 calories (23% from fat, 18% from protein, 60% from carb); 5 g protein; 3 g total fat; 0 g saturated fat; 2 g monounsaturated fat; 0 g polyunsaturated fat; 16 g carb; 5 g fiber; 2 g sugar; 82 mg phosphorus; 38 mg calcium; 1 mg iron; 86 mg sodium; 314 mg potassium; 1,948 IU vitamin A; 14 mg vitamin C; 0 mg cholesterol

Glycemic Index: Low

Kidney Bean Stew

This is not your traditional bean soup. It's more closely related to soups like minestrone, with its tomatoes and other vegetables. But the seasoning is simple and American.

1 tablespoon (15 ml) olive oil

1½ cup (240 g) onion, sliced

1 cup (150 g) red bell pepper, seeded and chopped

¾ cup (98 g) carrot, sliced

1½ cup (180 g) zucchini, sliced

1 cup (100 g) celery, sliced

8 ounces (225 g) mushrooms, washed and sliced

2 cups (360 g) tomatoes, peeled and quartered

½ cup (125 g) dried kidney beans, soaked, cooked, and drained

½ teaspoon paprika

Black pepper, fresh ground

Heat the oil in a large saucepan and add the onion, red pepper, carrots, zucchini, and celery. Cook gently for 10 minutes, covered, and then add the mushrooms, tomatoes, kidney beans, paprika, and pepper to taste. Continue to cook, covered, for a another 10–15 minutes. Check the seasoning and serve.

Yield: 4 servings

Each with: 314 g water; 141 calories (24% from fat, 17% from protein, 59% from carb); 6 g Protein; 4 g total fat; 1 g saturated fat; 3 g monounsaturated fat; 1 g polyunsaturated fat; 23 g carb; 7 g fiber; 7 g sugar; 157 mg phosphorous; 62 mg calcium; 2 mg iron; 56 mg sodium; 876 mg potassium; 6025 IU vitamin A; 0 mg ATE vitamin E; 83 mg vitamin C; 0 mg cholesterol

Glycemic Index: Low

Spicy Bean Soup

If you like your bean soup with a little kick, this could be the recipe for you. (If not, just replace the spicy V8 with regular V8 and leave out the Tabasco.)

6 cups (1.4 L) water

1 cup (250 g) dried beans, assorted (navy, red, pinto, etc.)

1 cup (160 g) diced onion

1 cup (130 g) diced carrot

½ cup (75 g) diced green bell pepper

6 ounces (275 ml) vegetable juice such as V8, spicy flavor

¼ teaspoon Tabasco sauce

¾ cup (90 g) diced celery

1 teaspoon black pepper

1 cup (150 g) diced ham

Combine all ingredients in a large pot. Simmer for at least 3 hours.

Yield: 6 servings

Each with: 348 g water; 182 calories (12% from fat, 28% from protein, 60% from carb); 13 g protein; 2 g total fat; 1 g saturated fat; 1 g monounsaturated fat; 0 g polyunsaturated fat; 27 g carb; 7 g fiber; 4 g sugar; 205 mg phosphorus; 73 mg calcium; 2 mg iron; 425 mg sodium; 699 mg potassium; 3,779 IU vitamin A; 16 mg vitamin C; 10 mg cholesterol

Glycemic Index: Low

Fish Stew

Here's a hearty fish stew with a few unusual ingredients (like the sweet potato).

3 slices low-sodium bacon, cut into pieces

¾ cup (120 g) onion, chopped

1 clove garlic, minced

¾ teaspoon cumin

¼ teaspoon red pepper flakes

2 tablespoons (16 g) flour

4 cups (940 ml) low-sodium chicken broth

14 ounces (397 g) no-salt-added tomatoes

½ cup (120 ml) dry white wine

½ cup (75 g) green bell pepper, seeded and chopped

1 cup (133 g) sweet potatoes, peeled and cut
   into ½-inch (1 cm) cubes

½ pound (225 g) cod, cut into bite sized chunks

¾ cup (123 g) frozen corn kernels

1½ teaspoons lime juice

Pepper to taste

Fresh parsley or cilantro for garnish (if desired)

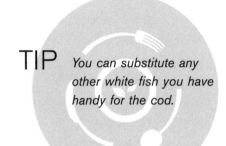

TIP *You can substitute any other white fish you have handy for the cod.*

Sauté bacon in large saucepan over medium heat until crisp. Stir in onion, garlic, cumin, and pepper flakes. Sauté five minutes or until onions are soft. Remove from heat and stir in flour. Cook one minute, stirring constantly. Gradually whisk in chicken broth. Stir in tomatoes, wine, peppers, and sweet potatoes. Bring to a boil and reduce heat and simmer 10 minutes or until sweet potatoes are soft. Add fish and corn. Simmer 2 to 3 minutes or until fish flakes with a fork. Season with lime juice and pepper. Spoon into bowls and garnish with parsley or cilantro if desired.

Yield: 4 servings

Each with: 531 g water; 280 calories (17% from fat, 31% from protein, 53% from carb); 21 g Protein; 5 g total fat; 1 g saturated fat; 2 g monounsaturated fat; 1 g polyunsaturated fat; 36 g carb; 5 g fiber; 10 g sugar; 310 mg phosphorous; 89 mg calcium; 3 mg iron; 188 mg sodium; 1027 mg potassium; 13236 IU vitamin A; 7 mg ATE vitamin E; 40 mg vitamin C; 31 mg cholesterol

Glycemic Index: Low

Fish Chowder

My daughter picked this one rainy, cold night. Since she isn't a fish lover, I figure it must be the amount of wine in it that appealed to her. It turns out to be a fairly liberal modification of the original recipe in a *Better Homes and Gardens* soup cookbook. It turned out quite well. And even she had to admit that fish isn't bad this way. You could use whatever fish you have on hand or that you prefer; the salmon and perch just happened to be what was in the freezer. If you leave out the potatoes, which weren't in the original recipe, you'd have an entrée that was low in carbs and potassium too.

1 pound (455 g) salmon

1 pound (455 g) perch

4 slices low-sodium bacon

1 onion, chopped

½ cup (50 g) chopped celery

1 clove garlic, minced

1½ cups (355 ml) white wine

1½ cups (355 ml) water

2 potatoes, cubed (optional)

¼ teaspoon thyme

1 teaspoon parsley

3 tablespoons (24 g) flour

3 tablespoons (42 g) unsalted butter, softened

½ cup (120 ml) skim milk

Thaw fish if frozen and cube. Cook bacon in Dutch oven. Crumble and set aside. Drain most of grease from pan. Sauté onion, celery, and garlic until tender. Add wine, water, potatoes (if using), and spices. Simmer until potatoes are almost done, about 20 minutes. Add fish, cover, and simmer 10 minutes more. Mix together flour and butter to form a paste. Stir into soup and simmer until thickened. Stir in milk and reserved bacon.

Yield: 8 servings

Each with: 246 g water; 336 calories (40% from fat, 34% from protein, 26% from carb); 26 g protein; 13 g total fat; 5 g saturated fat; 4 g monounsaturated fat; 3 g polyunsaturated fat; 20 g carb; 2 g fiber; 1 g sugar; 337 mg phosphorus; 106 mg calcium; 1 mg iron; 191 mg sodium; 710 mg potassium; 262 IU vitamin A; 9 mg vitamin C; 73 mg cholesterol

Glycemic Index: Low

Classic Chili

I keep experimenting with chili recipes. This is the current favorite. Sautéing the spices seems to give it a deeper, more complex flavor.

1 pound (455 g) dried kidney beans

2 pounds (900 g) beef chuck

2 onions, coarsely chopped

2 cloves garlic

1 green bell pepper, coarsely chopped

2 tablespoons (30 ml) olive oil

2 tablespoons (15 g) chili powder

1 tablespoon (7 g) cumin

1 teaspoon oregano

1 teaspoon cilantro

½ teaspoon black pepper

1 jalapeño pepper, chopped

1 can (28 ounces or 800 g) no-salt-added tomato puree

2 cups (480 g) no-salt-added canned tomatoes

Soak kidney beans overnight. Drain and add fresh water. Simmer until tender. Coarsely grind beef (or chop into cubes no bigger than ½ inch or 1 cm). Sauté beef, onion, garlic, and bell pepper in oil until beef is browned on all sides. Add spices and continue sautéing an additional 5 minutes. Transfer to slow cooker. Stir in tomato puree and tomatoes. Drain beans and add to slow cooker. Stir to mix, cover, and cook on low 4 to 5 hours.

Yield: 8 servings

Each with: 263 g water; 389 calories (59% from fat, 23% from protein, 18% from carb); 23 g protein; 26 g total fat; 9 g saturated fat; 12 g monounsaturated fat; 1 g polyunsaturated fat; 18 g carb; 4 g fiber; 9 g sugar; 73 mg calcium; 6 mg iron; 93 mg sodium; 1,031 mg potassium; 1,268 IU vitamin A; 39 mg vitamin C; 83 mg cholesterol

Glycemic Index: Low

Black Bean Chili

This makes a rather mild chili, but you can easily add more chili powder or some red pepper flakes to spice it up if that's the way you like your chili.

1 pound (455 g) ground turkey

1 tablespoon (15 ml) olive oil

½ onion, chopped

½ green bell pepper, seeded and chopped

2 cloves garlic, minced

4 cups (960 g) no-salt-added canned black beans, rinsed and drained

2 cups (480 g) no-salt-added stewed tomatoes

8 ounces (225 g) no-salt-added tomato sauce

1 cup (235 ml) dark beer or low-sodium beef broth

1 tablespoon (7 g) chili powder

1 tablespoon (7 g) ground cumin

1 teaspoon ground coriander

1 teaspoon crushed dried oregano

Heat large heavy saucepan or Dutch oven to medium-high. Brown the meat until cooked through. Drain meat and set aside. In the skillet, add the oil and bring to medium heat. Add the onion, bell pepper, and garlic, and cook until vegetables are tender, about 5 to 6 minutes. Return meat to pan. Add remaining ingredients. Bring chili to a boil; then reduce heat and simmer for 30 to 45 minutes or until thickened, stirring occasionally. Taste and adjust seasonings if necessary.

Yield: 6 servings

Each with: 259 g water; 350 calories (18% from fat, 40% from protein, 42% from carb); 35 g protein; 7 g total fat; 2 g saturated fat; 3 g monounsaturated fat; 2 g polyunsaturated fat; 36 g carb; 14 g fiber; 3 g sugar; 126 mg calcium; 5 mg iron; 71 mg sodium; 962 mg potassium; 552 IU vitamin A; 24 mg vitamin C; 58 mg cholesterol

Glycemic Index: Low

White Chili

White chili is made with chicken and white beans and without the typical tomatoes. This tends to give it a more subtle flavor than tomato chili, which many people seem to prefer once they've tried it.

1 pound (455 g) navy beans

1 tablespoon (15 ml) olive oil

4 garlic cloves, chopped

2 teaspoons (5 g) ground cumin

¼ teaspoon cloves

6 cups (1.4 L) low-sodium chicken broth

2 pounds (900 g) boneless chicken breasts

1 cup (160 g) onions, chopped

2 cans (4 ounces or 115 g) green chili peppers, chopped

1½ teaspoons dried oregano

¼ teaspoon cayenne pepper

2 cups (230 g) Monterey jack cheese, shredded

Place beans in a heavy large pot. Add enough cold water to cover by at least 3 inches and soak overnight. Place chicken in heavy large saucepan. Add cold water to cover and bring to simmer. Cook until just tender, about 15 minutes. Drain and cool. Cut chicken into cubes. Drain beans. Heat oil in same pot over medium high heat. Add onions and sauté until translucent, about 10 minutes. Stir in garlic, chilies, cumin, oregano, cloves, and cayenne and sauté 2 minutes. Add beans and stock and bring to boil. Reduce heat and simmer until beans are very tender, stirring occasionally, about 2 hours. Add chicken and one cup cheese to chili and stir until cheese melts. Serve with remaining cheese, sour cream, salsa, and cilantro.

Yield: 8 servings

Each with: 345 g water; 386 calories (34% from fat, 45% from protein, 21% from carb); 43 g Protein; 15 g total fat; 7 g saturated fat; 5 g monounsaturated fat; 1 g polyunsaturated fat; 20 g carb; 7 g fiber; 1 g sugar; 516 mg phosphorous; 325 mg calcium; 4 mg iron; 391 mg sodium; 758 mg potassium; 347 IU vitamin A; 70 mg ATE vitamin E; 10 mg vitamin C; 95 mg cholesterol

Glycemic Index: Low

Real Man Chili

This is a guy's kind of chili. It's spicy and full of just meat, with none of those beans for fillers.

3 pounds (1⅓ kg) beef round steak

2 tablespoons (30 ml) canola oil

2 cups (475 ml) low-sodium beef broth

8 ounces (225 g) no-salt-added tomato sauce

2 cups (480 g) no-salt-added canned tomatoes

6 ounces (177 ml) beer

4 ounces (115 g) canned chile peppers

2 tablespoons (15 g) chili powder

1 teaspoon garlic powder

1 tablespoon (7 g) onion powder

1 teaspoon Tabasco sauce

1 tablespoon (7 g) cumin

Sauté beef in oil until done and drain well; put beef and broth in a large pot and bring to a slow simmer; add tomato sauce, tomatoes, beer, chile peppers, spices, and Tabasco; simmer slowly for about 1 hour and 30 minutes or until meat is tender.

Yield: 10 servings

Each with: 209 g water; 370 calories (27% from fat, 58% from protein, 15% from carb); 52 g protein; 11 g total fat; 3 g saturated fat; 5 g monounsaturated fat; 2 g polyunsaturated fat; 14 g carb; 5 g fiber; 7 g sugar; 362 mg phosphorus; 45 mg calcium; 7 mg iron; 129 mg sodium; 921 mg potassium; 3,599 IU vitamin A; 12 mg vitamin C; 122 mg cholesterol

Glycemic Index: Low

Vegetable Chili

The flavor definitely says chili, but the ingredients are not what you would usually expect. A wide assortment of vegetables joins the beans for a warming, filling, flavorful bowl.

½ cup (125 g) dried kidney beans

¼ cup (35 g) bulgur

½ cup (120 ml) olive oil

1 cup (160 g) red onion, diced

½ cup (80 g) onion, diced

1½ tablespoons (15 g) garlic, minced

½ cup (50 g) celery, sliced

½ cup (65 g) carrot, sliced

2 tablespoons (15 g) chili powder

2 tablespoons (14 g) cumin

½ teaspoon cayenne pepper

1 tablespoon (2.5 g) fresh basil

1 tablespoon (4 g) fresh oregano

1 cup (120 g) yellow squash, cubed

1 cup (120 g) zucchini, cubed

1 cup (150 g) green bell pepper, cubed

1 cup (150 g) red bell pepper, cubed

8 ounces (225 g) mushroom, sliced

½ cup (90 g) tomatoes, diced

½ cup (130 g) no-salt-added tomato paste

¾ cup (175 ml) dry white wine

Pepper to taste

Soak beans in cold water to cover overnight. Drain off water. Add 3 cups (720 ml) fresh water to beans and cook over medium heat until tender, about 45 minutes. Drain beans, reserving cooking liquid. Bring ½ cup (120 ml) water to boil. Pour over bulgur in bowl. Let stand 30 minutes to soften wheat (the water will be absorbed). Heat olive oil in large saucepan. Add red and white onions and sauté until tender. Add garlic, celery, and carrots. Sauté until softened. Add chili powder, cumin, cayenne, basil, and oregano. Cook over low heat until carrots are almost tender.

Add squash, zucchini, peppers, and mushrooms and cook 4 minutes. Stir in bulgur, kidney beans, tomatoes, and reserved cooking liquid from beans. Cook 30 minutes or until vegetables are tender. Mix tomato paste with white wine until smooth and then stir into vegetable mixture.

Yield: 6 servings

Each with: 237 g water; 311 calories (57% from fat, 9% from protein, 35% from carb); 7 g Protein; 20 g total fat; 3 g saturated fat; 14 g monounsaturated fat; 2 g polyunsaturated fat; 27 g carb; 8 g fiber; 9 g sugar; 164 mg phosphorous; 95 mg calcium; 4 mg iron; 77 mg sodium; 905 mg potassium; 4087 IU vitamin A; 0 mg ATE vitamin E; 74 mg vitamin C; 0 mg cholesterol

Glycemic Index: Low

Quick Black Bean and Corn Chili

Canned sauce and beans make this chili one of the quickest meals you'll find. But don't let that fool you; the flavor is still full and well developed.

16 ounces (455 g) picante sauce

15 ounces (420 g) black beans, undrained

8 ounces (225 g) no-salt-added tomato sauce

1 cup (164 g) frozen corn

½ teaspoon cumin

1 cup (115 g) cheddar, shredded

2 tablespoons (30 g) sour cream

In medium saucepan, combine picante sauce, beans, tomato sauce, corn, and cumin. Bring to boil; reduce heat; simmer 5 minutes. Divide among serving bowls; top with cheese and sour cream.

Yield: 4 servings

Each with: 274 g water; 369 calories (31% from fat, 22% from protein, 46% from carb); 21 g Protein; 13 g total fat; 8 g saturated fat; 4 g monounsaturated fat; 1 g polyunsaturated fat; 44 g carb; 11 g fiber; 7 g sugar; 368 mg phosphorous; 303 mg calcium; 3 mg iron; 665 mg sodium; 695 mg potassium; 1035 IU vitamin A; 93 mg ATE vitamin E; 16 mg vitamin C; 38 mg cholesterol

Glycemic Index: Low

11

Salads and Salad Dressings

Salads fit perfectly into our low-GI lifestyle with their emphasis on vegetables and their typically low carbohydrate contents. This chapter includes a selection of both side-dish salads and main-dish salad meals. We try to have at least one salad meal a week during the summer when fresh vegetables are plentiful and we don't feel like cooking. There also are a couple of salad dressing recipes. Most commercial salad dressing is not that bad nutritionally, but these are some we like that are a little different from the ones in the grocery store.

Creamy Asian Dressing

This is a creamy salad dressing with Asian flavorings. But you may find that you like it well enough to use every day.

8 ounces (225 g) tofu

¼ teaspoon dried oregano

¼ teaspoon marjoram

1 clove garlic, minced

3 tablespoons (45 ml) balsamic vinegar

2 tablespoons (30 ml) Dick's Reduced Sodium Soy Sauce (see recipe in chapter 2)

¼ cup (25 g) green onions, chopped

2 tablespoon (30 ml) lemon juice

¼ cup (60 ml) water

Place tofu slices in a blender or a food processor fitted with the metal blade. Add remaining ingredients and only as much water as needed to make desired consistency. Process until smooth.

Yield: 32 servings

Each with: 12 g water; 5 calories (34% from fat, 32% from protein, 35% from carb); 0 g Protein; 0 g total fat; 0 g saturated fat; 0 g monounsaturated fat; 0 g polyunsaturated fat; 0 g carb; 0 g fiber; 0 g sugar; 6 mg phosphorous; 3 mg calcium; 0 mg iron; 1 mg sodium; 19 mg potassium; 9 IU vitamin A; 0 mg ATE vitamin E; 1 mg vitamin C; 0 mg cholesterol

Glycemic Index: Low

Balsamic Vinaigrette

This dressing has a more distinct flavor than many of the balsamic dressing sold commercially. The mustard seems to raise it to a higher level.

1 tablespoon (11 g) Dijon mustard

¼ cup (60 ml) balsamic vinegar

2 tablespoons (30 ml) water

2 tablespoons (30 ml) fresh lemon juice

¼ teaspoon pepper

¼ teaspoon dried tarragon

1 clove garlic, minced

¼ cup (60 ml) olive oil

In a jar, combine the mustard, vinegar, water, lemon juice, pepper, tarragon, and garlic. Shake well to combine. Add oils and shake again. Chill before serving.

Yield: 12 servings

Each with: 11 g water; 42 calories (96% from fat, 1% from protein, 3% from carb); 0 g Protein; 5 g total fat; 1 g saturated fat; 3 g monounsaturated fat; 0 g polyunsaturated fat; 0 g carb; 0 g fiber; 0 g sugar; 2 mg phosphorous; 2 mg calcium; 0 mg iron; 15 mg sodium; 9 mg potassium; 4 IU vitamin A; 0 mg ATE vitamin E; 1 mg vitamin C; 0 mg cholesterol

Glycemic Index: Low

Buttermilk Dill Dressing

This is a good dressing when you are having fish or chicken.

¼ cup (60 g) low-sodium mayonnaise

½ cup (120 ml) buttermilk

1 tablespoon (10 g) minced onion

2 teaspoons (2 g) dill

1 teaspoon basil

1 tablespoon (4 g) parsley

¼ teaspoon garlic powder

Dash cayenne pepper

Combine ingredients in a blender or food processor and process until smooth. Refrigerate several hours or overnight before serving to allow flavor to develop.

Yield: 6 servings

TIP *Replace one teaspoon of the dill with oregano or Italian seasoning for a good ranch-type dressing.*

Each with: 21 g water; 79 calories (84% from fat, 5% from protein, 11% from carb); 1 g protein; 7 g total fat; 1 g saturated fat; 2 g monounsaturated fat; 3 g polyunsaturated fat; 2 g carb; 0 g fiber; 1 g sugar; 37 mg calcium; 0 mg iron; 25 mg sodium; 68 mg potassium; 115 IU vitamin A; 2 mg vitamin C; 6 mg cholesterol

Glycemic Index: Low

Sun-Dried Tomato Vinaigrette

This dressing has a nice flavor, but it also contains a fair amount of fat, which I've not made any attempt to reduce.

3 tablespoons (45 ml) white wine vinegar

¼ cup (14 g) chopped sun-dried tomatoes

1 teaspoon Worcestershire sauce

1 clove garlic, minced

½ teaspoon sugar

¼ tablespoon white pepper

⅓ cup (80 ml) olive oil

Shake ingredients together in a jar with a tight-fitting lid.

Yield: 8 servings

(continued on page 294)

Each with: 7 g water; 70 calories (91% from fat, 1% from protein, 8% from carb); 0 g protein; 7 g total fat; 1 g saturated fat; 5 g monounsaturated fat; 1 g polyunsaturated fat; 1 g carb; 0 g fiber; 0 g sugar; 6 mg phosphorus; 3 mg calcium; 0 mg iron; 16 mg sodium; 63 mg potassium; 45 IU vitamin A; 5 mg vitamin C; 0 mg cholesterol

Glycemic Index: Low

Poppy Seed Dressing

This dressing is good on just about any kind of salad, but it seems to be particularly good on cabbage or cauliflower.

¼ cup (40 g) onion, chopped

¾ cup (175 ml) white wine vinegar

2 tablespoon (30 ml) olive oil

2½ tablespoons (22.5 g) poppy seeds

1 tablespoon (13 g) sugar

1 teaspoon dry mustard

¾ cup (175 ml) olive oil

Combine first 6 ingredients in container of electric blender; blend well. Slowly add ¾ cup (175 ml) oil, continuing to blend until thick. Pour into a jar with a tight-fitting lid and chill. Shake well before serving.

Yield: 12 servings

Each with: 17 g water; 158 calories (94% from fat, 1% from protein, 5% from carb); 0 g Protein; 17 g total fat; 2 g saturated fat; 12 g monounsaturated fat; 2 g polyunsaturated fat; 2 g carb; 0 g fiber; 2 g sugar; 18 mg phosphorous; 29 mg calcium; 0 mg iron; 2 mg sodium; 30 mg potassium; 0 IU vitamin A; 0 mg ATE vitamin E; 0 mg vitamin C; 0 mg cholesterol

Glycemic Index: Low

Oriental Coleslaw

Coleslaw gets an Asian makeover in this recipe featuring Chinese cabbage and a dressing flavored with soy sauce, rice wine vinegar, and sesame oil.

2 cups (140 g) bok choy, finely shredded

¼ cup (38 g) green bell pepper, chopped

¼ cup (28 g) carrot, coarsely shredded

3 tablespoons (45 ml) rice wine vinegar

2 teaspoons (1 g) sugar substitute, such as Splenda

2 teaspoons (5.4 g) sesame seeds, toasted

2 teaspoons (10 ml) Dick's Reduced Sodium Soy Sauce (see recipe in chapter 2)

1 teaspoon sesame oil

⅛ teaspoon red pepper flakes

Toss first three ingredients together. Mix remaining ingredients. Pour over vegetables and toss to coat.

Yield: 4 servings

Each with: 76 g water; 45 calories (38% from fat, 8% from protein, 53% from carb); 1 g Protein; 2 g total fat; 0 g saturated fat; 1 g monounsaturated fat; 1 g polyunsaturated fat; 6 g carb; 1 g fiber; 1 g sugar; 27 mg phosphorous; 35 mg calcium; 1 mg iron; 136 mg sodium; 108 mg potassium; 1426 IU vitamin A; 0 mg ATE vitamin E; 10 mg vitamin C; 0 mg cholesterol

Glycemic Index: Low

Barbecue Coleslaw

This slaw comes with the barbecue flavor already in it, so it's great for topping barbecue sandwiches. It's also good on burgers or just as a side dish.

2 cups (140 g) cabbage, grated

½ cup (50 g) celery, grated

(continued on page 296)

1 cup (150 g) green bell pepper, grated

½ cup (80 g) onion, minced

¾ cup (180 g) low-sodium catsup

¼ cup (60 ml) cider vinegar

2 tablespoons (2 g) brown sugar substitute, such as Splenda

1½ tablespoons (25 ml) Worcestershire sauce

1 tablespoon (11 g) prepared mustard

¼ teaspoon red pepper flakes

½ teaspoon liquid smoke

Combine all vegetable ingredients in a large bowl. Mix all other ingredients into the bowl. Chill and serve.

Yield: 6 servings

Each with: 102 g water; 59 calories (5% from fat, 10% from protein, 85% from carb); 2 g Protein; 0 g total fat; 0 g saturated fat; 0 g monounsaturated fat; 0 g polyunsaturated fat; 14 g carb; 2 g fiber; 10 g sugar; 33 mg phosphorous; 29 mg calcium; 1 mg iron; 57 mg sodium; 293 mg potassium; 476 IU vitamin A; 0 mg ATE vitamin E; 43 mg vitamin C; 0 mg cholesterol

Glycemic Index: Low

Dilled Cucumbers

Dilled cucumbers just seem to go well with fish, but you can serve them with any meat, and you won't be disappointed.

2 medium cucumbers, peeled and sliced

1 large onion, sliced

2 tablespoons (8 g) fresh dill, chopped

1 teaspoon sugar substitute, such as Splenda

½ cup (120 ml) white vinegar

½ teaspoon freshly ground black pepper

In medium bowl, combine cucumbers, onion, and dill. Stir sugar substitute into vinegar to dissolve. Add to the cucumber mixture; season with pepper. Cover and refrigerate several hours or overnight.

Yield: 10 servings

Each with: 83 g water; 20 calories (5% from fat, 13% from protein, 82% from carb); 1 g Protein; 0 g total fat; 0 g saturated fat; 0 g monounsaturated fat; 0 g polyunsaturated fat; 4 g carb; 1 g fiber; 2 g sugar; 24 mg phosphorous; 26 mg calcium; 1 mg iron; 4 mg sodium; 142 mg potassium; 100 IU vitamin A; 0 mg ATE vitamin E; 3 mg vitamin C; 0 mg cholesterol

Glycemic Index: Low

Pasta and Artichoke Heart Salad

Artichoke hearts give this pasta salad a flavor boost and lift it above the "ordinary" pasta salads. The overall effect is sort of Mediterranean.

2 cups (210 g) elbow macaroni

¾ pound (340 g) marinated artichoke hearts

1 cup (150 g) green bell pepper, chopped

½ cup (55 g) carrot, coarsely grated

½ cup (50 g) sliced black olives

¼ cup (60 ml) red wine vinegar

½ teaspoon basil

¼ teaspoon pepper

Cook pasta until al dente. Rinse with cool water. Drain and put in mixing bowl. Chop artichokes into bite-sized pieces. Add to pasta. Add the rest of the ingredients. Mix well and allow to stand for 2 hours in the refrigerator.

Yield: 4 servings

Each with: 153 g water; 274 calories (9% from fat, 15% from protein, 76% from carb); 10 g Protein; 3 g total fat; 0 g saturated fat; 1 g monounsaturated fat; 1 g polyunsaturated fat; 53 g carb; 8 g fiber; 4 g sugar;

(continued on page 298)

188 mg phosphorous; 76 mg calcium; 4 mg iron; 244 mg sodium; 545 mg potassium; 3060 IU vitamin A; 0 mg ATE vitamin E; 40 mg vitamin C; 0 mg cholesterol

Glycemic Index: Low

Pasta and Kidney Bean Salad

This is really an easy salad to put together, especially if you're like me and tend to cook a whole pound of kidney beans while you are doing it, and then wonder what to do with the leftovers.

2 cups (270 g) rotini or other medium sized pasta

2 cups (200 g) red kidney beans, cooked

1 cup (120 g) zucchini, diced

1 cup (150 g) green bell pepper, diced

1 cup (180 g) tomato, chopped

⅓ cup (34 g) green olives, chopped

1 cup (225 g) mayonnaise

½ teaspoon chili powder

½ teaspoon coriander

½ teaspoon paprika

¼ teaspoon sage

TIP *You can enhance the Mediterranean feel of this salad by crumbling a little feta cheese over it.*

Cook pasta until al dente. Rinse and drain. Put in large bowl and add rest of the ingredients. Mix thoroughly and serve at room temperature.

Yield: 6 servings

Each with: 130 g water; 383 calories (69% from fat, 8% from protein, 24% from carb); 8 g Protein; 30 g total fat; 5 g saturated fat; 8 g monounsaturated fat; 16 g polyunsaturated fat; 23 g carb; 8 g fiber; 2 g sugar; 129 mg phosphorous; 65 mg calcium; 3 mg iron; 423 mg sodium; 436 mg potassium; 641 IU vitamin A; 29 mg ATE vitamin E; 28 mg vitamin C; 14 mg cholesterol

Glycemic Index: Low

Chicken, Bean and Corn Salad

If you increase the serving size, this salad makes a great meal in itself.

1 cup (140 g) cooked chicken breast, cut in 1-inch (2½ cm) strips

15 ounce (420 g) kidney beans, rinsed and drained

10 ounces (280 g) frozen corn, thawed

½ cup (50 g) green onion, thinly sliced

1 tablespoon (15 ml) red wine vinegar

2 teaspoons (10 ml) olive oil

2 tablespoons (2 g) cilantro, chopped

In medium bowl, combine chicken and remaining ingredients. Serve on a bed of lettuce, if desired.

Yield: 4 servings

Each with: 655 g water; 783 calories (7% from fat, 18% from protein, 75% from carb); 40 g Protein; 7 g total fat; 1 g saturated fat; 3 g monounsaturated fat; 2 g polyunsaturated fat; 164 g carb; 27 g fiber; 22 g sugar; 636 mg phosphorous; 114 mg calcium; 6 mg iron; 69 mg sodium; 1622 mg potassium; 244 IU vitamin A; 2 mg ATE vitamin E; 26 mg vitamin C; 30 mg cholesterol

Glycemic Index: Low

Dried Bean and Cashew Salad

This makes a hearty salad that is a great side dish with a piece of grilled meat, or it can stand alone for lunch.

1 cup (202 g) dried lima beans, cooked

1 cup (167 g) black-eyed peas, cooked

¼ cup (25 g) celery, finely chopped

½ cup (50 g) red bell pepper, seeded and finely chopped

2 tablespoons (18 g) cashews, roasted

(continued on page 300)

¼ cup (25 g) green onions, chopped

1 tablespoon (15 ml) tomato sauce

1 garlic clove, crushed

¼ teaspoon cumin

3 tablespoons (45 ml) balsamic vinegar

6 tablespoons (90 ml) olive oil

In a large bowl, mix the beans and peas with the celery and sweet pepper. Roast the cashew nuts in a dry frying pan until browned. Put on paper towels and allow to cool. When cool, toss into the beans with the green onions. Mix the tomato sauce, garlic, cumin, vinegar, and olive oil together well. Pour over the beans and mix well. Allow to stand for about an hour before serving.

Yield: 6 servings

Each with: 69 g water; 212 calories (63% from fat, 9% from protein, 28% from carb); 5 g Protein; 15 g total fat; 2 g saturated fat; 11 g monounsaturated fat; 2 g polyunsaturated fat; 15 g carb; 4 g fiber; 3 g sugar; 90 mg phosphorous; 24 mg calcium; 2 mg iron; 29 mg sodium; 310 mg potassium; 531 IU vitamin A; 0 mg ATE vitamin E; 19 mg vitamin C; 0 mg cholesterol

Glycemic Index: Low

Spinach and Black-Eyed Pea Salad

This is a tasty salad of marinated black-eyed peas over spinach.

½ pound (225 g) black-eyed peas

1 cup (160 g) chopped onion

½ teaspoon minced garlic

4 cups (950 ml) water

14 ounces (395 g) artichoke hearts

1 tablespoon (15 g) Dijon mustard

1 tablespoon (15 ml) Worcestershire sauce

½ pound (225 g) spinach leaves

4 slices bacon, cooked and crumbled

Sort and wash peas; place in a Dutch oven with next 3 ingredients. Bring to a boil; reduce heat and simmer 40 minutes or until peas are tender. Drain. Keep peas warm. Drain artichoke hearts, reserving juice. Chop artichoke hearts and add to black-eyed peas. Combine reserved artichoke juice, mustard, and Worcestershire; pour over peas and toss gently. Arrange spinach leaves on individual salad plates; spoon salad onto spinach. Sprinkle with crumbled bacon and serve warm.

Yield: 6 servings

Each with: 302 g water; 132 calories (20% from fat, 25% from protein, 56% from carb); 9 g protein; 3 g total fat; 1 g saturated fat; 1 g monounsaturated fat; 1 g polyunsaturated fat; 20 g carb; 7 g fiber; 4 g sugar; 147 mg phosphorus; 73 mg calcium; 3 mg iron; 249 mg sodium; 622 mg potassium; 3,688 IU vitamin A; 21 mg vitamin C; 6 mg cholesterol

Glycemic Index: Low

Marinated Vegetable Salad

I really like marinated vegetables, especially in the summer when you can just add them to some lettuce to make a refreshing and filling salad.

½ cup (56 g) sliced zucchini

½ cup (90 g) sliced yellow squash

½ cup (36 g) broccoli florets

½ cup (50 g) cauliflower florets

¼ cup (33 g) sliced carrot

¼ cup (40 g) thinly sliced red onion

15 cherry tomatoes, halved

4 ounces (115 g) mushrooms, sliced

Marinade

1 cup (235 ml) olive oil

½ cup (120 ml) red wine vinegar

¼ cup (60 ml) lemon juice

1 teaspoon oregano

(continued on page 302)

1 teaspoon dry mustard

1 teaspoon minced onion

½ teaspoon pressed garlic

Mix vegetables in a bowl. Combine marinade ingredients and pour over vegetables. Refrigerate for several hours or overnight.

Yield: 8 servings

Each with: 71 g water; 265 calories (91% from fat, 2% from protein, 7% from carb); 1 g protein; 27 g total fat; 4 g saturated fat; 20 g monounsaturated fat; 3 g polyunsaturated fat; 5 g carb; 2 g fiber; 1 g sugar; 29 mg phosphorus; 16 mg calcium; 1 mg iron; 10 mg sodium; 228 mg potassium; 1,046 IU vitamin A; 21 mg vitamin C; 0 mg cholesterol

Glycemic Index: Low

Marinated Green Beans

These beans make a great ingredient to liven up an otherwise ordinary salad. They also can be used as a side dish or for nibbling.

2 cups (200 g) fresh green beans

½ cup (80 g) onion, sliced

2 tablespoons (30 ml) olive oil

1 tablespoon (1.5 ml) white wine vinegar

1 teaspoon Dijon mustard

2 garlic cloves, pressed

Wash the beans; cut off the ends and break in half. Steam them for a few minutes but do not let them lose their crunchiness. Drain. Place in a salad bowl with the onions. Combine the rest of the ingredients in a jar and shake well. Pour over the beans. Serve either hot or cold.

Yield: 2 servings

Each with: 144 g water; 173 calories (68% from fat, 6% from protein, 26% from carb); 3 g Protein; 14 g total fat; 2 g saturated fat; 10 g monounsaturated fat; 2 g polyunsaturated fat; 12 g carb; 5 g fiber; 3 g sugar; 57 mg phosphorous; 52 mg calcium; 1 mg iron; 37 mg sodium; 297 mg potassium; 762 IU vitamin A; 0 mg ATE vitamin E; 21 mg vitamin C; 0 mg cholesterol

Glycemic Index: Low

Oriental Vegetable Toss

This is a great side dish with a plain piece of meat marinated in a little more of the dressing.

½ pound (225 g) shredded lettuce

4 ounces (115 g) snow peas

½ cup (65 g) sliced carrot

1 cup (70 g) shredded cabbage

4 ounces (115 g) mushrooms, sliced

½ cup (75 g) sliced red bell pepper

4 ounces (115 g) mung bean sprouts

Dressing

¼ cup (60 ml) Dick's Reduced-Sodium Soy Sauce (see recipe in chapter 2)

2 tablespoons (30 ml) rice vinegar

2 tablespoons (30 ml) mirin wine

½ teaspoon ginger

1 tablespoon (8 g) sesame seeds

Toss all salad ingredients. Spoon dressing over top.

Yield: 6 servings

Each with: 122 g water; 39 calories (6% from fat, 24% from protein, 71% from carb); 2 g protein; 0 g total fat; 0 g saturated fat; 0 g monounsaturated fat; 0 g polyunsaturated fat; 7 g carb; 2 g fiber; 4 g sugar; 29 mg calcium; 1 mg iron; 16 mg sodium; 269 mg potassium; 1,822 IU vitamin A; 34 mg vitamin C; 0 mg cholesterol

Glycemic Index: Low

Italian Marinated Tomatoes

These tasty tomatos make a nice cool starting point for an Italian meal. They are also just as good with grilled or roasted meat.

6 slices tomatoes

6 slices red onion

1 tablespoon (2.5 g) fresh basil, sliced

2 tablespoons (30 ml) Italian salad dressing

Place tomato slices in shallow dish; top each with an onion slice. Sprinkle with basil. Pour salad dressing over tomato and onion. Cover and refrigerate 1 hour.

Yield: 6 servings

Each with: 61 g water; 34 calories (38% from fat, 7% from protein, 54% from carb); 1 g Protein; 2 g total fat; 0 g saturated fat; 0 g monounsaturated fat; 1 g polyunsaturated fat; 5 g carb; 1 g fiber; 2 g sugar; 19 mg phosphorous; 16 mg calcium; 0 mg iron; 86 mg sodium; 136 mg potassium; 267 IU vitamin A; 0 mg ATE vitamin E; 12 mg vitamin C; 0 mg cholesterol

Glycemic Index: Low

Italian Salad

Try this salad with your next Italian meal. Or you can add some tuna or salami and make it a meal in itself.

2 cups (110 g) romaine lettuce, torn into bite-size pieces

2 cups (110 g) iceberg lettuce, torn into bite-size pieces

1 cup (160 g) red onion, separated into rings

1 can (14 ounces or 395 g) artichoke hearts, drained and separated

1 cup (71 g) broccoli florets

1 cup (115 g) shredded mozzarella cheese

½ cup (120 ml) Italian salad dressing

Toss all ingredients together.

Yield: 4 servings

Each with: 191 g water; 227 calories (57% from fat, 16% from protein, 26% from carb); 10 g protein; 15 g total fat; 5 g saturated fat; 4 g monounsaturated fat; 4 g polyunsaturated fat; 16 g carb; 4 g fiber; 6 g sugar; 176 mg phosphorus; 188 mg calcium; 1 mg iron; 706 mg sodium; 419 mg potassium; 2,375 IU vitamin A; 29 mg vitamin C; 22 mg cholesterol

Glycemic Index: Low

Marinated Mushrooms

Serve these mushrooms over lettuce leaves for a tasty salad or heat them and serve with grilled beef or chicken.

1 pound (455 g) small mushrooms, cleaned

3 tablespoons (45 ml) olive oil

2 tablespoons (30 ml) lemon juice

½ teaspoon salt

½ teaspoon thyme

2 garlic cloves, chopped

½ teaspoon black pepper

2 tablespoons (8 g) fresh parsley

Slice off mushroom stems; leave the caps whole. Place in a pot with a small amount of water and cook gently for 15 minutes. Drain. Combine the remaining ingredients. Place mushrooms in the marinade and let sit for at least 2 hours in the refrigerator, stirring occasionally.

Yield: 4 servings

Each with: 113 g water; 118 calories (74% from fat, 11% from protein, 15% from carb); 4 g Protein; 11 g total fat; 1 g saturated fat; 7 g monounsaturated fat; 1 g polyunsaturated fat; 5 g carb; 1 g fiber; 2 g sugar; 100 mg phosphorous; 10 mg calcium; 1 mg iron; 302 mg sodium; 385 mg potassium; 165 IU vitamin A; 0 mg ATE vitamin E; 9 mg vitamin C; 0 mg cholesterol

Glycemic Index: Low

Dilled Carrots

These carrots make a nice addition to a salad, adding a little different flavor, but they are also good to just nibble on as a healthy snack.

1 pound (455 g) carrots, cut into 4-inch (10 cm) julienne strips

1 teaspoon (235 ml) mustard seed

1 cup (235 ml) cider vinegar

1 cup (235 ml) water

1½ teaspoons dill seed

1 clove garlic, cut in half

2 tablespoon (3 g) sugar substitute, such as Splenda

Cook carrots, covered, in 1-inch (2½ cm) of boiling water 3–4 minutes until tender-crisp. Place in jar. In small saucepan, bring remaining ingredients to boil. Reduce heat and simmer 5 minutes. Pour over carrots. Store in refrigerator.

Yield: 4 servings

Each with: 216 g water; 71 calories (9% from fat, 9% from protein, 82% from carb); 1 g Protein; 1 g total fat; 0 g saturated fat; 0 g monounsaturated fat; 0 g polyunsaturated fat; 14 g carb; 3 g fiber; 7 g sugar; 55 mg phosphorous; 61 mg calcium; 1 g iron; 83 mg sodium; 423 mg potassium; 19065 IU vitamin A; 0 mg ATE vitamin E; 7 mg vitamin C; 0 mg cholesterol

Glycemic Index: Low

Tomato, Cucumber, and Red Onion Salad with Mint

Mint adds a refreshing note to the salad.

2 large English hothouse cucumbers

⅓ cup (80 ml) red wine vinegar

1 tablespoon (13 g) sugar

1 teaspoon salt

3 large tomatoes, seeded and coarsely chopped

2/3 cup (107 g) coarsely chopped red onion

½ cup (48 g) chopped fresh mint

3 tablespoons (45 ml) olive oil

Cut cucumbers in half lengthwise and scrape out the seeds. Cut the halves diagonally into ½-inch-wide (1 cm wide) pieces and place in a large bowl. Add vinegar, sugar, and salt and let stand at room temperature for 1 hour, tossing occasionally. Add tomatoes, red onion, mint, and oil to the cucumbers and toss to blend. Season to taste with salt and pepper.

Yield: 6 servings

Each with: 201 g water; 110 calories (55% from fat, 6% from protein, 39% from carb); 2 g protein; 7 g total fat; 1 g saturated fat; 5 g monounsaturated fat; 1 g polyunsaturated fat; 11 g carb; 2 g fiber; 7 g sugar; 53 mg phosphorus; 44 mg calcium; 1 mg iron; 402 mg sodium; 395 mg potassium; 1,034 IU vitamin A; 15 mg vitamin C; 0 mg cholesterol

Glycemic Index: Low

Spinach, Orange, and Mushroom Salad

We've been trying to add a little more fruit into our diet, and this salad is one solution that everyone really liked.

6 cups (180 g) fresh spinach

1 orange, peeled and coarsely chopped

¼ cup (25 g) green onions, chopped

½ cup (35 g) mushrooms, sliced

1 tablespoon (15 ml) lemon juice

3 tablespoons (45 ml) olive oil

¼ teaspoon black pepper

¾ cup (83 g) toasted slivered almonds

(continued on page 308)

Place spinach in a large salad bowl. Add orange, mushrooms, and onions. Mix together lemon juice, oil, garlic powder, and pepper. Pour over salad and add almonds. Toss gently.

Yield: 4 servings

Each with: 311 g water; 362 calories (56% from fat, 18% from protein, 26% from carb); 18 g Protein; 25 g total fat; 3 g saturated fat; 16 g monounsaturated fat; 5 g polyunsaturated fat; 26 g carb; 15 g fiber; 7 g sugar; 286 mg phosphorous; 529 mg calcium; 7 mg iron; 278 mg sodium; 1189 mg potassium; 34541 IU vitamin A; 0 mg ATE vitamin E; 34 mg vitamin C; 0 mg cholesterol

Glycemic Index: Low

Pizza Salad

If you have a taste for pizza but are trying to get your recommended vegetables in for the day, this salad topped pizza may be the solution you are looking for.

3 large tomatoes

½ cup (60 g) mozzarella cheese, shredded

2 tablespoons (10 g) parmesan cheese, grated

1 pizza crust, unbaked

2 cups (110 g) romaine lettuce, shredded

½ cup (75 g) red bell peppers, chopped

¼ cup (25 g) ripe olives, sliced

2 tablespoons (30 ml) Italian salad dressing

Preheat oven to 450°F (230°C, gas mark 8). Core tomatoes; slice into ¼-inch-thick (0.6 cm thick) slices and set aside. Sprinkle mozzarella and Parmesan cheeses evenly over pizza shell; top with tomato slices, slightly overlapping. Bake about 8 minutes or until cheese melts. Meanwhile, in medium bowl, combine romaine, peppers, and olives; sprinkle with Italian dressing; toss to coat. Remove pizza from oven; top with romaine mixture. Cut into wedges and serve immediately.

Yield: 6 servings

Each with: 108 g water; 297 calories (25% from fat, 14% from protein, 61% from carb); 10 g Protein; 8 g total fat; 3 g saturated fat; 3 g monounsaturated fat; 2 g polyunsaturated fat; 45 g carb; 2 g fiber; 1 g sugar; 75 mg phosphorous; 85 mg calcium; 1 mg iron; 779 mg sodium; 243 mg potassium; 1857 IU vitamin A; 19 mg ATE vitamin E; 39 mg vitamin C; 9 mg cholesterol

Glycemic Index: Low

Asian Chicken Pasta Salad

This Asian flavored salad is really a full meal, and it's full of flavor.

8 ounces (225 g) orzo or other small pasta

3 tablespoons (45 ml) red wine vinegar

1½ tablespoons (30 g) chili sauce (see recipe in chapter 2)

1 tablespoon (15 ml) Dick's Reduced Sodium Soy Sauce (see recipe in chapter 2)

1 tablespoon (15 ml) sesame oil

1 tablespoon (8 g) gingerroot, peeled and grated

2 teaspoons (10 ml) Dick's Reduced-Sodium Teriyaki Sauce (see recipe in chapter 2)

2 cups (280 g) cooked chicken breast, cubed

4 ounces (115 g) fresh spinach, sliced into strips

½ cup (25 g) bean sprouts

½ cup (75 g) red bell pepper, cut into strips

¼ cup (25 g) green onion, sliced

3 tablespoons (21 g) slivered almonds, toasted

Prepare pasta according to package directions; drain and transfer to bowl. Meanwhile, in small bowl, mix together vinegar, chili sauce, soy sauce, oil, ginger, and teriyaki sauce; whisk well. To pasta in bowl, add chicken, spinach, sprouts, bell pepper, and green onions; toss to combine. Toss dressing with pasta mixture; refrigerate 2 hours or until ready to serve. Sprinkle with almonds.

Yield: 4 servings

(continued on page 310)

Each with: 136 g water; 423 calories (22% from fat, 31% from protein, 46% from carb); 33 g Protein; 10 g total fat; 2 g saturated fat; 4 g monounsaturated fat; 3 g polyunsaturated fat; 49 g carb; 4 g fiber; 4 g sugar; 335 mg phosphorous; 95 mg calcium; 4 mg iron; 115 mg sodium; 525 mg potassium; 4174 IU vitamin A; 4 mg ATE vitamin E; 27 mg vitamin C; 60 mg cholesterol

Glycemic Index: Low

Curried Rice Salad

This rice salad actually makes a great lunch or light dinner, as well as serving as a side dish.

3 cups (495 g) rice, regular, cooked, cold

1 cup (164 g) frozen corn, cooked and cooled

1 cup (25 g) celery, thinly sliced

¼ cup (38 g) green bell pepper, chopped

¼ cup (25 g) olives, sliced

3 tablespoons (30 g) onion, minced

¼ cup (30 g) dill pickles, chopped

Black pepper, to taste

¼ teaspoon curry powder

2 tablespoons chutney (see recipe in chapter 2)

⅓ cup (80 ml) French dressing

Combine first 8 ingredients. Stir curry powder and chutney into French dressing; pour over salad. Toss lightly and chill until serving time. To serve, mound on crisp salad greens. Garnish with slices of hard-cooked eggs, if desired.

Yield: 6 servings

Each with: 117 g water; 214 calories (30% from fat, 6% from protein, 64% from carb); 3 g Protein; 7 g total fat; 1 g saturated fat; 2 g monounsaturated fat; 3 g polyunsaturated fat; 35 g carb; 2 g fiber; 4 g sugar; 60 mg phosphorous; 29 mg calcium; 1 mg iron; 234 mg sodium; 152 mg potassium; 245 IU vitamin A; 0 mg ATE vitamin E; 7 mg vitamin C; 0 mg cholesterol

Glycemic Index: Low

Chick Pea and Rice Salad

I really like the flavor of this salad, but perhaps that's because I like the taste of cumin, which is the main spice in the dressing.

¾ cup (123 g) chick peas, cooked

1 cup (165 g) rice, cooked

½ cup (75 g) red bell pepper, diced

½ cup (75 g) green bell pepper, diced

½ cup (75 g) yellow bell pepper, diced

¼ cup (25 g) green onions, sliced

2 teaspoons (5.4 g) sesame seeds, toasted

1 teaspoon sesame oil

½ teaspoon cumin

2 tablespoons (30 ml) lemon juice

1 tablespoon (15 ml) olive oil

Toss together chick peas, rice, bell peppers, and onions in a large bowl. Whisk together all the remaining ingredients. Toss with salad.

Yield: 4 servings

Each with: 136 g water; 176 calories (32% from fat, 11% from protein, 57% from carb); 5 g Protein; 6 g total fat; 1 g saturated fat; 3 g monounsaturated fat; 2 g polyunsaturated fat; 26 g carb; 4 g fiber; 3 g sugar; 102 mg phosphorous; 49 mg calcium; 2 mg iron; 7 mg sodium; 312 mg potassium; 820 IU vitamin A; 0 mg ATE vitamin E; 129 mg vitamin C; 0 mg cholesterol

Glycemic Index: Low

Warm Potato Salad

When most people think of warm potato salads they think of the German variety, with its sweet and sour boiled dressing. This is a simpler version, with potatoes and a few veggies in a simple vinaigrette.

(continued on page 312)

1 pound (455 g) potatoes, cubed

1 cup (150 g) green bell pepper

½ tablespoon dill

½ tablespoon rosemary, crushed

2 tablespoons (30 ml) olive oil

1 tablespoon (15 ml) malt vinegar

3 tablespoons (30 g) onion, finely chopped

In a medium pot, cook quartered potatoes in salted water until tender. Meanwhile, combine remaining ingredients in a small bowl. Drain potatoes, add to the bowl, and toss gently. Serve warm.

Yield: 4 servings

Each with: 137 g water; 152 calories (40% from fat, 7% from protein, 53% from carb); 3 g Protein; 7 g total fat; 1 g saturated fat; 5 g monounsaturated fat; 1 g polyunsaturated fat; 21 g carb; 3 g fiber; 2 g sugar; 81 mg phosphorous; 25 mg calcium; 1 mg iron; 9 mg sodium; 609 mg potassium; 175 IU vitamin A; 0 mg ATE vitamin E; 40 mg vitamin C; 0 mg cholesterol

Glycemic Index: Low

Mexican Potato Salad

We like this potato salad full of Mexican flavors with a burger that also has had the Mexican treatment.

2 pounds (900 g) red potatoes, cooked and cooled

2 cups (225 g) cheddar, shredded, divided

⅔ cup (100 g) red bell pepper, diced

⅔ cup (115 g) black beans, drained

½ cup (50 g) celery, sliced

½ cup (65 g) jicama, sliced

⅓ cup (34 g) green onion, thinly sliced

2 tablespoons (2 g) fresh cilantro, chopped

¾ cup (175 ml) ranch dressing

½ cup (130 g) salsa

In large bowl, combine potatoes, 1½ cups (170 g) cheese, red bell pepper, beans, celery, jicama, green onions, cilantro, and salt. In small bowl, combine dressing and salsa; pour over potato mixture. Toss gently to coat. Chill at least 1 hour before serving. Top with the remaining ½ cup (55 g) cheese; garnish with cilantro sprigs, if desired.

Yield: 12 servings

Each with: 85 g water; 317 calories (35% from fat, 12% from protein, 53% from carb); 10 g Protein; 12 g total fat; 5 g saturated fat; 3 g monounsaturated fat; 3 g polyunsaturated fat; 43 g carb; 8 g fiber; 3 g sugar; 215 mg phosphorous; 197 mg calcium; 6 mg iron; 287 mg sodium; 568 mg potassium; 629 IU vitamin A; 59 mg ATE vitamin E; 23 mg vitamin C; 27 mg cholesterol

Glycemic Index: Low

Beet and Potato Salad

This was an experiment that turned out well. Our garden produced lots of beets this year, and I was looking for a new way to use them. Since we like them with mayonnaise, I thought of this nontraditional salad.

4 medium beets

2 large red potatoes

2 tablespoons (28 g) mayonnaise

1 tablespoon (11 g) prepared yellow mustard

Fill a large pot with water and add beets. Bring to a boil over medium-high heat and cook for about 30 minutes. Add potatoes to the water, and continue to cook until both beets and potatoes are soft, about 30 minutes more. Drain and let the vegetables cool until cool enough to handle. Cut into cubes and place them in a bowl. Stir in mayonnaise and mustard until well coated. Serve either warm or cold.

Yield: 6 servings

Each with: 58 g water; 103 calories (36% from fat, 8% from protein, 56% from carb); 2 g protein; 4 g total fat; 1 g saturated fat; 1 g monounsaturated fat; 2 g polyunsaturated fat; 15 g carb; 3 g fiber; 4 g sugar; 26 mg calcium; 2 mg iron; 48 mg sodium; 303 mg potassium; 34 IU vitamin A; 5 mg vitamin C; 3 mg cholesterol

Glycemic Index: Low

Mexican Deviled Eggs

This is a different kind of deviled egg, and one that is sure to please.

6 hard-boiled eggs

⅓ cup (87 g) salsa

2 slices bacon, cooked and crumbled

1 tablespoon (14 g) mayonnaise

Sliced black olives for garnish (optional)

Fresh parsley or cilantro for garnish (optional)

Peel and cut eggs in half lengthwise. Mash the yolks and mix with salsa, bacon, and mayonnaise. Fill the egg whites with the yolk mixture and chill. Garnish with olive slices or small sprigs of parsley or cilantro and serve on a lettuce-lined tray.

Yield: 6 servings

Each with: 56 g water; 115 calories (67% from fat, 29% from protein, 4% from carb); 8 g protein; 9 g total fat; 2 g saturated fat; 3 g monounsaturated fat; 2 g polyunsaturated fat; 1 g carb; 0 g fiber; 1 g sugar; 122 mg phosphorus; 32 mg calcium; 1 mg iron; 234 mg sodium; 91 mg potassium; 336 IU vitamin A; 1 mg vitamin C; 241 mg cholesterol

Glycemic Index: Low

Citrus Salad

This is a refreshing salad to serve with chicken or fish.

12 ounces (340 g) mandarin orange, drained

6 cups (330 g) Bibb lettuce, torn into small pieces

3 pink grapefruits peeled, seeded, and coarsely chopped

Combine mandarin oranges, grapefruit sections, and lettuce in a large salad bowl; toss lightly.

Yield: 6 servings

Each with: 254 g water; 81 calories (3% from fat, 9% from protein, 88% from carb); 2 g Protein; 0 g total fat; 0 g saturated fat; 0 g monounsaturated fat; 0 g polyunsaturated fat; 20 g carb; 3 g fiber; 17 g sugar; 37 mg phosphorous; 45 mg calcium; 1 mg iron; 6 mg sodium; 437 mg potassium; 3844 IU vitamin A; 0 mg ATE vitamin E; 79 mg vitamin C; 0 mg cholesterol

Glycemic Index: Low

Double Apple Salad

This salad has crispy apples and lots of other good things. It's hard to believe that it's actually good for you.

1 large Golden Delicious apple, diced

1 large Red Delicious apple, diced

1 teaspoon lemon juice

1 can pineapple (21 ounces or 588 g) tidbits, drained

1 cup (50 g) miniature marshmallows

2/3 cup (60 g) flaked coconut

½ cup (60 g) chopped walnuts

¼ cup (110 g) raisins

¼ cup (60 g) mayonnaise

2 tablespoons (15 g) thinly sliced celery

In a bowl, toss apples with lemon juice. Add remaining ingredients and mix well. Cover and chill for at least 1 hour.

Yield: 10 servings

Each with: 56 g water; 160 calories (52% from fat, 5% from protein, 43% from carb); 2 g protein; 10 g total fat; 2 g saturated fat; 2 g monounsaturated fat; 5 g polyunsaturated fat; 18 g carb; 1 g fiber; 13 g sugar; 48 mg phosphorus; 17 mg calcium; 1 mg iron; 39 mg sodium; 149 mg potassium; 46 IU vitamin A; 5 mg vitamin C; 2 mg cholesterol

Glycemic Index: Low

12

Side Dishes

S ide dishes can be either good news or bad news from a GI standpoint. You'll want to limit the number of high-GI items like potatoes that you eat. But lots of great low-GI choices can be made. Having two vegetable dishes rather than a veggie and a starch will lower the total GI count of a meal significantly. Make that second dish a nice creamy casserole and you won't even miss the potatoes. But you don't need to give up starches completely. There also are some rice and grain dishes here that can fit into your low-GI diet, as long as you are careful with quantities.

Quick Summer Squash

When you're looking for ways to use the zucchini and yellow squash that the garden has started producing, this recipe is quick to fix and tastes great.

1 pound (455 g) shredded yellow squash

1 tablespoon (14 g) unsalted butter

1 teaspoon low-sodium chicken bouillon

½ teaspoon garlic powder

½ teaspoon onion powder

1 teaspoon parsley

½ teaspoon oregano

Yield: 6 servings

Place squash in a 1-quart (1L) casserole. Melt butter, stir in remaining ingredients. Stir to mix. Cover and microwave on high until crisp-tender, about 3 to 4 minutes, stirring once in the middle of the cooking time.

Each with: 29 calories (59% from fat, 10% from protein, 31% from carb); 1 g protein; 2 g total fat; 1 g saturated fat; 1 g monounsaturated fat; 0 g polyunsaturated fat; 2 g carb; 1 g fiber; 1 g sugar; 12 mg calcium; 0 mg iron; 6 mg sodium; 150 mg potassium; 10 mg vitamin C; 5 mg cholesterol

Glycemic Index: Low

Scalloped Zucchini

Here's another of those old-time sorts of recipes. We sometimes make a meal of this by adding a pound of browned ground turkey to the mixture.

4 cups (496 g) chopped zucchini

½ cup (80 g) chopped onion

2 tablespoons (30 ml) olive oil

(continued on page 318)

½ cup (50 g) grated Parmesan cheese

½ cup (36 g) cracker crumbs

2 eggs

Cook zucchini until nearly done. Drain, reserving ½ cup (120 ml) of liquid, and chop coarsely. Cook onion in oil until soft. Stir all ingredients together and turn into a 1½-quart (1½ L) baking dish coated with nonstick vegetable oil spray. Bake at 350°F (180°C, gas mark 4) until set, about 40 minutes.

Yield: 8 servings

Each with: 82 g water; 111 calories (49% from fat, 21% from protein, 29% from carb); 6 g protein; 6 g total fat; 2 g saturated fat; 3 g monounsaturated fat; 1 g polyunsaturated fat; 8 g carb; 1 g fiber; 2 g sugar; 102 mg phosphorus; 102 mg calcium; 1 mg iron; 179 mg sodium; 250 mg potassium; 208 IU vitamin A; 11 mg vitamin C; 6 mg cholesterol

Glycemic Index: Low

Mexican Zucchini Oven Fries

These make a great alternative to french fries with a burger or other grilled meat.

2 cups (226 g) zucchini

1 tablespoon (4 g) oregano

1 tablespoon (7 g) cumin

Cut zucchini into ¼ inch by 3 inch (½ cm by 7½ cm) sticks, like French fries. Preheat oven to 500°F (250°C, gas mark 10). Arrange zucchini on nonstick baking sheet. Coat zucchini with nonstick vegetable oil spray. Combine spices and sprinkle over the zucchini fries. Place in very hot oven and cook 15 to 18 minutes. Serve hot with low-sodium taco sauce or salsa for dipping.

Yield: 4 servings

Each with: 59 g water; 18 calories (21% from fat, 20% from protein, 59% from carb); 1 g protein; 1 g total fat; 0 g saturated fat; 0 g monounsaturated fat; 0 g polyunsaturated fat; 3 g carb; 1 g fiber; 1 g sugar; 33 mg phosphorus; 35 mg calcium; 2 mg iron; 9 mg sodium; 202 mg potassium; 195 IU vitamin A; 11 mg vitamin C; 0 mg cholesterol

Glycemic Index: Low

Zucchini Pancakes

These make a great side dish with almost any kind of meat, but I have to admit to having them for breakfast a time or two also. Maybe that's just because I get desperate when the garden is really producing zucchini.

4 cups (452 g) shredded zucchini

4 eggs

½ cup (64 g) flour

⅛ teaspoon pepper

¼ teaspoon garlic powder

¼ cup (15 g) chopped fresh parsley

3 tablespoons (45 ml) canola oil

Wash zucchini and trim the ends. Grate or grind into a bowl. Squeeze dry. In a bowl, combine the zucchini and all the other ingredients except the oil. Heat the oil in a heavy skillet over medium heat. Drop zucchini mixture by heaping tablespoons into hot oil. Flatten them a little, and fry until golden brown on bottom. Turn and brown second side. Drain on paper towels. (If mixture is thin, add more flour.)

Yield: 6 servings

Each with: 110 g water; 168 calories (58% from fat, 16% from protein, 26% from carb); 7 g protein; 11 g total fat; 2 g saturated fat; 6 g monounsaturated fat; 3 g polyunsaturated fat; 11 g carb; 1 g fiber; 2 g sugar; 116 mg phosphorus; 37 mg calcium; 2 mg iron; 62 mg sodium; 293 mg potassium; 560 IU vitamin A; 17 mg vitamin C; 158 mg cholesterol

Glycemic Index: Low

Broccoli with Lemon Sauce

I always drizzled just a little lemon juice over broccoli before steaming it, but this slightly sweet sauce is so much better.

4 cups (284 g) broccoli florets

1 tablespoon (15 ml) lemon juice

1 teaspoon sugar substitute, such as Splenda

1 tablespoon (15 ml) water

Clean and trim broccoli. Cut stalks and florets into about 3-inch (7½ cm) pieces. Steam until crisp tender. Drain. Mix lemon juice, water, and sweetener. Drizzle over broccoli.

Yield: 4 servings

Each with: 88 g water; 33 calories (8% from fat, 26% from protein, 66% from carb); 3 g Protein; 0 g total fat; 0 g saturated fat; 0 g monounsaturated fat; 0 g polyunsaturated fat; 7 g carb; 2 g fiber; 2 g sugar; 60 mg phosphorous; 43 mg calcium; 1 mg iron; 30 mg sodium; 292 mg potassium; 567 IU vitamin A; 0 mg ATE vitamin E; 83 mg vitamin C; 0 mg cholesterol

Glycemic Index: Low

Asian Three Bean Salad

The ingredients aren't typically Asian, but the flavor certainly is. This makes a good lunch or light dinner with some added leftover chicken.

⅔ cup (114 g) pinto beans, cooked drained

⅔ cup (109 g) chick peas, cooked, drained

1½ cups (150 g) green beans, sliced, steamed

½ cup (50 g) celery, diced

¼ cup (40 g) red onion, diced

¼ cup (48 g) pimentos, diced

¼ cup (15 g) fresh parsley, chopped

2 tablespoons (30 ml) rice vinegar

1 tablespoon (15 ml) Dick's Reduced Sodium Soy Sauce (see recipe in chapter 2)

4 teaspoons (20 ml) olive oil

¼ teaspoon ginger

¼ teaspoon freshly ground pepper

In salad bowl, combine all ingredients. Chill. Serve on lettuce leaves.

Yield: 4 servings

Each with: 103 g water; 224 calories (23% from fat, 19% from protein, 58% from carb); 11 g Protein; 6 g total fat; 1 g saturated fat; 4 g monounsaturated fat; 1 g polyunsaturated fat; 33 g carb; 9 g fiber; 4 g sugar; 209 mg phosphorous; 80 mg calcium; 4 mg iron; 25 mg sodium; 717 mg potassium; 984 IU vitamin A; 0 mg ATE vitamin E; 25 mg vitamin C; 0 mg cholesterol

Glycemic Index: Low

Green Beans with Cashews

Cashews are one of my favorite nuts. Here they add flavor and texture to fresh green beans.

1 pound (455 g) fresh green beans

3 tablespoons (45 ml) olive oil

3 ounces (85 g) cashews

1 clove garlic, chopped

1 tablespoon (4.3 g) thyme

Slice beans. Boil them until just tender. Drain. Heat oil in a skillet over medium heat. Put in the cashew nuts and stir until they are golden brown. Remove from the skillet. Increase the heat. Put in the beans and garlic. Stir until the garlic begins to brown. Mix in the nuts and thyme and remove from the heat.

Yield: 4 servings

(continued on page 322)

Each with: 103 g water; 249 calories (68% from fat, 8% from protein, 23% from carb); 5 g Protein; 20 g total fat; 3 g saturated fat; 13 g monounsaturated fat; 3 g polyunsaturated fat; 16 g carb; 5 g fiber; 3 g sugar; 149 mg phosphorous; 66 mg calcium; 3 mg iron; 11 mg sodium; 363 mg potassium; 811 IU vitamin A; 0 mg ATE vitamin E; 19 mg vitamin C; 0 mg cholesterol

Glycemic Index: Low

Italian Green Beans

This has got to be the easiest recipe ever for spicing up the flavor of green beans and lifting them out of the ordinary, bland vegetable category.

2 cups (200 g) fresh green beans

1 tablespoon (15 ml) lemon juice

¼ teaspoon oregano

1 teaspoon pimento, chopped

Dash garlic powder

Cook green beans in boiling water until just tender; drain. Combine lemon juice, oregano, pimento, and garlic powder. Pour over beans.

Yield: 5 servings

Each with: 42 g water; 15 calories (3% from fat, 19% from protein, 78% from carb); 1 g Protein; 0 g total fat; 0 g saturated fat; 0 g monounsaturated fat; 0 g polyunsaturated fat; 3 g carb; 2 g fiber; 1 g sugar; 17 mg phosphorous; 17 mg calcium; 0 mg iron; 3 mg sodium; 97 mg potassium; 308 IU vitamin A; 0 mg ATE vitamin E; 9 mg vitamin C; 0 mg cholesterol

Glycemic Index: Low

Caraway Carrots

Here's another unusual flavor combination that works very well. Serve this as a side with pork.

1 pound (445 g) carrots

1 tablespoon (14 g) unsalted butter, melted

1 tablespoon (8 g) flour

1 tablespoon (6.7 g) caraway seeds

Peel carrots and slice into rounds or sticks. Cook, covered, in 1 cup of water about 10 minutes or until just tender; drain and reserve juice. Melt butter and add flour. Gradually add carrot water. Add caraway. Cook until slightly thickened. Add carrots back into pan and serve.

Yield: 6 servings

Each with: 67 g water; 56 calories (34% from fat, 7% from protein, 59% from carb); 1 g Protein; 2 g total fat; 1 g saturated fat; 1 g monounsaturated fat; 0 g polyunsaturated fat; 9 g carb; 3 g fiber; 4 g sugar; 35 mg phosphorous; 33 mg calcium; 0 mg iron; 53 mg sodium; 259 mg potassium; 12772 IU vitamin A; 16 mg ATE vitamin E; 5 mg vitamin C; 5 mg cholesterol

Glycemic Index: Low

Broiled Tomatoes

Broiled tomatoes with just a little cheese and fresh parsley make a great side dish for almost any meal. I could eat these at least 4 days a week (and sometimes do when the garden is producing).

3 medium tomatoes, halved

2 tablespoons (8 g) parsley, fresh, chopped

¼ teaspoon black pepper

2 tablespoons (10 g) Romano cheese, grated

2 tablespoons (28 g) unsalted butter

Sprinkle cut side of tomato halves with pepper. Broil 5 minutes, about 4 inches (10 cm) from heat. Place 1 teaspoon (5 g) butter, 1 teaspoon (1.3g) parsley, and 1 teaspoon (1.7g) cheese on each; broil until cheese melts.

Yield: 6 servings

(continued on page 324)

Each with: 73 g water; 46 calories (51% from fat, 18% from protein, 31% from carb); 2 g Protein; 3 g total fat; 2 g saturated fat; 1 g monounsaturated fat; 0 g polyunsaturated fat; 4 g carb; 1 g fiber; 0 g sugar; 55 mg phosphorous; 56 mg calcium; 0 mg iron; 64 mg sodium; 178 mg potassium; 629 IU vitamin A; 15 mg ATE vitamin E; 21 mg vitamin C; 8 mg cholesterol

Glycemic Index: Low

Roasted Cherry Tomatoes

Have you got more cherry or grape tomatoes than you can use up in salads? They can also be cooked and make a great summer side dish with a simple piece of grilled meat.

30 cherry tomatoes

¼ teaspoon garlic powder

1 teaspoon fresh basil

Coat a baking sheet or roasting pan with nonstick vegetable oil spray. Place tomatoes in a resealable plastic bag and coat with a little more spray. Add garlic powder and basil. Shake to cover tomatoes. Place on prepared pan and roast at 400°F (200°C, gas mark 6) until skins begin to pop, about 5 to 10 minutes.

Yield: 2 servings

Each with: 0 g water; 56 calories (11% from fat, 14% from protein, 76% from carb); 2 g protein; 1 g total fat; 0 g saturated fat; 0 g monounsaturated fat; 0 g polyunsaturated fat; 12 g carb; 3 g fiber; 0 g sugar; 3 mg phosphorus; 20 mg calcium; 1 mg iron; 0 mg sodium; 582 mg potassium; 1,621 IU vitamin A; 49 mg vitamin C; 0 mg cholesterol

Glycemic Index: Low

Fried Tomatoes

Fried tomatoes are a southern classic. This is just one variation. Green tomatoes are traditional, but I prefer ones that are firm and underripe but not completely green.

¼ teaspoon black pepper

2 tomatoes, sliced ¼-inch (½ cm) thick

2 tablespoons (16 g) flour

1 egg

¼ cup (35 g) cornmeal

¼ cup (60 ml) olive oil

Sprinkle pepper over the tomato slices; dust lightly with flour. Dip slices in beaten egg, letting excess drip off, and then coat well with cornmeal. Fry in hot oil until browned, turning gently (about 3 minutes each side).

Yield: 4 servings

Each with: 84 g water; 200 calories (64% from fat, 7% from protein, 28% from carb); 4 g protein; 15 g total fat; 2 g saturated fat; 4 g monounsaturated fat; 8 g polyunsaturated fat; 14 g carb; 1 g fiber; 0 g sugar; 52 mg phosphorus; 14 mg calcium; 1 mg iron; 35 mg sodium; 238 mg potassium; 542 IU vitamin A; 19 mg vitamin C; 0 mg cholesterol

Glycemic Index: Low

Deviled Tomatoes

This recipe is a little livelier version of broiled tomatoes than the other one in this chapter. Two kinds of mustard and a generous helping of garlic give these a bit of a kick.

4 cloves garlic, mashed

½ teaspoon dry mustard

2 tablespoons (30 ml) olive oil

1 tablespoon (11 g) Dijon mustard

Black pepper, to taste

2 medium tomatoes, halved

(continued on page 326)

In bowl, combine garlic, Dijon mustard, and pepper to taste. Add oil, slowly whisking till smooth. Place tomatoes in buttered baking dish and spread with mustard mixture. Broil tomatoes 3 inches (7½ cm) from heat for 1 minute or until tops are bubbly and golden.

Yield: 4 servings

Each with: 73 g water; 78 calories (78% from fat, 4% from protein, 18% from carb); 1 g Protein; 7 g total fat; 1 g saturated fat; 5 g monounsaturated fat; 1 g polyunsaturated fat; 4 g carb; 1 g fiber; 0 g sugar; 22 mg phosphorous; 6 mg calcium; 0 mg iron; 49 mg sodium; 172 mg potassium; 467 IU vitamin A; 0 mg ATE vitamin E; 19 mg vitamin C; 0 mg cholesterol

Glycemic Index: Low

Christmas Cauliflower

This dish is full of festive veggies for your holiday meal.

1 cauliflower, broken into florets

¼ cup (38 g) chopped green bell pepper

¼ cup (38 g) chopped red bell pepper

4 ounces (115 g) sliced mushrooms

¼ cup (56 g) unsalted butter

⅓ cup (42 g) flour

2 cups (475 ml) skim milk

½ teaspoon paprika

In a large saucepan, cook cauliflower until crisp-tender. Drain. In a medium saucepan, sauté peppers and mushrooms in butter for 2 minutes. Add flour; gradually stir in milk. Cook until thickened and bubbly. Place cauliflower in a greased 2-quart (2 L) baking dish. Pour sauce over. Bake uncovered at 325°F (170°C, gas mark 3) for 20 minutes. Sprinkle with paprika.

Yield: 10 servings

Each with: 109 g water; 92 calories (47% from fat, 16% from protein, 37% from carb); 4 g protein; 5 g total fat; 1 g saturated fat; 2 g monounsaturated fat; 2 g polyunsaturated fat; 9 g carb; 2 g fiber; 1 g sugar; 88 mg phosphorus; 81 mg calcium; 0 mg iron; 38 mg sodium; 219 mg potassium; 499 IU vitamin A; 31 mg vitamin C; 1 mg cholesterol

Glycemic Index: Low

Cauliflower Au Gratin

This cheesy cauliflower dish is great with just about any meat. Baking allows the cheese flavor to soak even more deeply into the cauliflower.

2 cups (200 g) cauliflower, cut into pieces

1 teaspoon unsalted butter

1 teaspoon flour

1 cup (235 g) milk, cold

¼ cup (30 g) cheddar cheese, diced

½ teaspoon fresh ground pepper

Steam cauliflower until tender. Rinse with cold water. Melt butter in saucepan. Add remaining ingredients. Cook over low heat, stirring constantly, until slightly thickened. Place cauliflower in baking dish coated with vegetable cooking spray. Cover with cheese topping. Bake at 350°F (180°C, gas mark 4) for 20 minutes.

Yield: 4 Servings

Each with: 117 g water; 80 calories (44% from fat, 26% from protein, 31% from carb); 5 g Protein; 4 g total fat; 2 g saturated fat; 1 g monounsaturated fat; 0 g polyunsaturated fat; 6 g carb; 2 g fiber; 4 g sugar; 125 mg phosphorous; 148 mg calcium; 0 mg iron; 87 mg sodium; 196 mg potassium; 245 IU vitamin A; 67 mg ATE vitamin E; 28 mg vitamin C; 12 mg cholesterol

Glycemic Index: Low

Creamed Cabbage

If you find yourself with a little extra cabbage left over from a head or a couple of heads from the garden that need to be used, add a little flavor to them with a cream sauce.

3 cups (210 g) coarsely chopped cabbage

2 tablespoons (28 g) unsalted butter

2 tablespoons (16 g) flour

1 cup (235 ml) skim milk

½ teaspoon white pepper

Place the cabbage in a saucepan, cover with water, and cook until tender, about 15 minutes. Drain and set aside. Melt the butter in the same pan. Stir in flour and heat, stirring constantly, until well mixed. Add milk slowly and cook and stir until thickened. Stir in cabbage and pepper.

Yield: 4 servings

Each with: 105 g water; 104 calories (51% from fat, 13% from protein, 35% from carb); 4 g protein; 6 g total fat; 4 g saturated fat; 2 g monounsaturated fat; 0 g polyunsaturated fat; 9 g carb; 1 g fiber; 0 g sugar; 87 mg phosphorus; 116 mg calcium; 1 mg iron; 47 mg sodium; 247 mg potassium; 368 IU vitamin A; 28 mg vitamin C; 16 mg cholesterol

Glycemic Index: Low

Stir-Fried Cabbage

The toasted seeds in this will remind you of Indian flavors, but this dish goes with just about any kind of meal. Its great flavor will even win over people who don't think they like cabbage.

1 small cabbage

2 small onions

3 tablespoons (45 ml) olive oil

½ teaspoon cumin seeds, whole

½ teaspoon fennel seeds, whole

4 teaspoons (10.8 g) sesame seeds

Remove coarse outer leaves from cabbage; quarter and core. Cut into fine shred, either by hand or with food processor. Set aside. Peel onions; cut in half lengthwise. Cut crosswise into thin half rings; set aside. In large wok or large wide pot over medium heat, heat oil. When very hot, add the cumin and the fennel seeds. As soon as the seeds turn a shade darker (just a few minutes), add the sesame seeds. Stir for a few seconds before adding onions. Stir-fry 2 or 3 minutes or until browned on the edges. Add cabbage, cover, and turn heat to low. Cook 2–3 minutes or until cabbage wilts. Uncover and cook over high heat; stir-fry 5 minutes or until vegetables are very tender.

Yield: 6 servings

Each with: 102 g water; 108 calories (62% from fat, 6% from protein, 32% from carb); 2 g Protein; 8 g total fat; 1 g saturated fat; 5 g monounsaturated fat; 1 g polyunsaturated fat; 9 g carb; 3 g fiber; 4 g sugar; 45 mg phosphorous; 59 mg calcium; 1 mg iron; 14 mg sodium; 194 mg potassium; 62 IU vitamin A; 0 mg ATE vitamin E; 26 mg vitamin C; 0 mg cholesterol

Glycemic Index: Low

Grilled Eggplant

Eggplant can become a high calorie vegetable if fried because it can soak up a lot of fat. Here we hold down the fat content by grilling it and only using just enough butter to ensure that it grills properly.

1 eggplant

⅓ cup (75 g) unsalted butter, melted

½ teaspoon garlic powder

½ teaspoon Italian seasoning

⅛ teaspoon black pepper

Peel the eggplant and then cut into ¾-inch (2 cm) slices. Combine butter, garlic powder, and Italian seasoning; stir well. Brush eggplant slices with butter mixture and sprinkle with pepper. Place eggplant about 3 to 4 inches (7½ to 10 cm) from coals. Grill over medium coals 10 minutes or until tender, turning and basting occasionally.

(continued on page 330)

Yield: 6 servings

Each with: 73 g water; 110 calories (81% from fat, 3% from protein, 16% from carb); 1 g Protein; 10 g total fat; 7 g saturated fat; 3 g monounsaturated fat; 0 g polyunsaturated fat; 5 g carb; 3 g fiber; 2 g sugar; 23 mg phosphorous; 12 mg calcium; 0 mg iron; 3 mg sodium; 183 mg potassium; 342 IU vitamin A; 85 mg ATE vitamin E; 2 mg vitamin C; 27 mg cholesterol

Glycemic Index: Low

Baked Eggplant

This is kind of an Americanized version of typical Italian baked eggplant using tomato soup and cheddar cheese.

1 medium eggplant

1 cups onion

2 ounces (57 g) cheddar cheese, shredded

1 can (10¾ ounces or 305 g) reduced-sodium condensed tomato soup

4 teaspoons (9.3 g) dry bread crumbs

1 teaspoon thyme

½ teaspoon black pepper

Cook eggplant and onion in small amount of water until tender. Drain; reserve liquid. Place eggplant and onion in small baking dish. Top with cheese. Blend condensed soup, ½ cup (120 ml) of eggplant liquid, bread crumbs, thyme, and pepper. Pour over eggplant; cover. Bake at 350°F (180°C, gas mark 4) for 30 minutes.

Yield: 4 servings

Each with: 198 g water; 131 calories (36% from fat, 17% from protein, 47% from carb); 6 g Protein; 6 g total fat; 3 g saturated fat; 1 g monounsaturated fat; 1 g polyunsaturated fat; 16 g carb; 5 g fiber; 6 g sugar; 125 mg phosphorous; 135 mg calcium; 1 mg iron; 104 mg sodium; 407 mg potassium; 333 IU vitamin A; 40 mg ATE vitamin E; 21 mg vitamin C; 15 mg cholesterol

Glycemic Index: Low

Curried Eggplant

Eggplant is not a vegetable that most people associate with curry. However, this version with Indian spices and tomatoes will change their mind. It will perk up an otherwise boring meal very quickly.

½ pound (225 g) eggplant

2 tablespoons (28 g) unsalted butter

¾ cup (120 g) onion, chopped finely

1 clove garlic, sliced

½ teaspoon turmeric

1 bay leaf

1 cinnamon stick

¼ teaspoon cayenne pepper

1 slice gingerroot

1½ cups (270 g) tomatoes

1 teaspoon garam masala

Wash and slice eggplants. Heat butter and sauté the onion and garlic when hot for 2 to 3 minutes. Add turmeric, bay leaf, and cinnamon stick and sauté another 2 minutes, stirring frequently. Stir in sliced eggplant. Add salt, cayenne, and ginger. Blend together well. Cook for 10 minutes. Add tomatoes, cover pot, and cook for another 10 minutes. Sprinkle with garam masala and serve.

Yield: 2 servings

Each with: 266 g water; 179 calories (57% from fat, 6% from protein, 37% from carb); 3 g Protein; 12 g total fat; 7 g saturated fat; 3 g monounsaturated fat; 1 g polyunsaturated fat; 18 g carb; 6 g fiber; 5 g sugar; 78 mg phosphorous; 34 mg calcium; 1 mg iron; 17 mg sodium; 619 mg potassium; 1174 IU vitamin A; 95 mg ATE vitamin E; 36 mg vitamin C; 31 mg cholesterol

Glycemic Index: Low

Corn and Zucchini Bake

Here's something a little different in a vegetable side dish, with corn and zucchini contributing to a cheese-flavored custard.

3 cups (339 g) sliced zucchini

¼ cup (40 g) chopped onion

1 tablespoon (15 ml) olive oil

10 ounces (280 g) frozen corn, cooked

1 cup (115 g) shredded low-fat Swiss cheese

2 eggs

¼ cup (30 g) bread crumbs

2 tablespoons (10 g) grated Parmesan cheese

Cook zucchini in boiling water until soft. Drain and mash with fork. Sauté onion in oil until soft. Combine zucchini, onion, corn, cheese, and eggs. Turn into a 1-quart (1 L) casserole coated with nonstick vegetable oil spray. Combine bread crumbs and Parmesan; sprinkle over top. Place on a baking sheet and bake uncovered at 350°F (180°C, gas mark 4) until a knife inserted near the center comes out clean, about 40 minutes.

Yield: 6 servings

Each with: 132 g water; 154 calories (29% from fat, 31% from protein, 40% from carb); 12 g protein; 5 g total fat; 2 g saturated fat; 2 g monounsaturated fat; 1 g polyunsaturated fat; 16 g carb; 2 g fiber; 4 g sugar; 233 mg phosphorus; 267 mg calcium; 1 mg iron; 168 mg sodium; 347 mg potassium; 243 IU vitamin A; 12 mg vitamin C; 10 mg cholesterol

Glycemic Index: Low

Corn and Spinach Casserole

This unusual combination is excellent served with roast pork or chicken.

¼ cup (40 g) chopped onion

1 tablespoon (14 g) unsalted butter

3 cups (492 g) frozen corn

2 eggs, beaten

½ cup (120 ml) milk

¼ teaspoon black pepper, freshly ground

1 tablespoon white wine vinegar

½ pound (225 g) spinach, coarsely chopped

2 tablespoons (10 g) Parmesan cheese, grated

4 slices low-sodium bacon

¼ cup (30 g) bread crumbs

Spray an 8 x 8-inch (20 x 20 cm) pan or 1½ quart (1.5 L) casserole with nonstick vegetable oil spray. Sprinkle chopped onion in the pan. Add corn kernels. Mix eggs with milk and pour over the corn. In a bowl, add vinegar and pepper to chopped spinach and toss until well seasoned. Place spinach mixture on top of corn. Sprinkle with cheese. Cover with bacon slices. Top with bread crumbs and bake in a preheated oven at 375°F (190°C, gas mark 5) for 45 minutes.

Yield: 6 servings

Each with: 139 g water; 187 calories (33% from fat, 20% from protein, 46% from carb); 10 g Protein; 7 g total fat; 3 g saturated fat; 3 g monounsaturated fat; 1 g polyunsaturated fat; 23 g carb; 4 g fiber; 5 g sugar; 176 mg phosphorous; 131 mg calcium; 2 mg iron; 148 mg sodium; 346 mg potassium; 4765 IU vitamin A; 57 mg ATE vitamin E; 4 mg vitamin C; 92 mg cholesterol

Glycemic Index: Low

Okra with Tomatoes

This is a quick and simple side dish that goes well with almost anything.

1 pound (455 g) okra, trimmed and sliced

1 pound (455 g) tomatoes, peeled, quartered

½ cup (80 g) onion, sliced

2 tablespoons (30 ml) olive oil

2 tablespoons (2 g) fresh cilantro, chopped

(continued on page 334)

Heat oil in a wok. Add the onion. Cook until soft, but do not brown. Add the okra and tomatoes and cook for a few more minutes, stirring frequently. Be careful not to overcook. As soon as the vegetables are cooked, sprinkle with cilantro and serve.

Yield: 4 servings

Each with: 228 g water; 127 calories (47% from fat, 10% from protein, 43% from carb); 3 g Protein; 7 g total fat; 1 g saturated fat; 5 g monounsaturated fat; 1 g polyunsaturated fat; 15 g carb; 5 g fiber; 2 g sugar; 105 mg phosphorous; 103 mg calcium; 2 mg iron; 21 mg sodium; 632 mg potassium; 1220 IU vitamin A; 0 mg ATE vitamin E; 55 mg vitamin C; 0 mg cholesterol

Glycemic Index: Low

Greek Vegetable Casserole

This Mediterranean vegetable casserole is almost a meal in itself. It goes very well with fish or chicken.

1 eggplant

2 pounds (900 g) zucchini

4 medium potatoes

1 green bell pepper

1 red bell pepper

2 small onions

1 cup (235 ml) olive oil

4 medium tomatoes

2 cloves garlic

1 teaspoon sugar

Black pepper, to taste

Prepare the vegetables: Cut the eggplant, zucchini, and potatoes in bite sized chunks (do not peel the zucchini or the eggplant). Remove the stems and seeds from the peppers and slice them into strips. Peel and slice the onions. Dice the tomatoes. Sauté the vegetables except the tomatoes in the olive oil in small batches. Sauté each batch for 2 or 3 minutes and then remove from the pan, trying to drain some of the oil so that enough oil is left for the next batch. Place the sautéed vegetables in a baking dish and toss them briefly. Add the tomatoes into the pan and sauté for a couple of minutes. Crush the garlic and add to the tomatoes. Add the sugar and pepper to taste and simmer for another minute. Pour the tomato sauce on top of the vegetables.

Yield: 6 servings

Per Serving: 589 g water; 582 calories (55% from fat, 6% from protein, 39% from carb); 9 g Protein; 37 g total fat; 5 g saturated fat; 26 g monounsaturated fat; 4 g polyunsaturated fat; 60 g carb; 11 g fiber; 10 g sugar; 273 mg phosphorous; 71 mg calcium; 3 mg iron; 45 mg sodium; 2078 mg potassium; 1917 IU vitamin A; 0 mg ATE vitamin E; 132 mg vitamin C; 0 mg cholesterol

Glycemic Index: Low

Roasted Summer Vegetables

We tend to think of roasting winter vegetable more often than summer ones. Lightly seasoned with herbs, this dish cooks quickly and is excellent either served hot, at room temperature, or cold. It makes a great companion to a grilled steak instead of higher GI items like potatoes.

1 red bell pepper, cored, seeded, and cut into strips

1 yellow bell pepper, cored, seeded, and cut into strips

4 cloves garlic, peeled and thinly sliced

1 tablespoon (15 ml) olive oil

2 cups (320 g) red onion, peeled and cut into wedges

2 small summer squash, ends trimmed and cut into ½-inch (1 cm) thick strips

2 small zucchini, ends trimmed and cut into ½-inch (1 cm) thick strips

1 tablespoon (4 g) oregano, fresh, chopped

½ teaspoon black pepper

1 tablespoon (15 ml) balsamic vinegar

Preheat oven to 425°F (220°C, gas mark 7) . In a large bowl, toss together peppers, onions, squash, garlic, olive oil, oregano, and pepper. Spread the vegetables on a baking sheet or metal

(continued on page 336)

roasting pan and roast for 20 minutes or until tender, stirring several times. Transfer to a serving bowl and cool slightly. Add vinegar and toss until mixed.

Yield: 6 servings

Each with: 157 g water; 68 calories (31% from fat, 10% from protein, 58% from carb); 2 g Protein; 3 g total fat; 0 g saturated fat; 2 g monounsaturated fat; 0 g polyunsaturated fat; 11 g carb; 3 g fiber; 4 g sugar; 53 mg phosphorous; 35 mg calcium; 1 mg iron; 8 mg sodium; 364 mg potassium; 994 IU vitamin A; 0 mg ATE vitamin E; 103 mg vitamin C; 0 mg cholesterol

Glycemic Index: Low

Roasted Vegetables

Here's a simple but tasty way to cook vegetables.

3 potatoes, cubed

1 cup (130 g) carrot, sliced 1 inch (2½ cm) long

½ cup (75 g) green bell pepper, cut in chunks

½ cup (75 g) red bell pepper, cut in chunks

4 ounces (115 g) mushrooms

½ teaspoon onion powder

¼ teaspoon garlic powder

½ teaspoon thyme

Place vegetables in a single layer in a roasting pan. Coat with nonstick olive oil spray. Sprinkle with spices. Roast at 350°F (180°C, gas mark 4) until done, about 30 minutes, turning once.

Yield: 6 servings

Each with: 209 g water ; 149 calories (3% from fat, 12% from protein, 86% from carb); 5 g protein; 0 g total fat; 0 g saturated fat; 0 g monounsaturated fat; 0 g polyunsaturated fat; 34 g carb; 4 g fiber; 4 g sugar; 143 mg phosphorus; 31 mg calcium; 2 mg iron; 28 mg sodium; 1,020 mg potassium; 4,037 IU vitamin A; 43 mg vitamin C; 0 mg cholesterol

Glycemic Index: Low

Indian Carrots and Spinach

Whenever I'm looking for a little different flavor combination for a side dish, I usually start with Indian recipes. Somehow they just seem to think of vegetables differently than we do in the western hemisphere, and I for one am always glad for a new taste.

½ cup (50 g) green onion, sliced

2 cloves garlic, minced

½ teaspoon turmeric

2 tablespoons (30 ml) olive oil

3 cups (330 g) carrot, coarsely grated

¼ cup (25 g) celery, grated

½ cup (120 ml) low-sodium vegetable broth

1 teaspoon gingerroot, grated

½ teaspoon coriander

½ cup (40 g) coconut, grated

1¼ cups (225 g) frozen spinach, thawed and drained

Sauté onions, garlic, and turmeric in oil until onions are soft. Add remaining ingredients, simmer for 10 minutes, and serve.

Yield: 6 servings

Each with: 125 g water; 115 calories (52% from fat, 10% from protein, 39% from carb); 3 g Protein; 7 g total fat; 3 g saturated fat; 3 g monounsaturated fat; 1 g polyunsaturated fat; 12 g carb; 4 g fiber; 4 g sugar; 60 mg phosphorous; 97 mg calcium; 1 mg iron; 101 mg sodium; 405 mg potassium; 15639 IU vitamin A; 0 mg ATE vitamin E; 7 mg vitamin C; 0 mg cholesterol

Glycemic Index: Low

Curried Vegetables

This is another easy vegetable dish that could be served as is for a side dish with something like the Indian chicken.

3 cups (720 g) no-salt-added canned tomatoes

½ cup (80 g) coarsely chopped onion

1 cup (124 g) cubed zucchini

½ cup (75 g) coarsely chopped green bell peppers

¼ teaspoon garlic powder

1 tablespoon (6 g) curry powder

Combine all ingredients in a saucepan. Cook and stir until vegetables are softened.

Yield: 4 servings

Each with: 161 g water; 41 calories (10% from fat, 15% from protein, 75% from carb); 2 g protein; 1 g total fat; 0 g saturated fat; 0 g monounsaturated fat; 0 g polyunsaturated fat; 9 g carb; 3 g fiber; 5 g sugar; 29 mg calcium; 1 mg iron; 10 mg sodium; 417 mg potassium; 1,043 IU vitamin A; 28 mg vitamin C; 0 mg cholesterol

Glycemic Index: Low

Easy Curried Vegetables

Many Indian curry recipes involve frying the spices first to develop a richer flavor. This recipe uses a simpler preparation method but still gives you flavorful vegetables to go with whatever meat you are serving.

2 cups (480 g) no-salt-added canned tomatoes

2 cups (226 g) sliced zucchini

½ cup (80 g) coarsely chopped onion

1 tablespoon (6 g) curry powder

Combine ingredients in a saucepan. Cook over medium heat until onion and zucchini are tender.

Yield: 4 servings

Each with: 190 g water; 43 calories (9% from fat, 16% from protein, 75% from carb); 2 g protein; 1 g total fat; 0 g saturated fat; 0 g monounsaturated fat; 0 g polyunsaturated fat; 10 g carb; 3 g fiber; 5 g sugar; 58 mg phosphorus; 59 mg calcium; 2 mg iron; 23 mg sodium; 442 mg potassium; 280 IU vitamin A; 23 mg vitamin C; 0 mg cholesterol

Glycemic Index: Low

Fruit and Vegetable Curry

Don't worry about the number of ingredients here; most of them are spices. You could substitute a couple of tablespoons of curry powder and save yourself some measuring, but I enjoy seeing what each spice adds.

4 cups (640 g) onion, coarsely chopped

2 tablespoons (30 ml) olive oil

2 cloves garlic, minced

1 teaspoon gingerroot, minced

1½ tablespoons (10.5 g) cumin

1½ tablespoons (9 g) coriander

1½ teaspoons cinnamon

1 teaspoon turmeric

½ teaspoon cayenne

½ teaspoon fennel seeds

¼ teaspoon cardamom

¼ teaspoon ground cloves

3 cups (360 g) zucchini, quartered and sliced

1½ cups (355 ml) water

1 cup (100 g) fresh green beans

(continued on page 340)

2 apples, cored and cubed

½ cup (75 g) red bell pepper, diced

1 cup (130 g) dried apricots, chopped

½ cup (73 g) raisins

2 tablespoons (30 ml) fresh lemon juice

Sauté the onions in the oil for 10 minutes. Stir in the garlic, ginger, and spices and continue to sauté, stirring constantly for 3 minutes. Add the zucchini and water and stir well so that the spices won't stick to the pot. Cover and simmer for 10 minutes. Mix in the green beans, apple, peppers, and dried apricots. Simmer gently, covered for about 30 minutes. Stir occasionally and add a little more water if needed to prevent sticking. When the fruit and vegetables are quite tender, stir in the raisins and the lemon juice.

Yield: 6 servings

Each with: 320 g water; 195 calories (23% from fat, 7% from protein, 71% from carb); 4 g Protein; 5 g total fat; 1 g saturated fat; 4 g monounsaturated fat; 1 g polyunsaturated fat; 38 g carb; 6 g fiber; 23 g sugar; 104 mg phosphorous; 87 mg calcium; 3 mg iron; 21 mg sodium; 665 mg potassium; 1455 IU vitamin A; 0 mg ATE vitamin E; 47 mg vitamin C; 0 mg cholesterol

Glycemic Index: Low

Balsamic Onions

Balsamic vinegar is good on lots of meats and vegetable, providing flavor with less acidity than other vinegars. It's particularly good on onions, helping to mellow their strong flavor.

1 tablespoon (15 ml) olive oil

4 medium onions

¼ cup (60 ml) balsamic vinegar

Preheat oven to 375°F (190°C, gas mark 5). Lightly spray a shallow roasting pan with vegetable oil spray. Wash onions and remove any loose skins. Rub onions with olive oil. Bake until tender, about 45 minutes to 1 hour. Open onions by cutting in half; drizzle with balsamic vinegar. Serve hot.

Each with: 157 g water; 97 calories (32% from fat, 7% from protein, 61% from carb); 2 g Protein; 4 g total fat; 1 g saturated fat; 2 g monounsaturated fat; 0 g polyunsaturated fat; 15 g carb; 3 g fiber; 7 g sugar; 48 mg phosphorous; 38 mg calcium; 0 mg iron; 7 mg sodium; 245 mg potassium; 3 IU vitamin A; 0 mg ATE vitamin E; 12 mg vitamin C; 0 mg cholesterol

Glycemic Index: Low

Mashed Turnips

They probably aren't something you typically think about as a side dish, but mashed turnips make a nice alternative to potatoes, with a significantly lower GI count.

1½ pounds (680 g) small turnips, peeled and quartered

Black pepper, to taste

½ teaspoon garlic, roasted and peeled

1 tablespoon (14 g) unsalted butter

Skim milk (optional)

TIP *You can find jars of roasted garlic in many grocery stores, or use the recipe in chapter 2.*

Steam turnips over boiling water until fork tender, about 15 minutes. Drain turnips and place in a food processor or blender along with garlic and butter. Process until smooth, adding skim milk as needed.

Yield: 8 servings

Each with: 80 g water; 32 calories (40% from fat, 8% from protein, 52% from carb); 1 g Protein; 2 g total fat; 1 g saturated fat; 0 g monounsaturated fat; 0 g polyunsaturated fat; 4 g carb; 2 g fiber; 3 g sugar; 23 mg phosphorous; 29 mg calcium; 0 mg iron; 14 mg sodium; 152 mg potassium; 44 IU vitamin A; 12 mg ATE vitamin E; 10 mg vitamin C; 4 mg cholesterol

Glycemic Index: Low

Sweet Potato Latkes

They aren't exactly the traditional Jewish treat, but they are very tasty and sport a much lower GI index.

2 medium sweet potatoes, finely grated

3 eggs

1 teaspoon granulated sugar

4 tablespoons (24 g) almonds, finely ground

2 tablespoons (18 g) golden raisins

2 tablespoons (22 g) dates, chopped

¼ cup (28 g) pecans, chopped

In large bowl, combine sweet potatoes, eggs, sugar, and enough ground almonds to make thick batter. Mix well. Fold in raisins, dates, and pecans. In large skillet, heat ¼ inch (5 mm) oil to 375°F (190°C). Spoon a heaping tablespoon of potato mixture into oil, flattening with back of wet spoon. Brown on both sides, about 3 minutes per side. Drain on paper towels.

Yield: 6 servings

Each with: 63 g water; 168 calories (47% from fat, 14% from protein, 39% from carb); 6 g Protein; 9 g total fat; 1 g saturated fat; 5 g monounsaturated fat; 2 g polyunsaturated fat; 17 g carb; 3 g fiber; 9 g sugar; 117 mg phosphorous; 48 mg calcium; 1 mg iron; 55 mg sodium; 263 mg potassium; 8062 IU vitamin A; 39 mg ATE vitamin E; 7 mg vitamin C; 118 mg cholesterol

Glycemic Index: Low

Sweet Potato Pudding

The banana and rum extract give these sweet potatoes a slightly Caribbean flavor. They are great with chicken or pork.

2 large sweet potatoes, peeled, cooked, and cut into cubes

1 banana, mashed

3 teaspoons (15 g) brown sugar, firmly packed

2 tablespoons (28 g) unsalted butter

¼ teaspoon ground nutmeg

1 teaspoon rum extract

1 egg white

Preheat oven to 350°F (180°C, gas mark 4). In a large bowl, beat all ingredients except egg white until smooth. Add a small amount of water if necessary to get a smooth consistency. Beat egg white until stiff. Fold gently into sweet potato mixture. Spoon into a casserole that has been sprayed with nonstick vegetable oil spray. Bake, uncovered, 45 to 50 minutes until lightly browned.

Yield: 4 servings

Each with: 108 g water; 171 calories (31% from fat, 6% from protein, 63% from carb); 3 g Protein; 6 g total fat; 4 g saturated fat; 2 g monounsaturated fat; 0 g polyunsaturated fat; 28 g carb; 3 g fiber; 13 g sugar; 41 mg phosphorous; 31 mg calcium; 1 mg iron; 39 mg sodium; 374 mg potassium; 13591 IU vitamin A; 48 mg ATE vitamin E; 15 mg vitamin C; 15 mg cholesterol

Glycemic Index: Low

Squash and Yams in Coconut Milk

Here's another one of those "island" dishes. This sweet combination is a perfect accompaniment to spicy grilled meats like jerk pork.

1 cup (160 g) onion, chopped

2 tablespoons (30 ml) olive oil

1 pound (445 g) acorn squash, pared and cut into 1-inch (2½ cm) pieces

3 cups (330 g) sweet potatoes, peeled and cubed

1 cup (235 ml) coconut milk

½ teaspoon ground cinnamon

¼ teaspoon ground cloves

(continued on page 344)

Cook onion in oil in 10-inch (25 cm) skillet over medium heat until tender. Stir in remaining ingredients. Heat to boiling. Reduce heat. Cover and simmer 10 minutes. Simmer, uncovered, stirring occasionally, until vegetables are tender, about 5 minutes longer.

Yield: 6 servings

Each with: 249 g water; 280 calories (39% from fat, 5% from protein, 55% from carb); 4 g Protein; 13 g total fat; 8 g saturated fat; 4 g monounsaturated fat; 1 g polyunsaturated fat; 41 g carb; 6 g fiber; 11 g sugar; 124 mg phosphorous; 85 mg calcium; 3 mg iron; 53 mg sodium; 762 mg potassium; 26092 IU vitamin A; 0 mg ATE vitamin E; 32 mg vitamin C; 0 mg cholesterol

Glycemic Index: Low

Curried Potatoes

These potatoes are a little bit spicy and a whole lot flavorful. You can vary the cayenne to make them as mild or hot as you like. They're great with grilled chicken rubbed with an Indian spicy mix.

1 pound (455 g) new potatoes, cut in half

1 tablespoon (14 g) unsalted butter

1 clove garlic, minced

1 cup (160 g) onion, chopped

1 teaspoon curry powder

1 tablespoon (4 g) fresh parsley, chopped

1 tablespoon (15 ml) lime juice

¼ teaspoon cayenne

Bring a large saucepan of water to a boil. Add potatoes and cook, covered, 15 to 20 minutes, until tender. Drain in a colander. In a large nonstick skillet, heat butter and sauté garlic and onion until softened. Stir in curry powder. Add parsley, lime juice, and cayenne and mix; add potatoes and toss.

Yield: 4 servings

Each with: 126 g water; 150 calories (18% from fat, 9% from protein, 73% from carb); 3 g Protein; 3 g total fat; 2 g saturated fat; 1 g monounsaturated fat; 0 g polyunsaturated fat; 28 g carb; 3 g fiber; 3 g sugar; 95 mg phosphorous; 32 mg calcium; 2 mg iron; 14 mg sodium; 686 mg potassium; 233 IU vitamin A; 24 mg ATE vitamin E; 16 mg vitamin C; 8 mg cholesterol

Glycemic Index: Low

Rosemary Roasted Potatoes

You want to be careful about potatoes because they have a fairly high GI rating. But these are too good not to have on those special occasions. They seem to go especially well with roast beef.

1½ pounds (680 g) potatoes, peeled and diced into 1-inch (2½ cm) chunks

1 teaspoon paprika

2 teaspoons (1.4 g) rosemary, crushed

1 teaspoon garlic, minced

3 tablespoons (45 ml) olive oil

Toss diced potatoes with olive oil, paprika, garlic, and half the rosemary. Place potatoes on a heavy baking tray, sprinkle with remaining rosemary and ½ teaspoon salt. Roast at 400°F (200°C, gas mark 6) for 1½ hours, turning often.

Yield: 4 servings

Each with: 138 g water; 212 calories (43% from fat, 6% from protein, 51% from carb); 3 g Protein; 10 g total fat; 1 g saturated fat; 7 g monounsaturated fat; 1 g polyunsaturated fat; 28 g carb; 3 g fiber; 2 g sugar; 107 mg phosphorous; 20 mg calcium; 1 mg iron; 11 mg sodium; 792 mg potassium; 323 IU vitamin A; 0 mg ATE vitamin E; 15 mg vitamin C; 0 mg cholesterol

Glycemic Index: Low

Barley Risotto

This may not be exactly like traditional risotto, but it's still a delightful side dish.

½ cup (100 g) pearl barley

1 teaspoon olive oil

3 tablespoons (25 g) minced carrots

3 tablespoons (30 g) minced onions

3 tablespoons (24 g) minced celery

1 teaspoon rosemary

1 bay leaf

½ teaspoon black pepper

1½ cups (355 ml) vegetable broth

Put barley in heavy skillet over low heat and toast. Shake pan frequently. When barley turns light brown and smells nutty, about 15 to 20 minutes, remove from skillet. Heat oil in skillet, add minced vegetables, and sauté for 3 minutes. Add barley and stir to coat grains. Add herbs and broth. Simmer, covered, until barley is tender and liquid is absorbed, about 35 minutes. Remove bay leaf before serving.

Yield: 4 servings

Each with: 108 g water; 138 calories (24% from fat, 11% from protein, 65% from carb); 4 g protein; 4 g total fat; 1 g saturated fat; 2 g monounsaturated fat; 1 g polyunsaturated fat; 23 g carb; 5 g fiber; 1 g sugar; 87 mg phosphorus; 27 mg calcium; 1 mg iron; 450 mg sodium; 187 mg potassium; 1041 IU vitamin A; 3 mg vitamin C; 0 mg cholesterol

Glycemic Index: Low

Bulgur and Vegetables

In this recipe, bulgur cooked with vegetables and just enough herbs to give it a great, rich flavor. It's perfect with any kind of simple meat.

1 cup (70 g) mushrooms, fresh sliced

1 cup (120 g) zucchini, sliced quartered

1 cup (235 ml) low-sodium chicken broth

½ cup (70 g) bulgur

⅓ cup (53 g) onion, chopped

⅓ cup (37 g) carrots, chopped

¼ cup (38 g) green pepper, chopped

1 clove garlic, minced

½ teaspoon basil, dried crushed

¼ teaspoon celery seed

¼ teaspoon thyme

Dash of pepper

½ cup (90 g) tomato, chopped

In a medium saucepan, combine mushrooms, zucchini, broth, bulgur wheat, onion, green pepper, garlic, basil, celery seed, thyme, and pepper. Bring to a boil. Reduce heat and stir in chopped tomato. Let stand 5 minutes or until all the liquid is absorbed. Fluff the bulgur wheat mixture with a fork.

Yield: 4 servings

Each with: 152 g water; 94 calories (7% from fat, 19% from protein, 74% from carb); 5 g Protein; 1 g total fat; 0 g saturated fat; 0 g monounsaturated fat; 0 g polyunsaturated fat; 19 g carb; 5 g fiber; 3 g sugar; 113 mg phosphorous; 29 mg calcium; 1 mg iron; 34 mg sodium; 380 mg potassium; 2057 IU vitamin A; 0 mg ATE vitamin E; 17 mg vitamin C; 0 mg cholesterol

Glycemic Index: Low

Bulgur and Lentil Pilaf

This bulgur and lentil dish makes a great side dish by itself, but it can also be the base for a vegetable-rich sauce, providing a lower GI option to rice or pasta.

1 cup (192 g) lentils

4 cups (945 ml) low-sodium vegetable broth

1 bay leaf

(continued on page 348)

3 tablespoons (42 g) unsalted butter

1 cup (160 g) onion, chopped

¼ teaspoon black pepper

1 cup (140 g) bulgur

Rinse the lentils and put in a pot with enough broth to cover. Add bay leaf, bring to a boil, and keep covered. Turn off heat and let stand for 30 minutes. While the lentils are soaking, melt butter in a heavy pot. Add chopped onion and pepper. Sauté until onions are tender and transparent. When onions are ready, keep heat at medium, stir in bulgur, and continue stirring until all the butter is absorbed. Lower heat to a simmer and add the rest of the broth and lentils in their broth. Bring to a boil, reduce heat again, cover tightly, and simmer until all the liquid has been absorbed. Add more liquid as needed until the bulgur and lentils are cooked. Remove bay leaf and serve.

Yield: 4 servings

Each with: 310 g water; 309 calories (30% from fat, 18% from protein, 52% from carb); 14 g Protein; 11 g total fat; 6 g saturated fat; 3 g monounsaturated fat; 1 g polyunsaturated fat; 41 g carb; 11 g fiber; 3 g sugar; 282 mg phosphorous; 107 mg calcium; 3 mg iron; 150 mg sodium; 598 mg potassium; 284 IU vitamin A; 74 mg ATE vitamin E; 4 mg vitamin C; 23 mg cholesterol

Glycemic Index: Low

Bulgur Wheat with Pecans

This is a simple recipe, but the pecans give an extra flavor boost to the bulgur, which is very plain if cooked by itself.

1 cup (140 g) bulgur, uncooked

½ teaspoon dried basil

⅛ teaspoon pepper

2 cups (475 ml) boiling water

¼ cup (28 g) pecan, chopped

Preheat oven to 350°F (180°C, gas mark 4). Lightly oil a 1-quart (1 L) baking dish or spray with a nonstick cooking spray. Place bulgur, basil, and pepper in prepared baking dish. Add boiling water and mix well. Cover and bake 20 minutes. Fluff with a fork, add pecans, and mix well. Serve hot.

Yield: 6 servings

Each with: 81 g water; 111 calories (27% from fat, 11% from protein, 62% from carb); 3 g Protein; 4 g total fat; 0 g saturated fat; 2 g monounsaturated fat; 1 g polyunsaturated fat; 18 g carb; 5 g fiber; 0 g sugar; 83 mg phosphorous; 15 mg calcium; 1 mg iron; 6 mg sodium; 117 mg potassium; 12 IU vitamin A; 0 mg ATE vitamin E; 0 mg vitamin C; 0 mg cholesterol

Glycemic Index: Low

Brown Rice with Mushrooms

Spice up your brown rice with onion soup and mushrooms without adding carbs. We love this with beef.

1 cup (190 g) brown rice

4 tablespoons (55 g) unsalted butter

1 can (14½ ounces or 410 g) low-sodium beef broth

1 can (10¾ ounces or 305 g) reduced-sodium onion soup

4 ounces (115 g) mushroom

Brown rice in butter. Add soups and mushrooms and bake 350°F (180°C, gas mark 4) until done, about an hour.

Yield: 4 servings

Each with: 344 g water; 207 calories (56% from fat, 12% from protein, 32% from carb); 6 g Protein; 13 g total fat; 8 g saturated fat; 4 g monounsaturated fat; 1 g polyunsaturated fat; 17 g carb; 2 g fiber; 3 g sugar; 95 mg phosphorous; 34 mg calcium; 1 mg iron; 334 mg sodium; 235 mg potassium; 356 IU vitamin A; 95 mg ATE vitamin E; 1 mg vitamin C; 31 mg cholesterol

Glycemic Index: Low

Country Rice

This recipe is very similar to a rice pilaf. I'd caution against adding too many other vegetables and ending up with jambalaya instead of a side dish.

1 cup (235 ml) low-sodium chicken broth

2/3 cup (67 g) chopped green onion

1/4 teaspoon black pepper

2/3 cup (130 g) uncooked rice

Bring the broth to a boil with the green onion and pepper. Add the rice, turn down to a simmer, cover, and cook for 20 minutes.

Yield: 4 servings

Each with: 91 g water; 48 calories (9% from fat, 19% from protein, 72% from carb); 2 g protein; 0 g total fat; 0 g saturated fat; 0 g monounsaturated fat; 0 g polyunsaturated fat; 9 g carb; 1 g fiber; 0 g sugar; 39 mg phosphorus; 20 mg calcium; 1 mg iron; 21 mg sodium; 114 mg potassium; 167 IU vitamin A; 3 mg vitamin C; 0 mg cholesterol

Glycemic Index: Low

Sun-Dried Tomato Rice

I guess I just get bored easily, but I'm always looking for a way to make things a little different. Don't get me wrong—I love plain rice. I could make a meal on a nice bowlful fresh from the steamer with nothing on it at all. But somehow that seems too plain for a meal. So we added a few Italian things to give you a different side dish. I served it with a grilled piece of fish that had been marinated in Italian dressing.

1/4 cup (40 g) chopped onion

1 cup (195 g) uncooked rice

2 tablespoons (30 ml) olive oil

1/4 teaspoon garlic powder

¼ cup (14 g) chopped sun-dried tomatoes

2¼ cups (535 ml) water

Sauté onion and rice in oil about 2 minutes or until rice begins to brown. Add remaining ingredients, cover, reduce heat, and simmer 20 minutes or until rice is tender.

Yield: 6 servings

Each with: 116 g water; 85 calories (55% from fat, 5% from protein, 40% from carb); 1 g protein; 5 g total fat; 1 g saturated fat; 4 g monounsaturated fat; 1 g polyunsaturated fat; 9 g carb; 1 g fiber; 0 g sugar; 23 mg phosphorus; 11 mg calcium; 1 mg iron; 16 mg sodium; 98 mg potassium; 59 IU vitamin A; 5 mg vitamin C; 0 mg cholesterol

Glycemic Index: Low

Spicy Rice

This dish is a family favorite. It's a quick and flavorful use for leftover rice.

1 cup (220 g) cooked brown rice

2 tablespoons (30 ml) olive oil

½ cup (80 g) chopped onion

¼ pound (115 g) shredded Cheddar cheese

1 jalapeño pepper, chopped

Brown rice in oil. Add remaining ingredients. Cover and simmer until heated through and cheese is melted.

Yield: 4 servings

Each with: 67 g water; 237 calories (63% from fat, 14% from protein, 23% from carb); 9 g protein; 17 g total fat; 7 g saturated fat; 8 g monounsaturated fat; 1 g polyunsaturated fat; 14 g carb; 1 g fiber; 1 g sugar; 192 mg phosphorus; 214 mg calcium; 1 mg iron; 179 mg sodium; 86 mg potassium; 312 IU vitamin A; 3 mg vitamin C; 30 mg cholesterol

Glycemic Index: Low

Mushroom Rice

This dish is just like the ones that come in the packaged mixes. It's almost as easy to cook and a lot healthier too.

8 ounces (225 g) mushrooms, sliced

2 tablespoons (28 g) unsalted butter

¼ teaspoon garlic powder

1 tablespoon (10 g) minced onion

1 tablespoon (4 g) parsley

1½ cups (293 g) uncooked rice

2 cups (475 ml) low-sodium chicken broth

1⅓ cups (315 ml) water

¼ cup (16 g) nonfat dry milk powder

In a large skillet, sauté the mushrooms in the butter until brown. Add the spices and rice and continue cooking until rice begins to brown, stirring occasionally. Add the chicken broth and water, cover, and return to boil. Lower heat and simmer until rice is tender and liquid absorbed, about 20 minutes. Stir in the milk powder.

Yield: 6 servings

Each with: 199 g water; 111 calories (33% from fat, 16% from protein, 52% from carb); 4 g protein; 4 g total fat; 2 g saturated fat; 1 g monounsaturated fat; 0 g polyunsaturated fat; 15 g carb; 1 g fiber; 3 g sugar; 56 mg calcium; 1 mg iron; 52 mg sodium; 271 mg potassium; 238 IU vitamin A; 3 mg vitamin C; 11 mg cholesterol

Glycemic Index: Low

13

Italian

Italian meals, with their emphasis on pasta, can be very high in GI. We need to learn to eat more like the Italians themselves do, thinking of the pasta as a side dish that is only a small part of the overall meal rather than the main part. These recipes will help you to do that with their focus on meats and vegetables. Help yourself further by choosing whole wheat pasta over the regular. This not only lowers the GI because it takes longer to digest, it also provides a nice boost in fiber.

Italian Grilled Beef Steak

This is steak with an Italian accent.

½ cup (120 ml) dry red wine

1 tablespoon (2 g) fresh rosemary, chopped *or*

2 teaspoons (2.4 g) dried rosemary

2 tablespoons (30 ml) Dick's Reduced-Sodium Soy Sauce (see recipe in chapter 2)

1 tablespoon (15 ml) Worcestershire sauce

2 garlic cloves, chopped

½ teaspoon garlic salt

1½ pounds (680 g) sirloin steak (1 inch or 2½ cm thick)

Mix all ingredients (except steak) in a glass baking dish. Add steak and turn to coat. Marinate 1 hour at room temperature or refrigerate up to 6 hours, turning occasionally. Prepare the grill or preheat broiler. Drain marinade into a small saucepan and boil for 1 minute and reserve to pass as sauce. Grill or broil steak to desired doneness, about 4 minutes per side for medium-rare. Transfer to platter and thinly slice across the grain. Serve with boiled marinade.

Yield: 4 servings

Each with: 127 g water; 499 calories (59% from fat, 39% from protein, 2% from carb); 46 g protein; 30 g total fat; 12 g saturated fat; 13 g monounsaturated fat; 1 g polyunsaturated fat; 3 g carb; 0 g fiber; 0 g sugar; 355 mg phosphorus; 35 mg calcium; 4 mg iron; 161 mg sodium; 631 mg potassium; 25 IU vitamin A; 7 mg vitamin C; 158 mg cholesterol

Glycemic Index: Low

Italian Cube Steak

In this dish, beef cube steak simmers in a tomato and vegetable sauce, providing a tender, flavorful result. It's good with pasta, but equally good all by itself for a lower GI dinner.

1 pound (455 g) beef cube steaks

2 tablespoons (16 g) flour

1/8 teaspoon pepper

2 tablespoons (30 ml) olive oil

1 cup (235 ml) low-sodium tomato juice

1/4 teaspoon garlic powder

1 teaspoon dried oregano

2 cups (240 g) zucchini, cut into julienne strips

1 cup (70 g) mushroom, sliced

2 tablespoons (10 g) Parmesan cheese, grated

Combine flour, salt, and pepper; dredge steaks in flour mixture and brown in oil in large frying pan to desired doneness. Pour off drippings. Combine tomato juice, garlic powder, and oregano; pour over steaks. Place zucchini and mushrooms over steaks. Cover tightly and cook slowly 20 minutes. Sprinkle with cheese before serving.

Yield: 4 servings

Each with: 200 g water; 338 calories (37% from fat, 53% from protein, 10% from carb); 44 g Protein; 14 g total fat; 3 g saturated fat; 7 g monounsaturated fat; 1 g polyunsaturated fat; 9 g carb; 1 g fiber; 4 g sugar; 334 mg phosphorous; 60 mg calcium; 5 mg iron; 112 mg sodium; 750 mg potassium; 431 IU vitamin A; 4 mg ATE vitamin E; 22 mg vitamin C; 105 mg cholesterol

Glycemic Index: Low

Italian Meatballs

These Italian-flavored meatballs are good over pasta, in a sandwich, or just as appetizers. We usually use a fairly plain marinara sauce, but they would be good in one of the vegetable sauces in this chapter too.

3/4 pound (340 g) lean ground beef

1/4 pound (115 g) ground pork

1 cup (115 g) bread crumbs

1/2 cup (50 g) parmesan cheese, grated

1 tablespoon (1.3 g) parsley flakes

1 clove garlic, minced

(continued on page 356)

½ cup (120 ml) milk

2 eggs, beaten

Pepper, to taste

2 tablespoons (30 ml) olive oil

1½ cups (370 g) low-sodium pasta sauce

Combine meats, crumbs, cheese, parsley, garlic, milk, eggs, and seasonings; mix thoroughly. Form into small balls; brown in oil. Add to sauce and cook over low heat 15 minutes.

Yield: 4 servings

Each with: 195 g water; 647 calories (55% from fat, 22% from protein, 23% from carb); 35 g Protein; 40 g total fat; 13 g saturated fat; 19 g monounsaturated fat; 3 g polyunsaturated fat; 37 g carb; 4 g fiber; 14 g sugar; 425 mg phosphorous; 283 mg calcium; 5 mg iron; 345 mg sodium; 851 mg potassium; 868 IU vitamin A; 73 mg ATE vitamin E; 11 mg vitamin C; 209 mg cholesterol

Glycemic Index: Low

Italian Stuffed Chicken Breast

These chicken rollups have great flavor and are a great start for any Italian meal. To cut the carbs, serve with fresh steamed green beans instead of pasta.

2 tablespoons (14 g) bread crumbs

1 tablespoon (5 g) Parmesan cheese

½ teaspoon dried oregano

8 ounces (225 g) boneless skinless chicken breast

½ cup (55 g) Swiss cheese

1 cup (245 g) no-salt-added tomato sauce

1 tablespoon unsalted butter, melted

Mix crumbs, Parmesan cheese, and oregano. Pound breasts thin. Cover with Swiss cheese. Roll up and brush with butter. Roll in crumb mixture. Bake at 350°F (180°C, gas mark 4) for 30 minutes. Add sauce and bake 10 minutes more.

Yield: 2 servings

Each with: 208 g water; 386 calories (42% from fat, 42% from protein, 16% from carb); 39 g Protein; 18 g total fat; 11 g saturated fat; 5 g monounsaturated fat; 1 g polyunsaturated fat; 15 g carb; 2 g fiber; 6 g sugar; 497 mg phosphorous; 399 mg calcium; 2 mg iron; 140 mg sodium; 801 mg potassium; 925 IU vitamin A; 128 mg ATE vitamin E; 17 mg vitamin C; 114 mg cholesterol

Glycemic Index: Low

Penne with Chicken

Poaching the chicken ahead of time ensures that it will be tender and flavorful. Once that is done, the rest of the preparation goes quickly, with the sauce simmering while the pasta cooks.

¾ pound (340 g) boneless skinless chicken breasts

1½ teaspoons olive oil

½ cup (50 g) green onion, chopped

3 garlic cloves, crushed

28 ounces (800 g) no-salt-added crushed tomatoes, with juice

2 tablespoons (5 g) fresh basil, chopped

½ teaspoon red pepper flakes, crushed

10 ounces (280 g) penne or other tube pasta

3 ounces (85 g) fresh mozzarella, diced

1 tablespoon (4 g) fresh parsley, chopped

½ cup Parmesan cheese, grated

In a large skillet, add enough water to the skinned chicken to cover it. Poach chicken in simmering water uncovered until chicken is no longer pink, about 8 minutes. Allow chicken to cool in poaching liquid. When cool, remove chicken from poaching liquid and chop it into bite-size pieces. Save the poaching liquid to add to the water you're going to cook the pasta in. Sauté the onion and garlic in heated olive oil until softened. Add hot pepper flakes and tomatoes and juice. Cook about 30 minutes over medium heat until sauce thickens. Cook penne in poaching liquid with additional water as needed. Combine chicken with the sauce mixture in serving bowl. Sprinkle with parsley and cheese.

(continued on page 358)

Yield: 4 servings

Each with: 282 g water; 504 calories (19% from fat, 32% from protein, 49% from carb); 42 g Protein; 11 g total fat; 5 g saturated fat; 4 g monounsaturated fat; 1 g polyunsaturated fat; 64 g carb; 3 g fiber; 5 g sugar; 588 mg phosphorous; 437 mg calcium; 6 mg iron; 412 mg sodium; 856 mg potassium; 801 IU vitamin A; 46 mg ATE vitamin E; 24 mg vitamin C; 74 mg cholesterol

Glycemic Index: Low

Chicken Florentine

These chicken breasts, cooked with spinach and then covered with a creamy mushroom sauce, make a great company meal. But the easy preparation and great taste make them the kind of thing you can have regularly just for the family too.

2 boneless skinless chicken breasts

½ cup (80 g) chopped onion

10 ounces (280 g) frozen chopped spinach thawed

2 tablespoons (14 g) Swiss cheese, shredded

½ cup (35 g) fresh mushrooms, sliced

⅛ teaspoon nutmeg

½ cup (120 ml) skim milk

½ cup (120 ml) low-sodium chicken broth

1 tablespoon (14 g) unsalted butter, melted

Flatten chicken to ¼ inch (5 mm). Set aside. Sauté onion in large skillet coated with nonstick vegetable cooking spray. Remove from heat, stir in spinach, cheese, and nutmeg. Divide mixture in half and shape into mounds. Transfer mounds to a 11 x 7-inch (27 x 18 cm) dish coated with cooking spray. Top each portion with a chicken breast half. Bake at 350°F (180°C, or gas mark 4) for 25 minutes or until chicken is done. Place mushrooms in skillet. Stir in milk and remaining ingredients and bring to a boil. Simmer 6 minutes, stirring frequently, until liquid is reduce and thickened. Spoon over chicken.

Yield: 2 servings

Each with: 348 g water; 261 calories (34% from fat, 43% from protein, 24% from carb); 29 g Protein; 10 g total fat; 6 g saturated fat; 3 g monounsaturated fat; 1 g polyunsaturated fat; 16 g carb; 6 g fiber; 3 g sugar; 375 mg phosphorous; 406 mg calcium; 4 mg iron; 242 mg sodium; 898 mg potassium; 17482 IU vitamin A; 107 mg ATE vitamin E; 8 mg vitamin C; 65 mg cholesterol

Glycemic Index: Low

Slow Cooker Italian Chicken Breasts

This made a great-tasting sauce with no extra work. And it's always nice to come home to a meal that's done and has filled the house with such an aroma.

1 cup (160 g) sliced onion

4 boneless chicken breasts

12 ounces (340 g) no-salt-added tomato paste

¼ teaspoon black pepper

½ teaspoon garlic powder

1 teaspoon oregano

1 teaspoon basil

¼ cup (60 ml) dry white wine

¼ cup (60 ml) water

Place onion in bottom of slow cooker. Place chicken on top. Combine remaining ingredients and pour over. Cook on low for 8 to 10 hours.

Yield: 6 servings

Each with: 119 g water; 119 calories (7% from fat, 46% from protein, 47% from carb); 14 g protein; 1 g total fat; 0 g saturated fat; 0 g monounsaturated fat; 0 g polyunsaturated fat; 14 g carb; 3 g fiber; 8 g sugar; 151 mg phosphorus; 39 mg calcium; 2 mg iron; 88 mg sodium; 752 mg potassium; 898 IU vitamin A; 15 mg vitamin C; 27 mg cholesterol

Glycemic Index: Low

Italian Breaded Pork Chops

You can easily vary the flavor of these chops by changing the seasonings. I was looking for a sort of Italian flavor, but you could just as easily make them southern, Mexican, barbecue, or whatever you want.

4 pork loin chops

½ cup (60 g) bread crumbs

1 tablespoon (4 g) parsley

1 tablespoon (4 g) Italian seasoning

1 teaspoon black pepper

1 teaspoon onion powder

Moisten chops with water. Combine bread crumbs and spices in a resealable plastic bag. Add chops and shake until evenly covered. Coat a baking sheet with nonstick vegetable oil spray. Place the chops on the sheet and coat the tops with more of the vegetable oil spray. Bake at 350°F (180°C, gas mark 4) until done, about 20 to 30 minutes depending on thickness of chops.

Yield: 4 servings

Each with: 76 g water; 189 calories (25% from fat, 51% from protein, 24% from carb); 23 g protein; 5 g total fat; 2 g saturated fat; 2 g monounsaturated fat; 1 g polyunsaturated fat; 11 g carb; 1 g fiber; 1 g sugar; 247 mg phosphorus; 55 mg calcium; 2 mg iron; 152 mg sodium; 430 mg potassium; 139 IU vitamin A; 3 mg vitamin C; 64 mg cholesterol

Glycemic Index: Low

Sausage and Eggplant Casserole

This hearty casserole is easy to make and is a nice alternative to pasta when you feel like something Italian. It's great with a little tomato sauce over it.

1 small eggplant

½ pound (225 g) sausage, bulk

1 cup (180 g) onion, chopped

1 egg, well beaten

1 teaspoon (5 g) unsalted butter, melted

¼ cup (30 g) cracker crumbs

Peel eggplant and cut into 1-inch (2.5 cm) cubes; cook in a small amount of boiling water 10 minutes or until tender. Drain. Let cool slightly. Cook sausage and onion until onion is tender and sausage is brown. Combine eggplant, sausage mixture, and egg. Mix well and spoon into a greased 1-quart (1 L) casserole. Combine butter and cracker crumbs; sprinkle over casserole. Bake at 350°F (180°C, or gas mark 4) for 25 minutes.

Yield: 4 servings

Each with: 178 g water; 296 calories (61% from fat, 18% from protein, 21% from carb); 13 g Protein; 21 g total fat; 7 g saturated fat; 9 g monounsaturated fat; 3 g polyunsaturated fat; 16 g carb; 5 g fiber; 5 g sugar; 165 mg phosphorous; 48 mg calcium; 2 mg iron; 501 mg sodium; 487 mg potassium; 145 IU vitamin A; 30 mg ATE vitamin E; 5 mg vitamin C; 99 mg cholesterol

Glycemic Index: Low

Italian Spaghetti Squash

Baking this spaghetti squash with tomato sauce gives the flavors a chance to mix and develop more than just pouring the sauce over. This is one of our favorite vegetarian meals.

2 cups (510 g) spaghetti squash, cooked and drained

8 ounces (225 g) no-salt-added tomato sauce

½ teaspoon dried oregano

⅛ teaspoon garlic powder

4 teaspoons (7 g) Parmesan cheese

Preheat oven to 375°F (190°C, or gas mark 5). Place squash in a casserole that has been sprayed with a nonstick cooking spray. Combine tomato sauce, oregano, and garlic powder and pour evenly over squash. Sprinkle with Parmesan cheese. Bake 20 minutes or until hot and bubbly.

(continued on page 362)

Yield: 4 servings

Each with: 97 g water; 46 calories (19% from fat, 16% from protein, 66% from carb); 2 g Protein; 1 g total fat; 0 g saturated fat; 0 g monounsaturated fat; 0 g polyunsaturated fat; 8 g carb; 1 g fiber; 2 g sugar; 40 mg phosphorous; 45 mg calcium; 1 mg iron; 47 mg sodium; 271 mg potassium; 240 IU vitamin A; 2 mg ATE vitamin E; 9 mg vitamin C; 2 mg cholesterol

Glycemic Index: Low

Ziti Salmon Salad

Pasta salad can be high in carbohydrates and GI rating, but this one holds the line by being more vegetables than pasta. Canned salmon makes it easy to fix as well as full of enough nutrition to make it a meal all by itself.

8 ounces (225 g) whole wheat pasta, such as ziti

16 ounces (455 g) salmon, drained, skin and bone removed

6 ounces (170 g) snow pea pods, thawed

1 cup (150 g) red bell peppers, chopped

1 yellow (150 g) bell peppers, chopped

½ cup (50 g) green onions, sliced

½ cup (120 ml) Italian dressing

Prepare ziti as package directs; drain. In large bowl, combine ziti and remaining ingredients; mix well. Cover; chill thoroughly. Stir before serving. Refrigerate leftovers.

Yield: 10 servings

Each with: 91 g water; 195 calories (28% from fat, 28% from protein, 44% from carb); 14 g Protein; 6 g total fat; 1 g saturated fat; 2 g monounsaturated fat; 2 g polyunsaturated fat; 22 g carb; 3 g fiber; 2 g sugar; 239 mg phosphorous; 137 mg calcium; 2 mg iron; 233 mg sodium; 309 mg potassium; 770 IU vitamin A; 8 mg ATE vitamin E; 64 mg vitamin C; 18 mg cholesterol

Glycemic Index: Low

Fish Fillets Italian

This dish features great tasting fish rollups, flavored with Italian herbs, cooked in tomato sauce, and topped with bread crumbs. Serve with fresh steamed broccoli for a really heart healthy meal.

1 pound (455 g) fish fillets, such as cod, flounder, perch, or sole

1 tablespoon (15 ml) olive oil

Black pepper, to taste

1 tablespoon (4 g) fresh parsley, chopped

1 teaspoon basil

¼ teaspoon oregano

1 cup (160 g) onion, sliced

8 ounces tomato sauce

1 tablespoon (14 g) unsalted butter, melted

¼ cup (30 g) dry bread crumbs

¼ cup (25 g) Parmesan cheese

Brush fillets with oil. Season with pepper to taste and with parsley, basil, and oregano. Roll up fillets. Spray an 8 x 8-inch (20 x 20 cm) baking dish with nonstick vegetable oil spray. Lay slices of onion on bottom of dish. Place rolled fillets, seam side down, on top of onions. Pour tomato sauce over fillets. Combine melted butter, bread crumbs, and cheese. Sprinkle on fillets. Bake at 400°F (200°C, or gas mark 6) for 20 minutes or until fish flakes easily with a fork.

Yield: 4 servings

Each with: 185 g water; 229 calories (37% from fat, 43% from protein, 20% from carb); 25 g Protein; 9 g total fat; 4 g saturated fat; 4 g monounsaturated fat; 1 g polyunsaturated fat; 11 g carb; 2 g fiber; 4 g sugar; 314 mg phosphorous; 122 mg calcium; 1 mg iron; 162 mg sodium; 695 mg potassium; 734 IU vitamin A; 45 mg ATE vitamin E; 13 mg vitamin C; 62 mg cholesterol

Glycemic Index: Low

Seafood Alfredo

This makes an elegant meal over spaghetti. It's good enough to serve to company.

8 ounces (225 g) shrimp

8 ounces (225 g) scallops

½ pound (225 g) salmon fillets, cubed

1 clove garlic

2 tablespoons (30 ml) olive oil

3 tablespoons (24 g) flour

1½ cups (355 ml) skim milk

1 teaspoon Italian seasoning

¼ cup (25 g) grated Parmesan cheese

TIP *We've also made this with all salmon instead of the shrimp and scallops. It's still a great meal.*

In a large saucepan, sauté shrimp, scallops, salmon, and garlic in olive oil until just cooked through. Shake together flour and milk in a jar. Add to pan along with Italian seasoning. Cook and stir until thickened and just beginning to boil. Stir in cheese. Serve over pasta.

Yield: 6 servings

Each with: 138 g water; 229 calories (41% from fat, 45% from protein, 14% from carb); 25 g protein; 10 g total fat; 2 g saturated fat; 5 g monounsaturated fat; 2 g polyunsaturated fat; 8 g carb; 0 g fiber; 0 g sugar; 166 mg calcium; 2 mg iron; 265 mg sodium; 436 mg potassium; 275 IU vitamin A; 4 mg vitamin C; 111 mg cholesterol

Glycemic Index: Low

Italian Portobello

These are pizza flavored snacks with Portobello mushroom "crusts." They proved to be an unexpected hit with young people.

5 ounces (140 g) frozen chopped spinach, thawed

6 ounces (165 g) part-skim mozzarella cheese, shredded

4 ounces (115 g) turkey pepperoni, coarsely chopped

1 teaspoon crushed dried basil

¼ teaspoon coarsely ground black pepper

12 portobello mushroom caps, 3 to 4 inch (7½ to 10 cm) diameter

2 tablespoons (30 ml) olive oil

Thaw spinach; press out liquid and finely chop. Combine spinach, cheese, pepperoni, basil, and pepper. Clean mushrooms; remove stems. Place open side up on lightly greased baking sheet; brush with olive oil. Spoon 2 tablespoons spinach mixture into each. Bake at 350°F (180°C, gas mark 4) for 12 minutes or broil 4 inches (10 cm) from heat for 3 to 4 minutes. Garnish with fresh basil.

Yield: 12 servings

Each with: 99 g water; 105 calories (47% from fat, 32% from protein, 20% from carb); 9 g protein; 6 g total fat; 2 g saturated fat; 3 g monounsaturated fat; 1 g polyunsaturated fat; 6 g carb; 2 g fiber; 2 g sugar; 180 mg phosphorus; 140 mg calcium; 1 mg iron; 280 mg sodium; 497 mg potassium; 1 1/203 IU vitamin A; 0 mg vitamin C; 21 mg cholesterol

Glycemic Index: Low

Zucchini and Eggplant Casserole

This is a meatless Italian meal, relatively low in the things most people should be avoiding anyway. Summer would probably be the best time for this when fresh vegetables are plentiful.

2 cups (164 g) sliced eggplant

1 cup (150 g) red bell peppers, cut in rings

1 cup (160 g) sliced onion

16 ounces (455 g) mushrooms, sliced

4 cups (452 g) sliced zucchini

2 tablespoons (30 ml) olive oil

3 cups (750 g) low-sodium spaghetti sauce

4 ounces (115 g) part-skim mozzarella cheese, shredded

(continued on page 366)

Brush veggies with olive oil. Grill or panfry until soft. Coat a 9 × 13-inch (23 × 33 cm) baking dish with nonstick vegetable oil spray. Spoon enough sauce in the bottom to cover. Layer veggies, adding sauce every couple of layers. Finish with sauce and then cheese. Bake at 400°F (200°C, gas mark 6) until heated through and cheese is browned.

Yield: 6 servings

Each with: 324 g water; 278 calories (43% from fat, 15% from protein, 42% from carb); 11 g protein; 14 g total fat; 3 g saturated fat; 8 g monounsaturated fat; 1 g polyunsaturated fat; 31 g carb; 7 g fiber; 20 g sugar; 250 mg phosphorus; 208 mg calcium; 2 mg iron; 169 mg sodium; 1,107 mg potassium; 1809 IU vitamin A; 64 mg vitamin C; 12 mg cholesterol

Glycemic Index: Low

Eggplant and Fresh Tomato Parmesan

This variation of eggplant parmesan alternates fresh tomato slices with breaded eggplant slices in a pinwheel fashion that makes a great presentation as well as a great tasting dish.

½ cup (60 g) bread crumbs

1 tablespoon (5 g) Parmesan cheese, shredded

1 teaspoon (15 ml) olive oil

1 clove garlic, crushed

6 eggplant slices, peeled and cut ¼-inch (5 mm) thick

1 egg white, beaten

1 cup (90 g) tomato, sliced

½ cup (60 g) fresh mozzarella cheese

2 tablespoons (5 g) fresh basil leaves, chopped

In medium bowl, combine bread crumbs, Parmesan cheese, oil, and garlic. Dip one eggplant slice in egg white; coat lightly with bread crumb mixture. Repeat with remaining slices. Spray large skillet with nonstick vegetable oil cooking spray; heat over medium-high heat. Cook eggplant slices in a single layer 6 minutes on each side, until lightly browned and tender. Arrange eggplant and tomato slices alternately in a 9-inch (23 cm) pie plate, overlapping slices. Sprinkle with mozzarella cheese. Cover with foil; bake at 400°F (200°C, or gas mark 6) for 20 minutes or until cheese is melted. Uncover; sprinkle with basil.

Yield: 2 servings

Each with: 1374 g water; 577 calories (19% from fat, 17% from protein, 64% from carb); 27 g Protein; 14 g total fat; 5 g saturated fat; 4 g monounsaturated fat; 2 g polyunsaturated fat; 102 g carb; 49 g fiber; 36 g sugar; 532 mg phosphorous; 362 mg calcium; 5 mg iron; 282 mg sodium; 3454 mg potassium; 1334 IU vitamin A; 52 mg ATE vitamin E; 40 mg vitamin C; 25 mg cholesterol

Glycemic Index: Low

Manicotti

When we were first married (many years ago), manicotti was THE meal that we made whenever we entertained. Over the years we somehow quit making it, maybe because the preparation does take a little more than you want to do when you are dealing with kids on a school night. But we recently made a batch on a snowy weekend, and now I wonder why we haven't done that more often. It's still as good as ever.

1 pound (455 g) lean ground beef

24 ounces (675 g) no salt added tomato sauce

6 ounces (170 g) no-salt-added tomato paste

¼ cup (60 ml) water

15 ounces (430 g) ricotta cheese

3 cups (450 g) fresh mozzarella cheese grated

1 egg, beaten

1 teaspoon parsley flakes

12 manicotti noodles, cooked, rinsed and drained

¼ cup (25 g) Parmesan cheese, grated

Brown beef and drain fat. Remove half and set aside. Stir in tomato sauce, tomato paste, and water into remaining meat and simmer 10 minutes. Meanwhile, combine other half of meat in a medium bowl with ricotta, 2 cups (300 g) Mozzarella, egg, and parsley. Into a greased 13 x 9 x 2-inch (33 x 23 x 5 cm) baking dish pour ⅓ sauce. Stuff manicotti noodles with ricotta mixture; place on top of sauce. Pour remaining sauce over filled noodles; top with remaining mozzarella. Sprinkle with Parmesan cheese. Bake, uncovered, at 350°F (180°C, or gas mark 4) for 20 minutes.

(continued on page 368)

Yield: 6 servings

Each with: 270 g water; 681 calories (46% from fat, 27% from protein, 28% from carb); 45 g Protein; 34 g total fat; 17 g saturated fat; 12 g monounsaturated fat; 2 g polyunsaturated fat; 47 g carb; 4 g fiber; 10 g sugar; 612 mg phosphorous; 567 mg calcium; 5 mg iron; 612 mg sodium; 1158 mg potassium; 1559 IU vitamin A; 192 mg ATE vitamin E; 21 mg vitamin C; 157 mg cholesterol

Glycemic Index: Low

Skillet "Calzone"

Are you looking for the flavor of calzone without the time and effort of making and shaping the bread dough? This recipes starts with sliced French bread that's topped with a beef and tomato mixture that gives you the same kind of flavor with much less work.

8 slices French bread, cut diagonally ½-inch (1 cm) thick

2 tablespoons (10 g) Parmesan cheese, grated

¾ pound (340 g) lean ground beef

1 tablespoon (15 ml) olive oil

1 cup (150 g) green bell peppers, sliced

1 clove garlic, finely chopped

14½ ounces (410 g) no-salt-added tomatoes undrained

8 ounces (225 g) pizza sauce

4 ounces (115 g) mushroom, sliced

Set oven control to broil. Place bread slices on ungreased cookie sheet. Spray bread with butter flavored cooking spray; sprinkle with cheese. Broil with tops 4 to 6 inches (10 to 15 cm) from heat for 1 to 2 minutes or until light brown; set aside. Heat oil in large nonstick skillet over medium-high heat. Cook beef, bell pepper, and garlic in oil, stirring occasionally, until beef is brown. Stir in tomatoes, pizza sauce, and mushrooms. Cook 2 to 4 minutes or until hot. Place 2 toasted bread slices on each of 4 serving plates; top with beef mixture.

Yield: 4 servings

Each with: 280 g water; 482 calories (38% from fat, 22% from protein, 39% from carb); 27 g Protein; 21 g total fat; 7 g saturated fat; 9 g monounsaturated fat; 2 g polyunsaturated fat; 48 g carb; 4 g fiber; 10 g sugar; 289 mg phosphorous; 113 mg calcium; 6 mg iron; 845 mg sodium; 902 mg potassium; 731 IU vitamin A; 4 mg ATE vitamin E; 48 mg vitamin C; 61 mg cholesterol

Glycemic Index: Low

Penne in Vodka Cream Sauce

I never really thought of vodka as being an Italian sort of thing. But vodka pasta sauces seem to be all the rage, so maybe I just don't know. At any rate, this is an incredibly rich sauce, with vodka, cream, and pureed peppers plus chopped fresh tomatoes. You could also make the sauce separately to serve over veggies or other kinds of pasta.

1 cup (150 g) red bell peppers

¾ cup (355 ml) vodka

⅔ cup (160 g) whipping cream

6 tablespoons (85 g) unsalted butter

6 ounces (170 g) plum tomato, peeled, seeded and chopped

1 pound (455 g) penne

½ cup (50 g) Parmesan cheese, grated

3 tablespoons (12 g) parsley, fresh, minced

Soak red peppers in vodka for 24 hours. Combine cream, butter, and tomatoes in heavy large saucepan. Simmer until reduced by ⅓, about 12 minutes. Cook pasta according to directions. Drain and add to sauce. Process pepper and vodka mixture until smooth. Add vodka to pasta. Simmer until sauce thickens, stirring constantly, about 3 minutes. Mix in Parmesan and parsley. Serve immediately.

Yield: 4 servings

Each with: 132 g water; 774 calories (36% from fat, 13% from protein, 51% from carb); 23 g Protein; 29 g total fat; 17 g saturated fat; 8 g monounsaturated fat; 2 g polyunsaturated fat; 90 g carb; 1 g fiber; 3 g sugar; 424 mg phosphorous; 214 mg calcium; 5 mg iron; 215 mg sodium; 480 mg potassium; 2547 IU vitamin A; 212 mg ATE vitamin E; 57 mg vitamin C; 79 mg cholesterol

Glycemic Index: Low

Tuscan Beans in Tomato Sauce

This is perhaps Florence's most famous dish. Some recipes call for tomato paste rather than tomatoes.

1 pound (455 g) great northern beans, or cannellini beans

2 sprigs fresh sage

6 tablespoons (90 ml) olive oil

½ teaspoon minced garlic

1 cup (180 g) Roma tomatoes, peeled and chopped

¼ teaspoon black pepper

Soak beans overnight. Drain the beans. Simmer in fresh water to cover, along with 1 sprig of sage and 1 tablespoon (15 ml) olive oil, for about 1½ hours or until tender. In a separate pan (large enough to hold the beans), heat the remaining oil on low heat with the garlic and the rest of the sage so that the flavors infuse. Do not brown the garlic. Add the tomatoes and simmer for 10 minutes. Then add the drained beans, season with pepper, and cook for another 15 minutes or so. There should be a good amount of sauce.

Yield: 6 servings

Each with: 211 calories (58% from fat, 11% from protein, 32% from carb); 6 g protein; 14 g total fat; 2 g saturated fat; 10 g monounsaturated fat; 2 g polyunsaturated fat; 17 g carb; 4 g fiber; 1 g sugar; 44 mg calcium; 1 mg iron; 5 mg sodium; 326 mg potassium; 4 mg vitamin C; 0 mg cholesterol

Glycemic Index: Low

Eggplant and Pepper Salad

This tasty salad features roasted vegetables for a nice flavor boost. You can serve it as is over lettuce leaves. It's equally good cold or at room temperature.

1 large eggplant

2 green bell peppers

2 celery stalks

5 tablespoons (75 ml) olive oil, divided

2 garlic cloves, minced

¼ cup (60 ml) red wine vinegar

1 teaspoon oregano

½ teaspoon black pepper

¼ cup (25 g) black olives, chopped

Preheat oven to 400°F (200°C, or gas mark 6). Place whole eggplant, unpeeled, on a rack in oven. Wrap the two peppers and celery stalks individually in aluminum foil and place them on the rack as well. Bake for 30 minutes. Remove peppers and celery and let cool. Bake eggplant for another 15 minutes. It should be very tender and have collapsed. When vegetables are cool enough to handle, peel eggplant, cut into several pieces, and drain in a colander for 20 minutes. Squeeze out some of the excess moisture. Chop peppers, removing stems and seeds. Leave in large pieces. Chop celery into ½-inch (1 cm) pieces. Dice eggplant and combine with peppers and celery in a large bowl. Heat 1 tablespoon of olive oil in a skillet and sauté the garlic until golden. Add to the bowl. Add remaining ingredients and mix thoroughly. Cover and let stand for 1 hour at room temperature before serving.

Yield: 6 servings

Each with: 127 g water; 136 calories (77% from fat, 4% from protein, 20% from carb); 1 g Protein; 12 g total fat; 2 g saturated fat; 9 g monounsaturated fat; 1 g polyunsaturated fat; 7 g carb; 4 g fiber; 3 g sugar; 30 mg phosphorous; 23 mg calcium; 1 mg iron; 59 mg sodium; 272 mg potassium; 231 IU vitamin A; 0 mg ATE vitamin E; 32 mg vitamin C; 0 mg cholesterol

Glycemic Index: Low

Easy Marinara

If you are in a hurry for pasta sauce, this is for you. It may not have the rich flavor that a sauce that's been simmered for hours has, but it is good. Be aware that some cans of crushed tomatoes have added salt and some don't.

28 ounces (800 g) crushed tomatoes

2 tablespoons (8 g) Italian seasoning

2 cloves garlic, minced

(continued on page 372)

Combine all ingredients in a saucepan and simmer 5 minutes.

Yield: 6 servings

Each with: 134 g water; 35 calories (10% from fat, 16% from protein, 74% from carb); 1 g protein; 0 g total fat; 0 g saturated fat; 0 g monounsaturated fat; 0 g polyunsaturated fat; 6 g carb; 2 g fiber; 4 g sugar; 31 mg calcium; 1 mg iron; 7 mg sodium; 345 mg potassium; 1,171 IU vitamin A; 18 mg vitamin C; 0 mg cholesterol

Glycemic Index: Low

Zucchini Pasta Sauce

I like spaghetti sauce with lots of vegetables in it. This one is great over any kind of pasta.

1 cup (160 g) onion, finely diced

3 tablespoons (12 g) fresh parsley, finely chopped

2 cloves garlic, crushed

¼ cup (60 g) olive oil

1½ pounds (680 g) zucchini, about 6

2 cups (490 g) no-salt-added tomato sauce

2 teaspoons (2.8 g) basil

Sauté onion, parsley, and garlic in oil about 10 minutes: Stir in zucchini and simmer about 5 minutes, stirring occasionally. Add tomato sauce and basil and simmer for 30 minutes, stirring occasionally.

Yield: 6 servings

Each with: 205 g water; 140 calories (58% from fat, 8% from protein, 34% from carb); 3 g Protein; 9 g total fat; 1 g saturated fat; 7 g monounsaturated fat; 1 g polyunsaturated fat; 13 g carb; 3 g fiber; 7 g sugar; 79 mg phosphorous; 42 mg calcium; 1 mg iron; 23 mg sodium; 656 mg potassium; 689 IU vitamin A; 0 mg ATE vitamin E; 35 mg vitamin C; 0 mg cholesterol

Glycemic Index: Low

Pork Pasta Sauce

Using ground pork instead of sausage gives this sauce a milder, more subtle flavor than typical sauces.

3 tablespoons (45 ml) olive oil, divided

½ cup (80 g) onion, diced

¼ cup (25 g) celery, minced

¼ cup (33 g) carrot, scraped and minced

½ pound (225 g) ground pork

28 ounces (795 g) no-salt-added tomatoes

¼ teaspoon dried thyme

2 tablespoons (8 g) fresh parsley, minced

Black pepper, freshly ground to taste

Heat 2 tablespoons (30 ml) of the oil in a 3 quart (3 L) nonaluminum saucepan. Add the onion, celery, and carrot and sauté over low heat until the vegetables just begin to color. Use a slotted spoon to remove the vegetables to a plate. Add the remaining tablespoon (15 ml) of oil to the pan and sauté the ground pork until it is lightly browned. Pour off and discard any excess fat from the pan and return the vegetables to the pan. Puree the tomatoes and add them to the saucepan along with the parsley and pepper. Bring to a boil, lower the heat, and simmer, uncovered, stirring occasionally, for 1½ hours.

Yield: 2 servings

Each with: 509 g water; 571 calories (69% from fat, 16% from protein, 15% from carb); 23 g Protein; 45 g total fat; 12 g saturated fat; 26 g monounsaturated fat; 5 g polyunsaturated fat; 22 g carb; 5 g fiber; 12 g sugar; 297 mg phosphorous; 166 mg calcium; 6 mg iron; 140 mg sodium; 1236 mg potassium; 3540 IU vitamin A; 2 mg ATE vitamin E; 47 mg vitamin C; 82 mg cholesterol

Glycemic Index: Low

Clam Sauce

Chicken broth is used to extend the recipe rather than the usual clam juice. I prefer a little thicker sauce that sticks to the pasta better than the traditional, so I usually add a teaspoon of cornstarch to the chicken broth before stirring it in.

½ teaspoon minced garlic

1 tablespoon (15 ml) olive oil

1 can (6½ ounces or 182 g) minced clams

½ cup (120 ml) low-sodium chicken broth

2 tablespoons (8 g) parsley

Sauté garlic in oil until lightly browned. Add clams, including juice. Simmer 2 minutes. Stir in chicken broth and parsley and simmer 1 minute longer.

Yield: 4 servings

Each with: 47 g water; 62 calories (58% from fat, 12% from protein, 30% from carb); 2 g protein; 4 g total fat; 1 g saturated fat; 3 g monounsaturated fat; 1 g polyunsaturated fat; 5 g carb; 0 g fiber; 0 g sugar; 54 mg phosphorus; 22 mg calcium; 0 mg iron; 143 mg sodium; 80 mg potassium; 172 IU vitamin A; 3 mg vitamin C; 9 mg cholesterol

Glycemic Index: Low

Sun-Dried Tomato Spaghetti Sauce

This is a flavor-packed sauce that has an extra boost from sun-dried tomatoes.

½ cup (28 g) sun-dried tomatoes

½ cup (80 g) coarsely chopped onion

½ cup (75 g) chopped green bell pepper

2 tablespoons (30 ml) olive oil

8 ounces (225 g) no-salt-added tomato sauce

½ teaspoon garlic powder

½ teaspoon oregano

1 teaspoon basil

½ teaspoon onion powder

1 teaspoon parsley

2 tablespoons (30 ml) vinegar

Soak the tomatoes in boiling water for 10 minutes. Drain. Sauté onion and pepper in oil until soft. Add remaining ingredients to skillet and simmer until sauce is desired thickness, about 30 minutes.

Yield: 4 servings

Each with: 65 g water; 53 calories (33% from fat, 11% from protein, 56% from carb); 2 g protein; 2 g total fat; 0 g saturated fat; 1 g monounsaturated fat; 0 g polyunsaturated fat; 8 g carb; 2 g fiber; 0 g sugar; 51 mg phosphorus; 24 mg calcium; 3 mg iron; 305 mg sodium; 446 mg potassium; 787 IU vitamin A; 20 mg vitamin C; 0 mg cholesterol

Glycemic Index: Low

Ultimate Pasta Sauce

This pasta sauce contains just a bit of everything. It isn't really difficult to make, but it is long simmered so you need to plan ahead to give it time.

½ pound (225 g) lean ground beef

4 ounces (115 g) mushroom, sliced

3 slices low-sodium bacon

1 teaspoon black pepper (or to taste)

½ pound (225 g) Italian sausage

¼ cup (60 ml) red wine

1 tablespoon (15 ml) olive oil

Dash cinnamon (or to taste)

Dash ground cloves (or to taste)

1 cup (160 g) onion, chopped

1 cup (150 g) green bell peppers, chopped

6 ounces (170 g) no-salt-added tomato paste

14 ounces (400 g) no-salt-added tomatoes undrained

(continued on page 376)

½ teaspoon basil

½ teaspoon oregano

1 bay leaf

2 cloves garlic, sliced

Sauté bacon in oil. Then add beef, sausage, green pepper, and onion. Cook until meat is browned. Then add mushrooms, tomatoes (with juice), bay leaf, and seasonings. Simmer for 1 hour. Add tomato paste and wine and simmer for another 30 minutes. Remove bay leaf before serving.

Yield: 4 servings

Each with: 300 g water; 487 calories (63% from fat, 21% from protein, 16% from carb); 25 g Protein; 34 g total fat; 12 g saturated fat; 16 g monounsaturated fat; 4 g polyunsaturated fat; 20 g carb; 5 g fiber; 11 g sugar; 295 mg phosphorous; 82 mg calcium; 5 mg iron; 557 mg sodium; 1200 mg potassium; 924 IU vitamin A; 1 mg ATE vitamin E; 53 mg vitamin C; 89 mg cholesterol

Glycemic Index: Low

Eggplant and Tomato Sauce

Here's another vegetable sauce. This one features eggplants and peppers.

1 teaspoon olive oil

¾ cup (175 ml) dry sherry

1 cup (160 g) onion, finely chopped

2 cloves garlic cloves, minced

¼ cup (25 g) celery, chopped

1 cup (82 g) eggplant, peeled and cubed

½ cup (75 g) red bell peppers, minced

½ teaspoon nutmeg

3 cups (540 g) no-salt-added tomatoes chopped

1 tablespoon (2.5 g) fresh basil

Pepper, to taste

In a large skillet, heat oil and sherry until bubbling. Add onion and cook for 5 minutes. Add garlic, eggplant, and pepper. Cover and cook for 2 minutes. Add nutmeg, basil, and tomatoes. Bring to a boil, lower heat and simmer, uncovered for 20 minutes. Season to taste.

Yield: 6 servings

Each with: 186 g water; 94 calories (14% from fat, 9% from protein, 76% from carb); 2 g Protein; 1 g total fat; 0 g saturated fat; 1 g monounsaturated fat; 0 g polyunsaturated fat; 13 g carb; 3 g fiber; 7 g sugar; 43 mg phosphorous; 57 mg calcium; 2 mg iron; 24 mg sodium; 373 mg potassium; 585 IU vitamin A; 0 mg ATE vitamin E; 30 mg vitamin C; 0 mg cholesterol

Glycemic Index: Low

Italian Bean Soup

This is a simple bean soup that's made more flavorful by the addition of Italian herbs.

1 cup (215 g) dried navy beans

2 quarts (1.9 L) water

1 cup (160 g) onion, chopped

1 cup (150 g) green pepper, chopped

1 cup (130 g) carrots, chopped

1½ teaspoon dried basil

1½ teaspoon oregano

¼ teaspoon dry mustard

2 cloves garlic, minced

24 ounces (675 g) no-salt-added tomato sauce

½ cup (53 g) whole wheat pasta, uncooked

Sort and wash beans; place in a Dutch oven. Cover with water 2 inches (5 cm) above beans. Bring to a boil. Cook over high heat 2 minutes. Remove from heat, cover, and let stand 1 hour. Drain beans. Add 2 quarts (1.9 L) water and all ingredients except macaroni. Cover and simmer 1½ hours or until beans are tender, stirring occasionally. Add macaroni and cook uncovered 10 minutes or until macaroni is tender.

Yield: 8 servings

(continued on page 378)

Each with: 377 g water; 105 calories (4% from fat, 17% from protein, 79% from carb); 5 g Protein; 1 g total fat; 0 g saturated fat; 0 g monounsaturated fat; 0 g polyunsaturated fat; 22 g carb; 5 g fiber; 6 g sugar; 93 mg phosphorous; 55 mg calcium; 2 mg iron; 29 mg sodium; 541 mg potassium; 3080 IU vitamin A; 0 mg ATE vitamin E; 29 mg vitamin C; 0 mg cholesterol

Glycemic Index: Low

Italian-Style Chicken Soup

This one is good either as a full meal or just to have on hand for lunches.

1 pound (455 g) boneless chicken breasts, cubed

1 can low-sodium chicken broth

1 can (14½ ounces or 410 g) low-sodium tomatoes

2 cups (475 ml) water

2 teaspoons (4 g) low-sodium chicken bouillon

4 ounces (115 g) mushrooms, sliced

½ cup (65 g) sliced carrot

½ cup (56 g) sliced zucchini

½ cup (62 g) frozen green beans

6 ounces (128 g) frozen spinach

½ teaspoon garlic powder

1 teaspoon basil

½ teaspoon oregano

Combine ingredients in slow cooker. Cover and cook on low 8–10 hours or high 4 to 5 hours.

Yield: 6 servings

Each with: 174 g water; 43 calories (12% from fat, 42% from protein, 46% from carb); 5 g protein; 1 g total fat; 0 g saturated fat; 0 g monounsaturated fat; 0 g polyunsaturated fat; 6 g carb; 2 g fiber; 2 g sugar; 69 mg phosphorus; 63 mg calcium; 1 mg iron; 76 mg sodium; 309 mg potassium; 5,433 IU vitamin A; 10 mg vitamin C; 7 mg cholesterol

Glycemic Index: Low

14

Mexican and Latin American

We love Mexican-and Latin American-flavored food. The recipes here offer a wide range of flavors, ingredients, and heat levels. Mexican cooking is also a good place to incorporate more beans. Beans are good because they are low in GI and very high in fiber.

Mexican Steak and Potatoes

This is a simple meat and potatoes dish, but it's livened up with the addition of tomato sauce and Mexican-style seasonings.

3 pounds (1⅓ kg) beef round steak, ½-inch (1 cm) thick

2 pounds (900 g) potatoes

8 ounces (225 g) no-salt-added tomato sauce

½ teaspoon ground pepper

½ teaspoon cumin

1 clove garlic, smashed

1 cup (235 ml) water

Cut round steak into cubes and brown in heavy skillet or Dutch oven. Peel and cube potatoes (approximately in ½-inch [1 cm] cubes). Once meat is slight browned, add potatoes and continue to brown. Add tomato sauce, pepper, cumin powder, and garlic. Add water and simmer until meat and potatoes are tender.

Yield: 6 servings

Each with: 329 g water; 572 calories (19% from fat, 62% from protein, 20% from carb); 85 g Protein; 12 g total fat; 4 g saturated fat; 4 g monounsaturated fat; 1 g polyunsaturated fat; 27 g carb; 3 g fiber; 3 g sugar; 618 mg phosphorous; 33 mg calcium; 9 mg iron; 117 mg sodium; 1591 mg potassium; 144 IU vitamin A; 0 mg ATE vitamin E; 18 mg vitamin C; 204 mg cholesterol

Glycemic Index: Low

Mexican Chicken

This is a quick and easy Mexican chicken dish that is great over rice or noodles. If you'd like it a little spicier, add a few shakes of Tabasco sauce to the tomato sauce mixture along with the spices.

8 ounces (225 g) no-salt-added tomato sauce

½ cup (120 ml) orange juice

½ cup (80 g) onion, finely chopped

½ teaspoon oregano, crushed

½ teaspoon chili powder

1 clove garlic, minced

12 ounces (340 g) boneless skinless chicken breast, cut into 1-inch (2½ cm) pieces

2 teaspoons (5.3 g) cornstarch

1 tablespoon (15 ml) water

¼ cup (15 g) fresh parsley, chopped

In a large skillet, combine tomato sauce, orange juice, onion, oregano, chili powder, and garlic. Bring to a boil: reduce heat. Cover and simmer 5 minutes. Stir in chicken; return to boiling. Cover and simmer 12–15 minutes more or until chicken is tender and no longer pink. Meanwhile, combine cornstarch and water. Stir into skillet. Cook and stir until thickened and bubbly. Cook and stir 2 minutes more.

Yield: 6 servings

Each with: 111 g water; 96 calories (9% from fat, 60% from protein, 31% from carb); 14 g Protein; 1 g total fat; 0 g saturated fat; 0 g monounsaturated fat; 0 g polyunsaturated fat; 7 g carb; 1 g fiber; 2 g sugar; 132 mg phosphorous; 22 mg calcium; 1 mg iron; 45 mg sodium; 363 mg potassium; 438 IU vitamin A; 3 mg ATE vitamin E; 17 mg vitamin C; 33 mg cholesterol

Glycemic Index: Low

Quick Mexican Chicken and Rice

This quick dish makes a complete meal all by itself.

8 ounces (225 g) no-salt-added tomato sauce

1 teaspoon cumin

¼ teaspoon onion powder

⅛ teaspoon garlic powder

¼ teaspoon cocoa

1 tablespoon (7.5 g) chili powder

2 boneless skinless chicken breast, cooked and chopped

1 cup (195 g) rice

1 cup (115 g) cheddar cheese, shredded

Prepare sauce in small saucepan by mixing ⅔ of the tomato sauce and spices. Add chopped, cooked chicken. Put sauce on low heat and stir occasionally. Prepare rice. When rice is done, add remaining ⅓ tomato sauce to rice and stir. To serve, place rice on plates, topped with chicken and sauce and then shredded cheese. Serve with sour cream, picante sauce, and chopped tomato if desired.

Yield: 2 servings

Each with: 233 g water; 506 calories (43% from fat, 30% from protein, 27% from carb); 37 g Protein; 24 g total fat; 14 g saturated fat; 7 g monounsaturated fat; 1 g polyunsaturated fat; 34 g carb; 4 g fiber; 6 g sugar; 567 mg phosphorous; 529 mg calcium; 3 mg iron; 509 mg sodium; 792 mg potassium; 2194 IU vitamin A; 175 mg ATE vitamin E; 18 mg vitamin C; 110 mg cholesterol

Glycemic Index: Low

Chicken with Black Bean Sauce

This quick cooking skillet chicken dish is topped with a black bean, corn, and salsa sauce which cooks in the same pan.

6 boneless skinless chicken breasts

2 teaspoons (5 g) ground cumin, divided

1 teaspoon garlic powder

1 tablespoon (15 ml) vegetable oil

1 cup (256 g) black beans, canned, rinsed, and drained

10 ounces (280 g) frozen corn

2/3 cup (173 g) salsa

½ cup (75 g) red bell pepper, diced

2 tablespoons (2 g) fresh cilantro, chopped

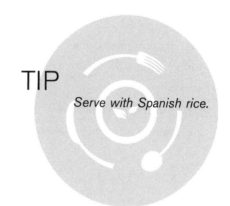

TIP

Serve with Spanish rice.

Sprinkle both sides of chicken with 1 teaspoon of the cumin and the garlic powder. Heat oil in 12-inch (30 cm) skillet over medium-high heat. Add chicken; cook 3 minutes. In medium bowl, combine beans, corn, salsa, red pepper, and remaining 1 teaspoon cumin. Turn chicken; spoon bean mixture evenly over chicken. Reduce heat to medium; cook uncovered 6–7 minutes or until chicken is cooked through. Push bean mixture off chicken into skillet. Transfer chicken to serving platter using a slotted spoon; keep warm. Cook bean mixture over high heat 2–3 minutes or until thickened, stirring frequently; spoon over chicken. Sprinkle with cilantro and serve.

Yield: 6 servings

Each with: 146 g water; 192 calories (19% from fat, 43% from protein, 38% from carb); 21 g Protein; 4 g total fat; 1 g saturated fat; 1 g monounsaturated fat; 2 g polyunsaturated fat; 19 g carb; 5 g fiber; 3 g sugar; 239 mg phosphorous; 32 mg calcium; 2 mg iron; 122 mg sodium; 544 mg potassium; 655 IU vitamin A; 4 mg ATE vitamin E; 21 mg vitamin C; 41 mg cholesterol

Glycemic Index: Low

Jerk Rotisserie Chicken

Here's a simple recipe for jerk-flavored chicken. You could also cook this on the grill or a rotisserie if desired. Make sure you use jerk seasoning without salt such as the one from Spice Hunter or make your own.

½ cup (80 g) chopped onion

1 roasting chicken

1 teaspoon paprika

2 teaspoons (6 g) garlic powder

3 tablespoons (12 g) jerk seasoning

Process the onion in a food processor or blender until very finely chopped. Rub it into the chicken, inside and out. Combine the paprika, garlic powder, and jerk seasoning. Rub all over the whole chicken and allow the chicken to marinate for at least 2 hours. Roast in oven at 350°F (180°C, gas mark 4) for 1 to 1½ hours until done.

Yield: 6 servings

Each with: 44 g water; 115 calories (62% from fat, 31% from protein, 8% from carb); 9 g protein; 8 g total fat; 2 g saturated fat; 3 g monounsaturated fat; 2 g polyunsaturated fat; 2 g carb; 0 g fiber; 1 g sugar; 90 mg phosphorus; 9 mg calcium; 1 mg iron; 34 mg sodium; 134 mg potassium; 266 IU vitamin A; 1 mg vitamin C; 36 mg cholesterol

Glycemic Index: Low

Chicken Mole

Chicken mole can be a long involved recipe. We shortened the time but kept the traditional flavor by using the microwave to prepare the sauce and cook the chicken.

2 teaspoons (4 g) cocoa powder, unsweetened

1½ teaspoon chili powder

½ teaspoon cumin, ground

½ teaspoon oregano, dried crushed

8 ounces (225 g) no-salt-added tomato sauce

¼ cup (40 g) onion, finely chopped

3 cloves garlic, minced

1 pound (455 g) boneless skinless chicken
   breast, cut into bite-sized pieces

4 ounces (115 g) green chili peppers, diced, drained

2 tablespoons (14 g) almonds, toasted sliced

4 flour tortillas

½ cup (90 g) tomato, chopped

½ cup (28 g) lettuce, shredded

1 avocado, sliced

TIP *Rather than rolling it in tortillas, you can also serve it over rice.*

In a 1-½ quart (1.5 L) microwave-safe casserole, combine cocoa powder, chili powder, cumin, oregano, and salt. Stir in tomato sauce, onion and garlic. Micro-cook, covered, on 100% power (high) for 2 to 3 minutes or until mixture is bubbly around edges, stirring once. Stir in chicken and chili peppers. Cover; cook on high for 8 to 10 minutes (10 to 12 minutes for low-wattage ovens) or until chicken is tender and no longer pink inside, stirring every 3 minutes. Garnish with almonds. To serve: warm tortillas, fill with chicken mixture, tomato, lettuce, and avocado.

Yield: 4 servings

Each with: 231 g water; 343 calories (31% from fat, 37% from protein, 32% from carb); 32 g Protein; 12 g total fat; 2 g saturated fat; 6 g monounsaturated fat; 2 g polyunsaturated fat; 28 g carb; 6 g fiber; 4 g sugar; 341 mg phosphorous; 97 mg calcium; 4 mg iron; 400 mg sodium; 891 mg potassium; 797 IU vitamin A; 7 mg ATE vitamin E; 26 mg vitamin C; 66 mg cholesterol

Glycemic Index: Low

Grilled Lime Fajitas

This dish features lime-flavored chicken with enough cayenne to have a little kick.

1 pound (455 g) flank steak or chicken breast

½ cup (120 ml) lime juice

¼ cup (4 g) chopped cilantro

¼ cup (60 ml) white vinegar

¼ cup (60 ml) olive oil

3 tablespoons (45 ml) balsamic vinegar

1 tablespoon (5 g) cayenne pepper

3 cloves garlic, minced

1 tablespoon (6 g) black pepper

Mix all ingredients except meat together. Marinate meat in mixture overnight. Preheat grill. Remove marinade and cook in saucepan till it boils. Set aside and let cool. Grill meat, basting with marinade until cooked. Cut into long, thin strips. Serve with hot tortillas, grilled sliced bell peppers, and onion, sour cream, guacamole, and salsa.

Yield: 4 servings

Each with: 127 g water; 361 calories (59% from fat, 36% from protein, 5% from carb); 32 g protein; 23 g total fat; 6 g saturated fat; 14 g monounsaturated fat; 2 g polyunsaturated fat; 5 g carb; 1 g fiber; 1 g sugar; 254 mg phosphorus; 34 mg calcium; 3 mg iron; 68 mg sodium; 499 mg potassium; 747 IU vitamin A; 11 mg vitamin C; 62 mg cholesterol

Glycemic Index: Low

Chicken Tequila

A generous helping of tequila ensures that this chicken will be both tender and flavorful. Serve over noodles or rice.

1 cup (235 ml) low-sodium chicken broth

9 ounces (255 g) no-salt-added tomatoes, undrained

3 cloves garlic, minced

2 boneless skinless chicken breasts

½ cup (120 ml) tequila

¼ cup (120 ml) lime juice

Dash cayenne pepper

1 teaspoon chili powder

1 teaspoon cumin

½ teaspoon coriander

1 tablespoon (15 ml) olive oil

Simmer the chicken breasts in the broth until tender. Remove and cube. Set aside, reserving broth. Sauté the garlic in olive oil. Add tomatoes (breaking up) and the remaining ingredients; simmer, covered ½ hour. Add chicken and reheat. If sauce becomes too thick, add the reserved broth.

Yield: 4 servings

Each with: 177 g water; 161 calories (40% from fat, 40% from protein, 20% from carb); 10 g Protein; 4 g total fat; 1 g saturated fat; 3 g monounsaturated fat; 1 g polyunsaturated fat; 5 g carb; 1 g fiber; 2 g sugar; 108 mg phosphorous; 36 mg calcium; 1 mg iron; 57 mg sodium; 305 mg potassium; 286 IU vitamin A; 2 mg ATE vitamin E; 12 mg vitamin C; 21 mg cholesterol

Glycemic Index: Low

Chicken and Mushroom Quesadillas

If you have an indoor grill like the George Foreman models, it is perfect for making these quesadillas. If not, place them on a baking sheet in an oven heated to 350°F (180°C, gas mark 4) until crisp.

1 tablespoon (15 ml) olive oil

2½ teaspoons (7.8 g) chili powder

½ teaspoon minced garlic

1 teaspoon oregano

8 ounces (225 g) mushrooms, sliced

1 cup (225 g) chicken breast, cooked and shredded

⅔ cup (106 g) finely chopped onion

½ cup (8 g) chopped fresh cilantro

1½ cups (173 g) shredded low-fat Monterey Jack cheese

16 corn tortillas, 5½ inch (14 cm)

TIP

Serve these with salsa and fat-free sour cream.

Heat olive oil in a large skillet over medium-high heat. Add chili powder, garlic, and oregano and sauté about 1 minute. Add mushrooms and sauté until tender, about 10 minutes. Remove from heat and mix in the chicken, onion, and cilantro. Cool for 10 minutes and then mix in the cheese. Coat one side of 8 of the tortillas with olive oil spray and place them oil side down on a baking sheet. Divide chicken mixture among tortillas, spreading to even thickness. Top with the remaining 8 tortillas and coat tops with olive oil spray. Grill quesadillas until heated through and golden brown, about 3 minutes per side. Cut into wedges to serve.

Yield: 12 servings

Each with: 57 g water; 122 calories (26% from fat, 32% from protein, 43% from carb); 10 g protein; 4 g total fat; 1 g saturated fat; 2 g monounsaturated fat; 1 g polyunsaturated fat; 13 g carb; 2 g fiber; 1 g sugar; 206 mg phosphorus; 97 mg calcium; 1 mg iron; 128 mg sodium; 181 mg potassium; 315 IU vitamin A; 2 mg vitamin C; 13 mg cholesterol

Glycemic Index: Low

Pork and Potatoes With Cumin

This pork stew is great over noodles or rice, but for a lower carbohydrate meal, just ladle it into bowls and eat.

2 pounds (900 g) pork shoulder roast boneless, cut in 1-inch (2½ cm) cubes

¼ cup (31 g) flour

½ cup (120 ml) olive oil

½ cup (80 g) onion, chopped, 1 medium

2 slices low-sodium bacon, cut up

½ cup (120 ml) water

2 tablespoons (30 ml) orange juice

2 tablespoons (30 ml) lime juice

2 tablespoons (14 g) cumin

1 teaspoon oregano

¼ teaspoon pepper

4 cups (720 g) tomatoes, chopped

2 medium potatoes, diced

½ cup (115 g) sour cream

Coat pork with the flour. Heat oil in 10-inch (20 cm) skillet until hot. Cook and stir pork in oil over medium heat until brown. Remove pork with slotted spoon and drain. Cook and stir onion and bacon in the same skillet until bacon is crisp. Stir in the pork and the remaining ingredients except the sour cream. Heat to boiling and then reduce heat. Cover and simmer until pork is done, about 45 minutes. Stir in sour cream and heat until hot.

Yield: 7 servings

Each with: 298 g water; 600 calories (64% from fat, 18% from protein, 18% from carb); 27 g Protein; 43 g total fat; 12 g saturated fat; 23 g monounsaturated fat; 5 g polyunsaturated fat; 28 g carb; 3 g fiber; 2 g sugar; 367 mg phosphorous; 76 mg calcium; 4 mg iron; 127 mg sodium; 1164 mg potassium; 653 IU vitamin A; 20 mg ATE vitamin E; 36 mg vitamin C; 101 mg cholesterol

Glycemic Index: Low

Mexican Roast Loin of Pork

An overnight marinating in citrus and spices makes this roast both tender and flavorful. A creamy orange sauce adds even more flavor to the final product.

5 pounds (2¼ kg) boneless pork loin roast

2 tablespoons (15 g) chili powder

½ cup (120 ml) lime juice

1 teaspoon cumin, ground

1 teaspoon oregano leaves, dried

½ teaspoon pepper

2 cloves garlic, crushed

6 ounces (170 g) orange juice concentrate thawed, divided

¼ cup (60 ml) white wine, dry

½ cup (115 g) sour cream

Place pork roast in a shallow glass or plastic dish. Mix chili powder, lime juice, cumin, oregano, pepper, garlic, and ¼ cup of orange juice concentrate and brush mixture onto the pork roast. Cover and refrigerate at least 8 hours. Heat oven to 325°F (170°C, or gas mark 3). Place pork, fat side up, on rack in a shallow roasting pan. Insert meat thermometer so that the tip is in the center of the thickest part of the roast and does not rest in fat. Roast uncovered until thermometer registers 170°F (77°C), 2 to 2½ hours. Remove pork and rack from the pan. Strain the drippings from the pan and set aside. Add enough water to remaining orange juice concentrate to measure ½ of a cup; stir juice and wine into the drippings Stir in sour cream. Serve with the pork roast.

Yield: 12 servings

Each with: 166 g water; 335 calories (38% from fat, 52% from protein, 9% from carb); 42 g Protein; 14 g total fat; 5 g saturated fat; 6 g monounsaturated fat; 1 g polyunsaturated fat; 8 g carb; 1 g fiber; 6 g sugar; 416 mg phosphorous; 33 mg calcium; 2 mg iron; 103 mg sodium; 948 mg potassium; 492 IU vitamin A; 14 mg ATE vitamin E; 24 mg vitamin C; 108 mg cholesterol

Glycemic Index: Low

Fish in Cilantro Sauce

If you're like me and love the flavor of cilantro, these fish fillets will be a favorite. If you're one of those people who don't love cilantro, substitute parsley and they will be just as good.

2 pounds (900 g) catfish fillets

1 cup (160 g) onion, sliced

1 clove garlic, small, minced

1 tablespoon (15 ml) olive oil

¼ cup (24 g) almonds, toasted, ground

2 tablespoons (30 ml) lime juice

2 tablespoons (30 g) green chilies

1 dash pepper

½ cup (8 g) fresh cilantro, snipped

Thaw the fish fillets if frozen. Cook onion and garlic in hot oil until tender but not brown. Add the almonds, lime juice, chilies, and pepper. Heat through. In a well greased 13 x 9 x 2-inch (33 x 23 x 5 cm) baking dish, arrange the fish fillets. Top with the onion mixture. Sprinkle evenly with the cilantro. Bake, covered, in a preheated 350°F (180°C, or gas mark 4) oven for about 30 minutes or until the fish flakes easily when tested with a fork.

Yield: 6 servings

Each with: 149 g water; 273 calories (56% from fat, 37% from protein, 7% from carb); 25 g Protein; 17 g total fat; 3 g saturated fat; 9 g monounsaturated fat; 3 g polyunsaturated fat; 4 g carb; 1 g fiber; 2 g sugar; 345 mg phosphorous; 37 mg calcium; 1 mg iron; 97 mg sodium; 561 mg potassium; 318 IU vitamin A; 23 mg ATE vitamin E; 7 mg vitamin C; 71 mg cholesterol

Glycemic Index: Low

Mexican Grilled Shrimp

We've made this recipe as a main dish a few times, and I'm planning on doing it for New Year's Eve. Shrimp has a fairly high natural sodium count, so you'll want to be careful not to overdo it.

1 pound (455 g) large shrimp, peeled

2 tablespoons (30 ml) lime juice

1 tablespoon (20 g) honey

½ teaspoon cilantro

½ teaspoon cumin

¼ teaspoon garlic powder

Combine all ingredients in a zipped plastic bag. Turn to coat shrimp well. Marinate at least 2 hours. Grill or sauté until done.

Yield: 4 servings

Each with: 94 g water; 140 calories (13% from fat, 68% from protein, 18% from carb); 23 g protein; 2 g total fat; 0 g saturated fat; 0 g monounsaturated fat; 1 g polyunsaturated fat; 6 g carb; 0 g fiber; 5 g sugar; 236 mg phosphorus; 63 mg calcium; 3 mg iron; 169 mg sodium; 228 mg potassium; 218 IU vitamin A; 5 mg vitamin C; 172 mg cholesterol

Glycemic Index: Low

Individual Mexican Quiche

Individual sausage and egg dishes can be easily made in whatever quantity is needed. This is good for breakfast or for a light dinner.

1 flour tortilla, 6-inch (15 cm) flour

1 ounce (28 g) sausage

1 egg

2 ounces (57 g) Monterey jack cheese

1 tablespoon (9 g) green pepper, chopped

¼ cup (60 ml) milk

Heat tortilla and place in small dish such as a soup bowl that has been sprayed with nonstick vegetable oil spray. Top with half of the cheese. Cook sausage and pepper and add to dish. Mix together remaining ingredients and pour over dish. Top with rest of cheese. Bake at 350°F (180°C, or gas mark 4) for 30 to 35 minutes.

Yield: 1 serving

Each with: 143 g water; 515 calories (62% from fat, 23% from protein, 16% from carb); 29 g Protein; 35 g total fat; 16 g saturated fat; 13 g monounsaturated fat; 3 g polyunsaturated fat; 20 g carb; 1 g fiber; 5 g sugar; 493 mg phosphorous; 571 mg calcium; 3 mg iron; 852 mg sodium; 340 mg potassium; 931 IU vitamin A; 235 mg ATE vitamin E; 7 mg vitamin C; 284 mg cholesterol

Glycemic Index: Low

Taco Quiche

This is a Mexican flavored quiche. Baking it without a crust reduces the fat content to less than half what it would be if you bought a premade pie crust.

½ pound (225 g) extra-lean ground beef, 93 percent lean

2 tablespoons (8 g) taco seasoning

½ cup (120 ml) water

½ cup (58 g) shredded low-fat Monterey Jack cheese

2 ounces (55 g) green chiles, seeded, diced

3 eggs

1 cup (235 ml) fat-free evaporated milk

Preheat oven to 375°F (190°C, gas mark 5). Brown beef in skillet. Drain. Stir in taco seasoning mix and water, cover, and simmer until thickened. Cool 10 minutes. Add cheese and chiles and mix well. Spoon into pie pan that has been coated with nonstick vegetable oil spray. Combine eggs and milk. Mix until smooth. Pour over meat mixture. Bake in preheated oven for 40 to 45 minutes or until custard is set. Allow pie to stand 5 minutes before serving.

Yield: 6 servings

Each with: 119 g water; 173 calories (30% from fat, 51% from protein, 19% from carb); 17 g protein; 4 g total fat; 2 g saturated fat; 2 g monounsaturated fat; 1 g polyunsaturated fat; 6 g carb; 0 g fiber; 5 g sugar; 229 mg phosphorus; 193 mg calcium; 2 mg iron; 321 mg sodium; 371 mg potassium; 451 IU vitamin A; 4 mg vitamin C; 30 mg cholesterol

Glycemic Index: Low

Chicken and Rice Skillet

This Mexican skillet meal may remind you of some of the boxed meal mixes. But the flavor is superior, and the nutrition is much better.

1 tablespoon (15 ml) olive oil

1 pound (455 g) boneless skinless chicken breasts, cubed

1 cup (160 g) onion, chopped

¾ cup (113 g) green bell peppers, chopped

10 ounces (280 g) frozen corn, thawed

1 cup (235 ml) low-sodium chicken broth

1 cup (260 g) mild salsa

1½ cups (293 g) instant rice

½ cup (58 g) cheddar, shredded

Heat oil in large skillet on medium-high heat. Add chicken, onion, and pepper; cook and stir until chicken is cooked through. Add corn, broth, and salsa; bring to boil. Stir in rice; cover. Remove from heat. Let stand 5 minutes. Fluff with fork. Sprinkle with cheese; cover. Let stand 2 minutes or until cheese melts.

Yield: 4 servings

Each with: 363 g water; 408 calories (26% from fat, 36% from protein, 39% from carb); 37 g Protein; 12 g total fat; 5 g saturated fat; 5 g monounsaturated fat; 1 g polyunsaturated fat; 40 g carb; 4 g fiber; 7 g sugar; 451 mg phosphorous; 171 mg calcium; 2 mg iron; 358 mg sodium; 869 mg potassium; 630 IU vitamin A; 49 mg ATE vitamin E; 33 mg vitamin C; 83 mg cholesterol

Glycemic Index: Low

Mexican Beans

These are good either by themselves or as an addition to chili or other dishes.

1 cup (250 g) dried black beans

1 cup (250 g) dried black-eyed peas

1 ham hock

3 cups (690 ml) low-sodium chicken broth

1½ tablespoons (11 g) chili powder

1 tablespoon (7 g) cumin

The night before, cover beans and peas with water and let stand to soften. Preheat oven to 275°F (140°C, gas mark 1). Combine beans, ham hock, and broth in a heavy 2-quart (2 L) ovenproof pot over medium heat. Cover, bring to a boil, and place in the oven. Check the beans every 30 minutes and add ½ cup (120 ml) more broth each time if all the liquid has been absorbed. Cook for 1½ hours or until beans are soft.

Yield: 6 servings

Each with: 155 g water; 113 calories (17% from fat, 28% from protein, 55% from carb); 8 g protein; 2 g total fat; 1 g saturated fat; 1 g monounsaturated fat; 1 g polyunsaturated fat; 17 g carb; 5 g fiber; 2 g sugar; 127 mg phosphorus; 34 mg calcium; 2 mg iron; 102 mg sodium; 376 mg potassium; 592 IU vitamin A; 2 mg vitamin C; 2 mg cholesterol

Glycemic Index: Low

Mexican Vegetable Casserole

This squash casserole gets a Mexican makeover with the addition of chilies and cheese. This makes a great side dish with simple grilled beef or chicken rubbed with Mexican spices.

4 cups (480 g) zucchini, sliced

1 cup (160 g) onion, chopped

3 tablespoons (45 ml) olive oil

2 cloves garlic

4 ounces (115 g) chopped green chilies

16 ounces (455 g) frozen corn

1 cup (120 g) cheddar, grated

Sauté squash and onion in oil until barely tender. Add garlic, chilies, corn, and cheese; mix well. Put in buttered 1-quart (1 L) casserole and bake at 400°F (200°C, or gas mark 6) for 20 minutes.

Yield: 6 servings

Each with: 185 g water; 241 calories (53% from fat, 15% from protein, 32% from carb); 9 g Protein; 15 g total fat; 6 g saturated fat; 7 g monounsaturated fat; 1 g polyunsaturated fat; 21 g carb; 4 g fiber; 5 g sugar; 221 mg phosphorous; 186 mg calcium; 1 mg iron; 232 mg sodium; 503 mg potassium; 567 IU vitamin A; 57 mg ATE vitamin E; 28 mg vitamin C; 23 mg cholesterol

Glycemic Index: Low

Black Bean and Pork Stew

The beans and squash provide a contrast in tastes and textures.

4 cups (940 ml) water

½ cup (125 g) dried black beans

2 ancho chilies

¾ pound (340 g) boneless pork shoulder

1½ cup (270 g) tomatoes, chopped

½ cup (80 g) onion, chopped

½ cup (120 ml) dry red wine

1 teaspoon dried sage

1 teaspoon dried marjoram

½ teaspoon ground cumin

¼ teaspoon ground cinnamon

1 clove garlic

2 cups (280 g) butternut squash, pared and cut in 1-inch (2½ cm) cubes

1 cup (150 g) red bell peppers, diced

2 tablespoons (2 g) fresh cilantro, chopped

Heat water, beans, and chilies to boiling in Dutch oven. Boil uncovered 2 minutes; remove from heat. Cover and let stand 1 hour. Remove chilies; reserve. Heat beans to boiling; reduce heat. Simmer covered for 1 hour. Seed and chop chilies. Trim fat from pork Cut pork into 1-inch (2½ cm) cubes. Stir pork, chilies, and remaining ingredients except squash, bell pepper, and cilantro into beans. Heat to boiling; reduce heat. Cover and simmer 30 minutes, stirring occasionally. Stir in squash. Cover and simmer 30 minutes, stirring occasionally, until squash is tender. Stir in bell pepper and cilantro. Cover and simmer about 5 minutes or until bell pepper is crisp-tender.

Yield: 4 servings

Each with: 506 g water; 260 calories (24% from fat, 35% from protein, 41% from carb); 22 g Protein; 7 g total fat; 2 g saturated fat; 2 g monounsaturated fat; 1 g polyunsaturated fat; 26 g carb; 7 g fiber; 4 g sugar; 294 mg phosphorous; 80 mg calcium; 4 mg iron; 93 mg sodium; 1106 mg potassium; 10813 IU vitamin A; 2 mg ATE vitamin E; 80 mg vitamin C; 55 mg cholesterol

Glycemic Index: Low

Mexican Beef Stew

This is a fairly traditional beef stew, with the flavor enhanced with Mexican spices. It's a great meal for a cold day.

4 tablespoons (60 ml) olive oil

3 tablespoons (45 ml) red wine vinegar

1½ pounds (680 g) beef stew meat

1 cup (235 ml) red wine

1 cup (180 g) onion, minced

1 bay leaf

1 clove garlic, minced

½ teaspoon oregano

1 teaspoon cumin

½ cup (123 g) no-salt-added tomato sauce

4 medium potatoes, cubed

½ cup (55 g) carrot, sliced

Pepper to taste

TIP *For even easier preparation, put everything in a slow cooker and cook on low for 8–10 hours.*

In Dutch oven, sauté onion and garlic in oil. Add everything else except potatoes and carrots. Cover tightly and simmer 1½ hours until meat is thoroughly tender. Half an hour before meat is ready, add carrots and potatoes. Remove bay leaf before serving.

Yield: 6 servings

Each with: 327 g water; 473 calories (31% from fat, 28% from protein, 41% from carb); 30 g Protein; 15 g total fat; 3 g saturated fat; 9 g monounsaturated fat; 1 g polyunsaturated fat; 45 g carb; 5 g fiber; 6 g sugar; 401 mg phosphorous; 56 mg calcium; 4 mg iron; 121 mg sodium; 1671 mg potassium; 1894 IU vitamin A; 0 mg ATE vitamin E; 30 mg vitamin C; 61 mg cholesterol

Glycemic Index: Low

Papaya-Pineapple Salsa

This fruity salsa is only mildly spicy, but it has great flavor. We like it best over fish, but try it with chicken or over a salad too.

¾ cup (135 g) ripe papaya, diced

¾ cup (120 g) fresh pineapple, diced

½ cup (65 g) jicama, diced

3 tablespoons (30 g) red onion

1 chili pepper, seeded and minced

1 clove garlic, minced

2 teaspoons (4 g) lime peel

2 tablespoons (30 ml) fresh lime juice

1 tablespoon (1 g) cilantro, minced

Combine papaya, pineapple, jicama, red onion, chili pepper, garlic, lime zest, lime juice, and cilantro. Cover and refrigerate until ready to serve. For best flavor and texture, do not make more than 2 hours before serving.

Yield: 8 servings

Each with: 46 g water; 23 calories (2% from fat, 5% from protein, 93% from carb); 0 g Protein; 0 g total fat; 0 g saturated fat; 0 g monounsaturated fat; 0 g polyunsaturated fat; 6 g carb; 1 g fiber; 4 g sugar; 6 mg phosphorous; 9 mg calcium; 0 mg iron; 1 mg sodium; 83 mg potassium; 196 IU vitamin A; 0 mg ATE vitamin E; 13 mg vitamin C; 0 mg cholesterol

Glycemic Index: Low

15

Asian

As I mentioned in the introduction, Asian food often has the reputation for being high in GI with its emphasis on rice and noodles. But it doesn't have to be that way. We have here a number of recipes that are low in GI. Many can stand on their own. Others can be combined with a reasonable quantity of rice and still fit within your diet.

Beef with Rice Noodles

This dish is traditional stir-fried beef and vegetable dish served with rice noodles, providing a quick and tasty meal.

1¾ pounds (795 g) beef round steak, boneless

4 tablespoons (60 ml) sake, or sherry, divided

1 tablespoon (6 g) finely chopped gingerroot

3 teaspoons (45 ml) vegetable oil, divided

1 clove garlic, crushed

4 ounces (115 g) rice noodles

2 cups (140 g) bok choy, thinly sliced

½ cup (50 g) green olives, thinly sliced

Trim fat from beef steak. Cut beef diagonally into ¼-inch (5 mm) strips. Mix beef, 2 tablespoons (30 ml) sake, the gingerroot, 2 teaspoons (10 ml) oil and garlic in medium glass or plastic bowl. Cover and refrigerate 30 minutes. Place rice noodles in large bowl. Cover with hot water. Let stand 10 minutes; drain well. Chop coarsely. Heat 1 teaspoon oil in wok. Add beef mixture; stir-fry about 5 minutes or until beef is done. Add rice noodles, bok choy, and onions. Stir-fry about 4 minutes or until bok choy is crisp-tender. Sprinkle mixture with 2 tablespoons (30 ml) sake. Serve over noodles.

Yield: 4 servings

Each with: 181 g water; 560 calories (25% from fat, 53% from protein, 22% from carb); 72 g Protein; 15 g total fat; 4 g saturated fat; 6 g monounsaturated fat; 3 g polyunsaturated fat; 29 g carb; 1 g fiber; 0 g sugar; 467 mg phosphorous; 45 mg calcium; 8 mg iron; 367 mg sodium; 712 mg potassium; 92 IU vitamin A; 0 mg ATE vitamin E; 2 mg vitamin C; 179 mg cholesterol

Glycemic Index: Low

Beef and Broccoli

I love Chinese food. I love it mostly because of the taste, but partly because dishes like this one can be prepared from start to finish in well under a half hour, making them great for weeknight dinners.

½ pound (225 g) beef round steak, boneless, cut into thin strips

1 dash white pepper

1 pound (455 g) broccoli

1 teaspoon cornstarch

1 teaspoon Dick's Reduced-Sodium Soy Sauce (see recipe in chapter 2)

1 teaspoon sesame oil

¼ cup (60 ml) low-sodium chicken broth

1 teaspoon vegetable oil

1 tablespoon (10 g) garlic finely chopped

1 teaspoon gingerroot, finely chopped

8 ounces (225 g) bamboo shoots

Trim fat from beef. Cut beef lengthwise into 2-inch (5 cm) strips. Cut strips crosswise into ⅛-inch slices. Toss beef with white pepper. Place broccoli in 1 inch (2½ cm) boiling water; heat to boiling. Cover and cook 2 minutes. Immediately rinse with cold water; drain. Mix cornstarch and soy sauce; stir in sesame oil and broth. Spray nonstick wok or 12-inch (30 cm) skillet with nonstick cooking spray; heat over medium-high heat until cooking spray starts to bubble. Add beef; stir-fry about 2 minutes or until brown. Remove beef from wok. Cool wok slightly. Wipe clean and re-spray. Add oil and rotate wok to coat sides. Heat over medium-high heat. Add garlic and ginger root; stir-fry 30 seconds. Add bamboo shoots; stir-fry 20 seconds. Stir in beef and broccoli. Stir in cornstarch mixture; cook and stir about 30 seconds or until thickened. Serve over rice.

Yield: 4 servings

Each with: 180 g water; 229 calories (27% from fat, 59% from protein, 14% from carb); 34 g Protein; 7 g total fat; 2 g saturated fat; 2 g monounsaturated fat; 2 g polyunsaturated fat; 8 g carb; 3 g fiber; 2 g sugar; 315 mg phosphorous; 64 mg calcium; 3 mg iron; 102 mg sodium; 693 mg potassium; 758 IU vitamin A; 15 mg ATE vitamin E; 101 mg vitamin C; 96 mg cholesterol

Glycemic Index: Low

Sesame Beef

Donna sent us this great recipe for sesame beef. It's one that those of you who love Chinese food will want to try.

2 tablespoons (30 ml) olive oil

2 tablespoons (26 g) sugar

2 tablespoons (30 ml) Dick's Reduced-Sodium Soy Sauce (see recipe in chapter 2)

2 cloves garlic

¼ cup (25 g) chopped green onions

Black pepper, to taste

1 pound (455 g) round steak, cut in strips

1 tablespoon (8 g) sesame seeds, toasted

Mix together 1 tablespoon (15 ml) of the oil, the sugar, soy sauce, garlic, green onions, and pepper. Marinate the meat in this mixture for at least 30 minutes. Heat the remaining oil in skillet or wok. Add meat and marinade and stir-fry. Serve over rice and top with sesame seeds.

Yield: 4 servings

Each with: 72 g water; 319 calories (45% from fat, 46% from protein, 9% from carb); 36 g protein; 15 g total fat; 4 g saturated fat; 5 g monounsaturated fat; 4 g polyunsaturated fat; 7 g carb; 0 g fiber; 6 g sugar; 13 mg calcium; 4 mg iron; 59 mg sodium; 372 mg potassium; 62 IU vitamin A; 2 mg vitamin C; 109 mg cholesterol

Glycemic Index: Low

Mongolian Beef

This dish is similar to what you get at Mongolian barbecue restaurants.

1 pound (455 g) flank steak

¼ teaspoon black pepper

2 tablespoons (30 ml) peanut oil

2 tablespoons (20 g) chopped garlic

2 green onions, slivered

Sauce

2 teaspoons (9 g) sugar

2 teaspoons (10 ml) Dick's Reduced-Sodium Soy Sauce (see recipe in chapter 2)

1 tablespoon (15 ml) oyster sauce

1 tablespoon (15 ml) wine (I suggest sherry.)

1½ tablespoons (12 g) cornstarch

¼ cup (60 ml) chicken stock

2 tablespoons (32 g) hoisin sauce

2 teaspoons (10 ml) ketchup

½ teaspoon crushed red chile pepper

Cut steak across the grain into strips about 2 inches (5 cm) long and very thin. Season with salt and pepper. In a separate bowl, combine sauce ingredients and mix well. Heat wok and then add oil. When hot, add garlic and cook quickly. Add beef and onions and stir-fry until tender. Add sauce mixture and cook about 1 minute while stirring. Serve over sticky rice or rice noodles.

Yield: 4 servings

Each with: 104 g water; 336 calories (46% from fat, 40% from protein, 14% from carb); 33 g protein; 17 g total fat; 5 g saturated fat; 7 g monounsaturated fat; 3 g polyunsaturated fat; 11 g carb; 0 g fiber; 5 g sugar; 261 mg phosphorus; 32 mg calcium; 2 mg iron; 1,150 mg sodium; 450 mg potassium; 116 IU vitamin A; 2 mg vitamin C; 63 mg cholesterol

Glycemic Index: Low

Chinese Stuffed Peppers

Stuffed peppers are given a decidedly Asian flavor with traditional oriental seasonings.

6 cups (900 g) green bell pepper

¼ cup (46 g) long grain rice

1 tablespoon (15 ml) vegetable oil

1 green onion, medium, chopped

1 tablespoon (6 g) fresh ginger, minced

1 garlic clove, minced

1½ pounds (680 g) ground pork

1 cup (130 g) frozen peas, thawed

3 tablespoons (45 ml) Dick's Reduced-Sodium Soy Sauce (see recipe in chapter 2)

3 tablespoons (45 ml) dry sherry

½ teaspoon pepper

1½ cup (355 ml) low-sodium beef broth

1 tablespoon (8 g) cornstarch

2 tablespoons (30 ml) water

Preheat oven to 375°F (190°C, or gas mark 5). Slice tops off peppers and scoop out seeds. Stand peppers in 9 x 9-inch (23 x 23 cm) square baking dish. In medium saucepan of boiling salted water, cook rice 7 minutes. Drain, rinse under cold water, and drain again. In medium skillet, heat oil. Add onion, ginger, and garlic. Cook over medium-high heat until vegetables are softened and fragrant but not browned, about 1 minute. Transfer to medium bowl. Add ground pork, peas, rice, 2 tablespoons (30 ml) soy sauce, 1 tablespoon (15 ml) sherry, and ½ teaspoon pepper to bowl. Mix gently but thoroughly to avoid crushing peas. Stuff peppers with meat mixture. In 2-cup (475 ml) glass measure, combine beef broth, remaining sherry, soy sauce, and pepper. Pour sauce over stuffed peppers and cover dish with foil. Bake 45 minutes. Remove foil from dish; reduce oven temperature to 350°F (180°C, or gas mark 4) and continue baking, basting a few times with sauce, for 15 minutes. Transfer peppers to serving platter. Place baking dish on top of stove. Dissolve cornstarch in 2 tablespoons (30 ml) water. Whisk into liquid in baking dish and cook over medium heat until sauce boils and thickens, about 2 minutes. Serve sauce with peppers.

Yield: 6 servings

Each with: 291 g water; 460 calories (53% from fat, 30% from protein, 18% from carb); 33 g Protein; 26 g total fat; 9 g saturated fat; 11 g monounsaturated fat; 4 g polyunsaturated fat; 20 g carb; 4 g fiber; 5 g sugar; 329 mg phosphorous; 54 mg calcium; 3 mg iron; 210 mg sodium; 777 mg potassium; 1129 IU vitamin A; 2 mg ATE vitamin E; 124 mg vitamin C; 107 mg cholesterol

Glycemic Index: Low

Chinese Meatballs

A place where I used to get lunch in the pre-diet days had a Chinese meatball entrée I was quite fond of. I've never been able to duplicate the flavor, but this is my favorite of the ways I've tried. They can be used in place of the meat in any of the Asian recipes.

1 pound (455 g) ground chicken breast

1 tablespoon (6 g) sodium-free beef bouillon

¼ teaspoon ginger

⅛ teaspoon garlic powder

⅛ teaspoon black pepper

1 tablespoon (15 ml) sherry

1 egg

Combine all ingredients. Shape into 1-inch (2½ cm) balls. Place in roasting pan that has been well coated with nonstick vegetable oil spray. Roast at 350°F (180°C, gas mark 4) until done, about 30 to 40 minutes, turning once.

Yield: 4 servings

Each with: 100 g water; 153 calories (14% from fat, 80% from protein, 6% from carb); 28 g protein; 2 g total fat; 1 g saturated fat; 1 g monounsaturated fat; 1 g polyunsaturated fat; 2 g carb; 0 g fiber; 1 g sugar; 245 mg phosphorus; 25 mg calcium; 1 mg iron; 123 mg sodium; 354 mg potassium; 90 IU vitamin A; 1 mg vitamin C; 66 mg cholesterol

Glycemic Index: Low

Five-Spice Chicken

This is a quick and simple recipe for chicken flavored with Chinese five-spice powder and other Asian ingredients. We sometimes place some fresh broccoli in the pan and let it all cook at the same time.

2 boneless skinless chicken breast halves

⅛ teaspoon fresh ginger, minced

2 tablespoons (12 g) orange zest

2 tablespoons (30 ml) orange juice

½ teaspoon five-spice powder

⅛ teaspoon rice wine vinegar

Mix together zest, juice, five-spice powder, ginger, and vinegar. Pour over chicken breasts placed in an 8 x 8-inch (20 x 20 cm) baking dish. Preheat oven to 350°F (180°C, or gas mark 4). Cover dish and bake for 40-45 minutes. Serve hot over rice with juices poured over each serving.

Yield: 2 servings

Each with: 45 g water; 105 calories (22% from fat, 70% from protein, 8% from carb); 18 g Protein; 2 g total fat; 1 g saturated fat; 1 g monounsaturated fat; 1 g polyunsaturated fat; 2 g carb; 0 g fiber; 0 g sugar; 130 mg phosphorous; 10 mg calcium; 1 mg iron; 41 mg sodium; 175 mg potassium; 24 IU vitamin A; 4 mg ATE vitamin E; 5 mg vitamin C; 47 mg cholesterol

Glycemic Index: Low

Sesame Chicken Teriyaki

These skewers of Asian sauced chicken with sesame seeds make a great appetizer or party food. But they are also easy enough to fix and so popular with both children and adults that you'll want to consider having them for dinner too.

2 tablespoons (30 ml) Dick's Reduced-Sodium Teriyaki Sauce (see recipe in chapter 2)

1 tablespoon (15 ml) water

2 cloves garlic, minced

¼ teaspoon ground ginger

6 ounces (170 g) boneless skinless chicken breasts, cut into ¾-inch (2 cm) wide strips

¼ teaspoon sesame seeds, toasted

For marinade, in a small mixing bowl combine teriyaki sauce, water, garlic, and ginger. Stir in chicken. Let stand 20 minutes at room temperature, stirring occasionally. Drain. Thread chicken, accordion-style, on two 10–12-inch (25–30 cm) skewers or four 6-inch (15 cm) skewers. Place on the unheated rack of a broiler pan. Broil 4–5-inch (10–13 cm) from heat for 3 minutes. Turn chicken and broil 2–3 minutes more or until chicken is tender and no longer pink. Sprinkle with toasted sesame seeds.

Yield: 2 servings

Each with: 71 g water; 96 calories (12% from fat, 87% from protein, 1% from carb); 20 g Protein; 1 g total fat; 0 g saturated fat; 0 g monounsaturated fat; 0 g polyunsaturated fat; 0 g carb; 0 g fiber; 0 g sugar; 169 mg phosphorous; 13 mg calcium; 1 mg iron; 56 mg sodium; 222 mg potassium; 18 IU vitamin A; 5 mg ATE vitamin E; 1 mg vitamin C; 49 mg cholesterol

Glycemic Index: Low

Glazed Chicken and Vegetables

This was the first dish we tried out of Merle Schell's Chinese cookbook, and it was a winner. We've made some changes since, but the inspiration was hers.

2 boneless chicken breasts, shredded

1 tablespoon (15 ml) low-sodium chicken broth

1 tablespoon (15 ml) sherry

1 egg white

2 tablespoons (16 g) cornstarch

2 cups (475 ml) low-sodium chicken broth

2 tablespoons (30 ml) Dick's Reduced-Sodium Soy Sauce (see recipe in chapter 2)

(continued on page 410)

1 teaspoon red wine vinegar

Black pepper, to taste

2 tablespoons (30 ml) sesame oil

½ cup (65 g) sliced carrot

1 teaspoon minced gingerroot

1 cup (71 g) broccoli florets

1 cup (70 g) sliced mushrooms

¼ cup (60 ml) water

1½ teaspoons dry mustard

¼ cup (25 g) sliced scallions

In a bowl, combine first 4 ingredients and 1 tablespoon (8 g) of the cornstarch, stir until blended, and set aside. In a second bowl, combine chicken broth, soy sauce, vinegar, and pepper. Set aside. Heat oil in wok. Add carrot, ginger, broccoli, and mushrooms and stir-fry 1 minute. Add chicken broth mixture, reduce heat, and simmer 1 minute. While mixture is cooking, combine remaining cornstarch, water, and mustard powder. Raise heat to medium. When sauce starts to bubble, add chicken mixture and scallions. Cook 1 minute or until chicken is white all over. Stir in cornstarch mixture and continue stirring until sauce is thickened.

Yield: 4 servings

Each with: 216 g water; 157 calories (47% from fat, 31% from protein, 22% from carb); 12 g protein; 8 g total fat; 1 g saturated fat; 3 g monounsaturated fat; 3 g polyunsaturated fat; 8 g carb; 1 g fiber; 2 g sugar; 35 mg calcium; 1 mg iron; 101 mg sodium; 377 mg potassium; 2,527 IU vitamin A; 20 mg vitamin C; 22 mg cholesterol

Glycemic Index: Low

HINT: Pay attention to the short times for stir-frying. It's easy to end up with the vegetables overcooked by the time you get the sauce thickened.

Chicken and Pepper Stir-Fry

Usually we think of pepper steak with beef and green pepper. Here we turn that around by using chicken and red peppers to create a delightful alternative.

1 pound (455 g) boneless skinless chicken breasts

3 tablespoons (45 ml) Dick's Reduced-Sodium Soy Sauce (see recipe in chapter 2)

1 tablespoon (15 ml) dry sherry

½ cup (80 g) onion, cut into wedges

1 cup (150 g) red peppers, thinly sliced

1½ cups (105 g) mushroom, sliced

1 tablespoon (15 ml) olive oil

1 teaspoon gingerroot, grated

8 ounces (225 g) bamboo shoots, drained

¼ cup (120 ml) low-sodium chicken broth

1 teaspoon cornstarch

¼ teaspoon pepper

Cut chicken into ½-inch (1 cm) pieces. place in a bowl; stir in soy sauce and sherry. Let stand 30 minutes. Spray a cold wok or large skillet with nonstick vegetable oil spray; preheat over medium-high heat. Add onion, stir-fry 2 minutes. Add peppers and stir-fry 1 minute. Add mushrooms and stir-fry about 1 minute more or until veggies are crisp-tender. Remove veggies from wok; set aside. Drain chicken, reserving the marinade. Add oil to wok. Add gingerroot; stir-fry 15 seconds. Add half the chicken and stir fry 3-4 minutes until no longer pink. Remove. Stir-fry remaining chicken 3-4 minutes. Return all chicken, veggies, and bamboo shoots to wok; push from center of wok. Stir broth, cornstarch, and pepper into reserved marinade; add to wok. Cook and stir until slightly thickened; toss gently to coat chicken mixture. Serve while hot.

Yield: 4 servings

Each with: 224 g water; 244 calories (25% from fat, 65% from protein, 11% from carb); 38 g Protein; 6 g total fat; 1 g saturated fat; 3 g monounsaturated fat; 1 g polyunsaturated fat; 6 g carb; 1 g fiber; 3 g sugar; 378 mg phosphorous; 30 mg calcium; 2 mg iron; 121 mg sodium; 644 mg potassium; 1248 IU vitamin A; 22 mg ATE vitamin E; 51 mg vitamin C; 111 mg cholesterol

Glycemic Index: Low

Chicken and Snow Peas

This is a fairly traditional Chinese-type recipe, similar to dishes like moo goo gai pan.

1 pound (455 g) boneless chicken breasts

2 tablespoons (16 g) cornstarch

1 egg white

1 tablespoon (15 ml) sherry

½ teaspoon white pepper

8 ounces (225 g) mushrooms, sliced

1½ cups (355 ml) low-sodium chicken broth

1 tablespoon (6 g) sliced gingerroot

5 tablespoons (75 ml) olive oil, divided

¼ cup (25 g) sliced green onion

¼ cup (25 g) sliced celery

4 ounces (115 g) snow peas

¼ cup (31 g) sliced water chestnuts

1 cup (70 g) coarsely shredded Napa cabbage

In a bowl, combine the chicken, 1 tablespoon (8 g) of the cornstarch, the egg white, sherry, and pepper. Marinate at least 15 minutes. Simmer mushrooms in broth 15 minutes. Drain and reserve liquid. Simmer gingerroot in broth until ready to use. Mix remaining cornstarch with 2 tablespoons (30 ml) water. Shake well to thoroughly dissolve. Heat 3 tablespoons (45 ml) of the olive oil in a wok or heavy skillet. Add chicken and cook, stirring, just until pieces separate and chicken is no longer pink. Drain into a sieve over a bowl. Add remaining olive oil to wok. Add onions, celery, snow peas, water chestnuts, mushrooms, and cabbage and stir-fry for 2 minutes. Remove ginger pieces from chicken broth. Add broth to wok. Bring to a boil. Return chicken to wok. Add water/cornstarch mixture. Cook, stirring, until thickened. Serve over steamed rice.

Yield: 4 servings

Each with: 235 g water; 251 calories (64% from fat, 16% from protein, 20% from carb); 10 g protein; 18 g total fat; 3 g saturated fat; 13 g monounsaturated fat; 2 g polyunsaturated fat; 13 g carb; 2 g fiber; 3 g sugar; 137 mg phosphorus; 38 mg calcium; 2 mg iron; 66 mg sodium; 474 mg potassium; 473 IU vitamin A; 21 mg vitamin C; 11 mg cholesterol

Glycemic Index: Low

Chicken and Cashews

This is a spicy variation of Kung Pao Chicken using cashews rather than the more common peanuts. Vary the red pepper flakes according to how hot you want it to be.

2 boneless skinless chicken breasts, cut into ¾-inch (2 cm) cubes

3 tablespoons (45 ml) Dick's Reduced-Sodium Soy Sauce, divided (see recipe in chapter 2)

1 tablespoon (15 ml) rice wine, or sherry

1 tablespoon (8 g) cornstarch

2 teaspoons (9 g) sugar

1 teaspoon white vinegar

¼ cup (60 ml) vegetable oil

½ teaspoon red pepper flakes

3 green onions, sliced

1 tablespoon (6 g) fresh ginger, minced

½ cup (70 g) unsalted cashews

Marinate chicken in 1 tablespoon (15 ml) soy sauce and rice wine for 30 minutes. Combine 2 tablespoons (30 ml) soy sauce, cornstarch, sugar, and vinegar and set aside. Heat oil in wok or skillet. Add red pepper to taste and cook until black. Add chicken and stir-fry for 2 minutes. Remove chicken. Add green onions and ginger and stir-fry for 1 minute. Return chicken to wok. Cook 2 minutes, stirring constantly; add soy sauce mixture and any remaining chicken marinade. Add cashews. Cook until thickened and bubbly. Serve over cooked rice.

Yield: 4 servings

Each with: 31 g water; 285 calories (69% from fat, 15% from protein, 15% from carb); 11 g Protein; 22 g total fat; 3 g saturated fat; 9 g monounsaturated fat; 9 g polyunsaturated fat; 11 g carb; 1 g fiber; 3 g sugar; 157 mg phosphorous; 14 mg calcium; 1 mg iron; 27 mg sodium; 214 mg potassium; 101 IU vitamin A; 2 mg ATE vitamin E; 1 mg vitamin C; 21 mg cholesterol

Glycemic Index: Low

Noodles with Peanut Sauce and Chicken

I used to be leery of Asian recipes that called for peanut butter. Then I tried this one and it was so good that I now actually consider finding a recipe with peanut butter a really good thing.

8 ounces (225 g) spaghetti

½ cup (130 g) peanut butter, creamy

2 tablespoons (30 ml) Dick's Reduced-Sodium Soy Sauce (see recipe in chapter 2)

1 teaspoon gingerroot, grated

½ cup (120 ml) low-sodium chicken broth

4 ounces (115 g) bean sprouts

1 cup (150 g) red bell peppers, sliced

2 green onion, sliced

1 pound (455 g) boneless skinless chicken breast

Cook spaghetti. Mix peanut butter, soy sauce, and gingerroot in saucepan. Add chicken broth. Add spaghetti, bean sprouts, bell pepper, and onion. Toss. Slice chicken into thin strips. Stir fry until no longer pink. Stir into spaghetti mixture.

Yield: 4 servings

Each with: 214 g water ; 403 calories (39% from fat, 37% from protein, 24% from carb); 38 g protein; 18 g total fat; 3 g saturated fat; 8 g monounsaturated fat; 5 g polyunsaturated fat; 25 g carb; 6 g fiber; 5 g sugar; 404 mg phosphorous; 43 mg calcium; 2 mg iron; 131 mg sodium; 669 mg potassium; 1194 IU vitamin A; 7 mg ATE vitamin E; 49 mg vitamin C; 66 mg cholesterol

Glycemic Index: Low

Chicken Fried Rice

This is our favorite recipe for fried rice. It's a little more work than some recipes, but I think the result is worth it.

1 pound (455 g) boneless skinless chicken breast

½ teaspoon cornstarch

1 dash white pepper

1 cup (50 g) bean sprouts

5 tablespoons (75 ml) vegetable oil

2 eggs, slightly beaten

2½ ounces (70 g) sliced mushrooms

3 cups (495 g) white rice

2 tablespoons (30 ml) Dick's Reduced-Sodium Soy Sauce (see recipe in chapter 2)

2 green onions with tops, sliced

Cut chicken into ¼-inch (5 mm) pieces. Toss together chicken, cornstarch, and dash white pepper. Heat wok until very hot. Add 1 tablespoon (15 ml) oil and coat sides. Add eggs. Cook and stir until eggs are thickened throughout but still moist. Remove eggs from wok. Wash and dry wok thoroughly. Reheat wok, add 2 tablespoons (30 ml) oil, and coat sides. Add chicken and stir-fry until chicken turns white. Add bean sprouts and mushrooms. Stir-fry 1 minute. Remove from wok and drain. Heat wok very hot, add 2 tablespoons oil, and coat sides. Add rice and stir-fry 1 minute. Stir in soy sauce. Add eggs, chicken mixture, and green onions and stir-fry 30 seconds.

Yield: 5 servings

Each with: 202 g water; 360 calories (44% from fat, 30% from protein, 26% from carb); 27 g Protein; 17 g total fat; 3 g saturated fat; 5 g monounsaturated fat; 8 g polyunsaturated fat; 23 g carb; 1 g fiber; 1 g sugar; 249 mg phosphorous; 28 mg calcium; 1 mg iron; 131 mg sodium; 324 mg potassium; 130 IU vitamin A; 37 mg ATE vitamin E; 1 mg vitamin C; 147 mg cholesterol

Glycemic Index: Low

Chinese Dumplings

This is a fairly traditional recipe for Chinese dumplings.

Dough

1 cup (125 g) flour

½ cup (120 ml) water, boiling

Filling

4 ounces (115 g) Napa cabbage, shredded

½ pound (225 g) ground pork loin

2 tablespoons (12 g) chopped green onion

½ tablespoon white wine

½ teaspoon cornstarch

½ teaspoon sesame oil

Dash white pepper

1 tablespoon (15 ml) olive oil

Cut the cabbage across into thin strips. In a large bowl, mix the cabbage, pork, green onions, wine, cornstarch, sesame oil, and the pepper. In a bowl, mix the flour and boiling water until a soft dough forms. Knead the dough on a lightly floured surface about 5 minutes or until smooth. Shape into a roll 12 inches (30 cm) long and cut into ½-inch (1 cm) slices. Roll 1 slice of dough into a 3-inch (7½ cm) circle and place 1 tablespoon pork mixture in the center of the circle. Lift up the edges of the circle and pinch 5 pleats up to create a pouch to encase the mixture. Pinch the top together. Repeat with the remaining slices of dough and filling. Heat a wok or nonstick skillet until very hot. Add 1 tablespoon (15 ml) olive oil, tilting the wok to coat the sides. Place 12 dumplings in a single layer in the wok and fry 2 minutes or until the bottoms are golden brown. Add ½ cup (120 ml) water. Cover and cook 6 to 7 minutes or until the water is absorbed. Repeat with the remaining dumplings.

Yield: 24 servings

Each with: 17 g water; 46 calories (33% from fat, 29% from protein, 37% from carb); 3 g protein; 2 g total fat; 0 g saturated fat; 1 g monounsaturated fat; 0 g polyunsaturated fat; 4 g carb; 0 g fiber; 0 g sugar; 28 mg phosphorus; 3 mg calcium; 0 mg iron; 6 mg sodium; 46 mg potassium; 18 IU vitamin A; 0 mg vitamin C; 8 mg cholesterol

Glycemic Index: Low

Bar-B-Q Pork Tenderloin

Pork tenderloins marinate in an Asian sauce before grilling and are then served with a short cut barbecue sauce that starts with a bottle of commercial sauce, and adds ingredients to give it an Asian flavor.

3 pounds (1⅓ kg) pork tenderloin (boneless)

⅔ cup (160 ml) Dick's Reduced-Sodium Soy Sauce (see recipe in chapter 2)

⅔ cup sesame oil

4 minced garlic cloves

1 tablespoon (5.5 g) ground ginger

19 ounces (535 g) barbecue sauce

Trim pork tenderloin of all fat. Combine ⅓ cup (80 ml) soy sauce, ⅓ cup (80 ml) sesame oil, 3 minced garlic cloves, and ginger, in a deep bowl and mix well. Place pork into marinade and place in refrigerator for 6 to 8 hours (overnight if you prefer). Remove pork from marinade and place on covered grill. Grill until done, turning occasionally. To prepare sauce, combine barbecue sauce, ⅓ cup (80 ml) sesame oil, ⅓ cup (80 ml) soy sauce, and 1 minced garlic clove in a bowl and mix well. Serve over sliced pork tenderloins.

Yield: 8 servings

Each with: 163 g water; 485 calories (45% from fat, 31% from protein, 24% from carb); 37 g Protein; 24 g total fat; 5 g saturated fat; 10 g monounsaturated fat; 8 g polyunsaturated fat; 29 g carb; 0 g fiber; 22 g sugar; 385 mg phosphorous; 9 mg calcium; 2 mg iron; 650 mg sodium; 632 mg potassium; 11 IU vitamin A; 3 mg ATE vitamin E; 2 mg vitamin C; 111 mg cholesterol

Glycemic Index: Low

Japanese Pork Chop Stir Fry

The microwave makes this meal extra quick, but the taste is every bit as good as if you'd slaved over it for hours.

10 ounces (280 g) frozen Japanese mixed vegetables, with seasoning

8 ounces (225 g) boneless pork loin chops cut into julienne strips

1 teaspoon olive oil

½ teaspoon cornstarch

2 teaspoons (30 ml) dry sherry

1 teaspoons Dick's Reduced-Sodium Soy Sauce (see recipe in chapter 2)

Empty frozen vegetables into a 1-quart (1 L) casserole; reserve seasoning packet. Add pork and oil to vegetables. Cover with lid or vented plastic wrap and microwave on high three minutes. Empty contents of seasoning packet into a small bowl. Stir in cornstarch; blend in sherry and soy sauce. Stir mixture into vegetables; re-cover. Microwave on high three to four minutes or until vegetables are crisp-tender and pork is no longer pink. Stir.

TIP

Serve this over rice.

Yield: 2 servings

Each with: 205 g water; 268 calories (25% from fat, 44% from protein, 31% from carb); 28 g Protein; 7 g total fat; 2 g saturated fat; 4 g monounsaturated fat; 1 g polyunsaturated fat; 20 g carb; 6 g fiber; 5 g sugar; 320 mg phosphorous; 51 mg calcium; 2 mg iron; 108 mg sodium; 664 mg potassium; 6071 IU vitamin A; 2 mg ATE vitamin E; 6 mg vitamin C; 71 mg cholesterol

Glycemic Index: Low

Teriyaki Fish

This recipe uses the soy sauce substitute, which is a separate recipe in chapter 2. You can use low-sodium soy sauce, but be aware of the extra sodium you are adding.

¼ cup (32 g) flour

⅛ teaspoon black pepper

2 catfish fillets, about 6 ounces (128 g) each, cut in 1-inch (2 ½-cm) pieces

2 tablespoons (30 ml) olive oil

¼ cup (60 ml) Dick's Reduced-Sodium Soy Sauce (see recipe in chapter 2)

¼ cup (50 g) sugar

½ teaspoon sesame oil

¼ cup (12 g) chopped chives

Combine the flour and pepper in a resealable plastic bag. Add the fish and shake to coat. Heat the olive oil in a large skillet. Add the fish and cook until done. Remove from skillet. Add the soy sauce and sugar to the pan. Cook and stir until the sugar is melted. Stir in the sesame oil. Add the fish and chives and stir to coat.

Yield: 4 servings

Each with: 64 g water; 251 calories (49% from fat, 21% from protein, 30% from carb); 13 g protein; 14 g total fat; 2 g saturated fat; 5 g monounsaturated fat; 5 g polyunsaturated fat; 19 g carb; 0 g fiber; 13 g sugar; 171 mg phosphorus; 12 mg calcium; 1 mg iron; 42 mg sodium; 256 mg potassium; 171 IU vitamin A; 2 mg vitamin C; 37 mg cholesterol

Glycemic Index: Low

Pineapple Rice

This makes not only a delicious version of fried rice but also a great presentation by using the hollowed out pineapple as a serving bowl.

1 fresh pineapple

2 cups (330 g) cooked rice

4 ounces (115 g) shrimp

1 boneless skinless chicken breast, cooked

2 green onions

¼ cup (33 g) peas

1 dash rice wine

2 teaspoons (10 ml) oil

Cut chicken into bite size pieces. Cut stem from pineapple. Cut pineapple in half. Hollow top and bottom portions of pineapple; set aside. Dice pineapple meat. Reserve ¼ cup of pineapple meat and save remainder for another dish or dessert. Heat 2 teaspoons (10 ml) of oil in wok, add rice and stir-fry a minute or two. Add shrimp and chicken, stir-fry another minute or two. Add peas, sliced green onions, and pineapple. Stir-fry another minute or two or until all is hot and well blended. Shake in a little rice wine. Heat pineapple shells in microwave. Serve rice mixture in pineapple.

Yield: 2 servings

Each with: 295 g water; 519 calories (29% from fat, 58% from protein, 13% from carb); 71 g Protein; 16 g total fat; 4 g saturated fat; 4 g monounsaturated fat; 6 g polyunsaturated fat; 16 g carb; 1 g fiber; 5 g sugar; 1111 mg phosphorous; 95 mg calcium; 3 mg iron; 380 mg sodium; 797 mg potassium; 1208 IU vitamin A; 234 mg ATE vitamin E; 41 mg vitamin C; 945 mg cholesterol

Glycemic Index: Low

Thai Style Shrimp and Chicken Soup

This soup is full of the complex flavors of Thai cooking and was a big hit around our house. It's also good served over rice.

2 boneless skinless chicken breasts

6 cups (1.4 L) water

1 small onion, peeled and chopped

1 bay leaf

2 sprigs parsley

½ teaspoon thyme

⅛ teaspoon pepper

1 garlic clove, crushed

2 teaspoons (4 g) coriander

1½ teaspoons chili powder

1 tablespoon (15 ml) Dick's Reduced-Sodium Soy Sauce (see recipe in chapter 2)

½ pound (225 g) shrimp

2 cups (140 g) mushrooms, sliced

6 scallions, with tops, sliced

⅓ cup cilantro, chopped fresh

Cut meat into strips. Place in large saucepan. Add water, onion, bay leaf, parsley, thyme, salt, and pepper. Bring to a boil. Lower heat and cook slowly, covered, 1 hour. Strain broth into a saucepan. Combine garlic, coriander, chili powder, and soy sauce. Stir into broth. Bring to a boil. Add chicken, shrimp, and mushrooms. Cook slowly, covered, about 5 minutes, until the shrimp turns pink and the chicken is tender. Stir in scallions and fresh cilantro. Remove and discard bay leaf. Serve in bowls over or with rice.

Yield: 6 servings

Each with: 307 g water; 75 calories (14% from fat, 76% from protein, 9% from carb); 14 g Protein; 1 g total fat; 0 g saturated fat; 0 g monounsaturated fat; 0 g polyunsaturated fat; 2 g carb; 1 g fiber; 0 g sugar; 148 mg phosphorous; 38 mg calcium; 2 mg iron; 88 mg sodium; 242 mg potassium; 432 IU vitamin A; 22 mg ATE vitamin E; 4 mg vitamin C; 71 mg cholesterol

Glycemic Index: Low

16

Cajun and Creole

Cajun dishes can be another good choice for a low-GI diet with their high flavor content and their reliance on vegetables and meat. We have all the classics here—gumbo, jambalaya, and étouffée—as well as a select set of other dishes and a great recipe for making your own Cajun sausage.

Smoked Chicken and Pepperoni Gumbo

This is an unusual gumbo made with pepperoni and smoked chicken breast. It's a good way to use up leftover smoked chicken. You can substitute smoked sausage for the pepperoni if desired.

¼ teaspoon white pepper

¼ teaspoon cayenne

½ teaspoon black pepper

½ teaspoon thyme

1 teaspoon dry parsley flakes

½ teaspoon file powder, optional

2 cups (320 g) onion

2 cups (300 g) green bell peppers

2 cups (200 g) celery

2 cups (280 g) cooked chicken breast, smoked

4 ounces (115 g) pepperoni, sliced

6 cups (1.4 L) low-sodium chicken broth

Cut vegetables into small pieces (about ½-inch [1 cm]). Cut smoked chicken breasts into bite size pieces. Cut pepperoni into slices about ⅛-inch (3 mm) thick (about twice as thick as presliced). Using cast iron Dutch oven or heavy covered skillet, sauté onions over medium high heat in the dry pan for about 3–4 minutes, stirring constantly. Then add the rest of the vegetables and cook for about 5 minutes more on medium heat, stirring frequently. Then add spices and stir to incorporate. Add the broth and the pepperoni slices. Turn heat down to medium low and simmer for at least ½ hour or until vegetables are tender and flavors are merged. About 5 minutes before serving, add the chicken breasts to the mixture.

Yield: 6 servings

Each with: 393 g water; 242 calories (40% from fat, 40% from protein, 20% from carb); 24 g Protein; 11 g total fat; 4 g saturated fat; 5 g monounsaturated fat; 1 g polyunsaturated fat; 12 g carb; 3 g fiber; 5 g sugar; 246 mg phosphorous; 55 mg calcium; 2 mg iron; 476 mg sodium; 646 mg potassium; 389 IU vitamin A; 3 mg ATE vitamin E; 45 mg vitamin C; 62 mg cholesterol

Glycemic Index: Low

Slow Cooker Sausage and Shrimp Jambalaya

This easy jambalaya cooks in the slow cooker while you are gone. When you get home, just toss in the shrimp and rice and dinner is ready in half an hour.

½ pound (225 g) shrimp, cooked and shelled

1 cup (150 g) green bell pepper, chopped

⅛ teaspoon cayenne

1 cup (160 g) onion, chopped

1½ cups (270 g) tomatoes, chopped

4 ounces (115 g) smoked sausage, sliced

1 cup (100 g) celery, chopped

8 ounces (225 g) chicken breast, cut in ½-inch (1 cm) cubes

1 clove garlic, crushed

2 cups (475 ml) low-sodium beef broth

1 tablespoon (4 g) parsley, minced

2 teaspoons (2.8 g) thyme

2 teaspoons (2.6 g) oregano, chopped

1 cup (165 g) rice, cooked

Shell shrimp; halve lengthwise. In slow cooker, combine all ingredients except shrimp and rice. Cover and cook on low 9–10 hours. Turn slow cooker on high and add cooked shrimp and cooked rice. Cover; cook on high 20–30 minutes.

Yield: 6 servings

Each with: 260 g water; 213 calories (25% from fat, 47% from protein, 28% from carb); 25 g Protein; 6 g total fat; 2 g saturated fat; 2 g monounsaturated fat; 1 g polyunsaturated fat; 15 g carb; 2 g fiber; 2 g sugar; 213 mg phosphorous; 62 mg calcium; 3 mg iron; 377 mg sodium; 441 mg potassium; 580 IU vitamin A; 23 mg ATE vitamin E; 37 mg vitamin C; 103 mg cholesterol

Glycemic Index: Low

Shrimp and Sausage Creole

This dish of sausage and shrimp in a cream sauce gives a nice combination of creaminess with some heat. It has a flavor that is very like the Creole dishes served in some of New Orleans's most expensive restaurants.

1 tablespoon (15 ml) olive oil

10 shrimp

4 ounces (115 g) andouille sausage, sliced

1 cup (70 g) sliced mushrooms

½ cup (120 ml) skim milk

2 teaspoons (10 ml) Worcestershire sauce

1 teaspoon Creole seasoning

1 tablespoon (4 g) parsley

Heat olive oil in a heavy, large skillet over medium-high heat. Add shrimp and sausage and sauté until shrimp just turn pink, about 3 minutes. Using slotted spoon, transfer shrimp and sausage to a plate. Add mushrooms to same skillet and sauté until tender, about 4 minutes. Stir in milk, Worcestershire sauce, and seasoning. Simmer until sauce thickens, about 3 minutes. Return shrimp and sausage to skillet and simmer until shrimp are cooked through, about 1 minute. Sprinkle parsley over top. Serve over pasta.

Yield: 2 servings

Each with: 137 g water; 349 calories (72% from fat, 20% from protein, 8% from Carb); 17 g protein; 28 g total fat; 8 g saturated fat; 15 g monounsaturated fat; 3 g polyunsaturated fat; 7 g carb; 0 g fiber; 1 g sugar; 108 mg calcium; 2 mg iron; 251 mg sodium; 429 mg potassium; 350 IU vitamin A; 14 mg vitamin C; 95 mg cholesterol

Glycemic Index: Low

Catfish Creole

A simple, Creole-style recipe. Any other white fish can be substituted for the catfish.

2 tablespoons (28 g) unsalted butter

1 cup (160 g) chopped onion

½ cup (50 g) chopped celery

½ cup (75 g) chopped green bell pepper

1 clove garlic, minced

1 can (14½ ounces or 410 g) no-salt-added tomatoes

1 lemon, sliced

1 tablespoon (15 ml) Worcestershire sauce

1 tablespoon (7 g) paprika

1 bay leaf

¼ teaspoon thyme

¼ teaspoon Tabasco sauce

2 pounds (900 g) catfish fillets

Melt the butter in a large skillet over medium heat. Add the onion, celery, bell pepper, and garlic. Cook until soft. Add tomatoes and their liquid. Break the tomatoes with a spoon. Add lemon slices, Worcestershire sauce, paprika, bay leaf, thyme, and Tabasco. Cook, stirring occasionally, for about 15 minutes or until the sauce is slightly thickened. Press fish pieces down into sauce and spoon some of the sauce over the top of the fish. Cover the pan and simmer gently until the fish flakes when prodded with a fork. Remove bay leaf and serve over hot cooked rice.

Yield: 6 servings

Each with: 169 g water; 142 calories (50% from fat, 26% from protein, 23% from carb); 10 g protein; 8 g total fat; 3 g saturated fat; 3 g monounsaturated fat; 1 g polyunsaturated fat; 9 g carb; 2 g fiber; 4 g sugar; 144 mg phosphorus; 47 mg calcium; 2 mg iron; 74 mg sodium; 454 mg potassium; 939 IU vitamin A; 31 mg vitamin C; 35 mg cholesterol

Glycemic Index: Low

Creole Pork Chops

Because they are only mildly spicy, these chops cooked in a Creole style sauce should be popular even with people who don't usually like Cajun and Creole food.

6 pork loin chops

3 tablespoons (45 ml) olive oil

1½ cups (240 g) onion, sliced

2 cloves garlic, minced

¼ cup (38 g) green bell pepper, chopped

½ cup (120 ml) dry white wine

14 ounces (400 g) no-salt-added tomatoes

3 tablespoons (45 ml) lemon juice

1½ tablespoons (25 ml) Worcestershire sauce

¼ teaspoon pepper

1 bay leaf

3 cups (495 g) rice, cooked

Brown pork chops on both sides in 1½ tablespoons (25 ml) hot oil in skillet; drain chops and discard drippings. Add remaining 1½ tablespoons (25 ml) oil. Sauté onions and garlic in skillet for 3 minutes. Add green pepper. Sauté for 1 minute. Add wine. Bring to a boil; stirring to deglaze skillet. Return chops to skillet; spoon sauce over chops. Add tomatoes, lemon juice, seasonings, and enough water to cover chops if necessary. Simmer, lightly covered, for 1 hour or until chops are tender, turning occasionally. Remove chops to warming platter. Remove bay leaf. Cook sauce over high heat until thickened to desired consistency. Spoon over chops.

Yield: 6 servings

Each with: 257 g water; 341 calories (32% from fat, 30% from protein, 38% from carb); 25 g Protein; 11 g total fat; 2 g saturated fat; 7 g monounsaturated fat; 1 g polyunsaturated fat; 31 g carb; 2 g fiber; 4 g sugar; 288 mg phosphorous; 54 mg calcium; 2 mg iron; 101 mg sodium; 649 mg potassium; 118 IU vitamin A; 2 mg ATE vitamin E; 25 mg vitamin C; 64 mg cholesterol

Glycemic Index: Low

Chicken Étouffée

This is a quick cooking Cajun dish, but the flavor is excellent.

1 cup (160 g) onion, chopped

½ cup (75 g) green bell peppers, chopped

½ cup (75 g) red bell peppers, chopped

½ cup (50 g) celery, chopped

1 clove garlic, minced

2 tablespoons (28 g) unsalted butter

2 tablespoons (16 g) flour

3 cups (420 g) cooked chicken breast chopped

¾ cup (175 g) water

½ teaspoon thyme

¼ teaspoon cayenne

1 dash Tabasco

2 cups (330 g) rice, cooked

Coat a large skillet with nonstick vegetable oil spray. Place over medium heat until hot. Add onion and other vegetables; sauté until tender. Remove from skillet; set aside. Place butter and flour in skillet; cook over low heat 5 minutes, stirring constantly, until mixture is color of a copper penny. Return vegetables to skillet. Add chicken and other ingredients except rice. Simmer 2 minutes or until thoroughly heated. Serve over hot, cooked rice.

Yield: 8 servings

Each with: 126 g water; 184 calories (25% from fat, 40% from protein, 35% from carb); 18 g Protein; 5 g total fat; 2 g saturated fat; 1 g monounsaturated fat; 1 g polyunsaturated fat; 16 g carb; 1 g fiber; 2 g sugar; 152 mg phosphorous; 24 mg calcium; 1 mg iron; 47 mg sodium; 235 mg potassium; 479 IU vitamin A; 27 mg ATE vitamin E; 21 mg vitamin C; 52 mg cholesterol

Glycemic Index: Low

Cajun Chicken Kabobs

The yogurt, while not traditionally a Cajun ingredient, helps to keep the chicken moist and limits the spiciness.

1 pound (455 g) boneless chicken breast halves, cubed

5½ ounces (155 g) plain fat-free yogurt

1 tablespoon (4 g) Cajun seasoning

2 teaspoons (4 g) coriander

½ teaspoon lemon juice

1 cup (150 g) diced red bell pepper

8 ounces (225 g) pineapple chunks

TIP *We usually serve this over rice, but they also are good as part of a main-dish salad.*

Place the chicken in a bowl. Mix the yogurt, Cajun seasoning, coriander, and lemon juice together and stir into the chicken. Refrigerate for 10 to 15 minutes. Thread onto 4 large skewers, alternating with the pepper and pineapple pieces. Place on a preheated grill or under the broiler and cook for 10 to 15 minutes, turning occasionally and basting with any remaining marinade.

Yield: 4 servings

Each with: 207 g water; 176 calories (9% from fat, 67% from protein, 24% from carb); 29 g protein; 2 g total fat; 0 g saturated fat; 0 g monounsaturated fat; 0 g polyunsaturated fat; 10 g carb; 1 g fiber; 9 g sugar; 297 mg phosphorus; 105 mg calcium; 1 mg iron; 106 mg sodium; 557 mg potassium; 1,233 IU vitamin A; 57 mg vitamin C; 67 mg cholesterol

Glycemic Index: Low

Baked Cajun Chicken

The preparation of this dish is not traditionally Cajun, but the flavor definitely is.

2 pounds (900 g) chicken breasts

2 tablespoons (30 ml) skim milk

2 tablespoons (13.8 g) onion powder

½ teaspoon thyme, crushed

¼ teaspoon garlic powder

¼ teaspoon white pepper

¼ teaspoon black pepper

Remove skin from chicken. Rinse chicken and pat dry. Spray a 13 x 9 x 2-inch (33 x 23 x 5 cm) baking dish with nonstick coating. Arrange the chicken, meaty sides up, in dish. Brush with milk. In small bowl, mix onion powder, thyme, garlic powder, white pepper, and black pepper. Sprinkle over chicken. Bake in a 375°F (190°C, or gas mark 5) oven for 45 to 55 minutes or until the chicken is tender and no longer pink.

Yield: 4 servings

Each with: 162 g water; 359 calories (18% from fat, 78% from protein, 4% from carb); 66 g Protein; 7 g total fat; 2 g saturated fat; 2 g monounsaturated fat; 2 g polyunsaturated fat; 4 g carb; 0 g fiber; 1 g sugar; 396 mg phosphorous; 56 mg calcium; 2 mg iron; 149 mg sodium; 475 mg potassium; 64 IU vitamin A; 18 mg ATE vitamin E; 1 mg vitamin C; 175 mg cholesterol

Glycemic Index: Low

Blackened Chicken

This give you a nice Cajun flavor right off the grill.

4 chicken thighs

2 tablespoons (28 g) unsalted butter, melted

5 teaspoons (15 g) Cajun blackening spice mix

Trim excess fat from the chicken. Cut slashes through the skin and ½ inch (1 cm) deep to allow spices to penetrate the meat. Brush the thighs with the melted butter and then rub the spice in. Cook on a medium grill for about 25 minutes.

Yield: 4 servings

Each with: 32 g water; 100 calories (67% from fat, 33% from protein, 0% from carb); 8 g protein; 7 g total fat; 4 g saturated fat; 2 g monounsaturated fat; 1 g polyunsaturated fat; 0 g carb; 0 g fiber; 0 g sugar; 71 mg phosphorus; 6 mg calcium; 0 mg iron; 36 mg sodium; 96 mg potassium; 204 IU vitamin A; 0 mg vitamin C; 49 mg cholesterol

Glycemic Index: Low

Hot Creole Turkey Sausage

These are moderately spicy sausages. You can vary the heat by adjusting the amount of cayenne.

1 jalapeño pepper, stems and seed removed, chopped

½ teaspoon cayenne pepper

1½ pounds (680 g) ground turkey

½ cup (80 g) finely chopped onion

½ teaspoon minced garlic

½ teaspoon freshly ground black pepper

1 tablespoon (4 g) minced fresh parsley

¼ teaspoon salt

¼ teaspoon thyme

1 bay leaf, crumbled

⅛ teaspoon allspice

⅛ teaspoon mace

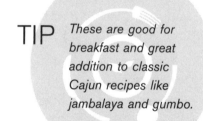 TIP *These are good for breakfast and great addition to classic Cajun recipes like jambalaya and gumbo.*

Combine all ingredients and mix well (running the mixture through a grinder helps to ensure thorough mixing). Stuff casings and form into links or make into patties as desired. Refrigerate up to 3 days for flavors to blend. Sausages may be grilled, panfried, or oven cooked.

Yield: 8 servings

(continued on page 432)

Each with: 66 g water; 151 calories (27% from fat, 70% from protein, 4% from carb); 25 g protein; 4 g total fat; 1 g saturated fat; 1 g monounsaturated fat; 1 g polyunsaturated fat; 1 g carb; 0 g fiber; 1 g sugar; 186 mg phosphorus; 26 mg calcium; 2 mg iron; 134 mg sodium; 280 mg potassium; 102 IU vitamin A; 2 mg vitamin C; 65 mg cholesterol

Glycemic Index: Low

Cajun Blackened Steak

OK, I'll be the first to admit that I usually prefer my steaks without added spices and embellishments, especially if it's a good cut like a rib eye. But every once in a while I'm looking for something a bit different, and this flavor combination is a winner that I've come back to several times.

4 tablespoons (55 g) unsalted butter, melted

1 teaspoon cayenne pepper

1 teaspoon black pepper

¼ teaspoon white pepper

1½ pounds (680 g) beef rib eye steaks

Heat a skillet to 350°F (180°C) and pour melted butter in. Combine seasoning in a small bowl. Dip steaks in melted butter and sprinkle with season mixture. Place steaks in skillet and cook each side for about 3½ minutes.

Yield: 4 servings

Each with: 120 g water; 379 calories (62% from fat, 37% from protein, 1% from carb); 34 g Protein; 26 g total fat; 13 g saturated fat; 9 g monounsaturated fat; 1 g polyunsaturated fat; 1 g carb; 0 g fiber; 0 g sugar; 339 mg phosphorous; 24 mg calcium; 4 mg iron; 109 mg sodium; 654 mg potassium; 540 IU vitamin A; 95 mg ATE vitamin E; 0 mg vitamin C; 131 mg cholesterol

Glycemic Index: Low

Okra Pilaf

This dish is a Cajun version of rice pilaf, with okra and tomatoes added. It makes a great side dish with blackened fish.

2 cups (200 g) thinly sliced okra

2 slices diced low-sodium bacon

1 cup (150 g) chopped green bell pepper

1 cup (160 g) chopped onion

1 cup (195 g) uncooked rice

2 cups (475 ml) low-sodium chicken broth

2 cups (480 g) no-salt-added canned tomatoes

In large skillet, sauté okra and bacon until lightly browned. Add bell pepper and onion; continue cooking until vegetables are crisp-tender. Add rice and chicken broth. Bring to a boil, stir once, cover, reduce heat, and simmer about 20 minutes or until rice is tender and liquid is absorbed. Add tomatoes; heat, and fluff with a fork.

Yield: 4 servings

Each with: 372 g water; 149 calories (16% from fat, 19% from protein, 64% from carb); 8 g protein; 3 g total fat; 1 g saturated fat; 1 g monounsaturated fat; 0 g polyunsaturated fat; 26 g carb; 4 g fiber; 6 g sugar; 152 mg phosphorus; 103 mg calcium; 3 mg iron; 100 mg sodium; 649 mg potassium; 468 IU vitamin A; 55 mg vitamin C; 4 mg cholesterol

Glycemic Index: Low

Cajun-Style Sweet Potatoes

Marti sent me this great-sounding recipe for sweet potatoes with a Cajun twist.

1½ teaspoons paprika

1 teaspoon brown sugar

¼ teaspoon black pepper

¼ teaspoon onion powder

¼ teaspoon thyme

¼ teaspoon rosemary

¼ teaspoon garlic powder

⅛ teaspoon cayenne pepper

2 sweet potatoes

1½ teaspoons olive oil

Preheat oven to 375°F (190°C, gas mark 5). In a small bowl, stir together paprika, brown sugar, black pepper, onion powder, thyme, rosemary, garlic powder, and cayenne pepper. Slice the sweet potatoes in half lengthwise. Brush each half with olive oil. Rub the seasoning mix over the cut surface of each half. Place sweet potatoes on a baking sheet or in a shallow pan. Bake in preheated oven until tender or about 1 hour.

Yield: 4 servings

Each with: 61 g water; 81 calories (21% from fat, 6% from protein, 73% from carb); 1 g protein; 2 g total fat; 0 g saturated fat; 1 g monounsaturated fat; 0 g polyunsaturated fat; 15 g carb; 2 g fiber; 6 g sugar; 29 mg phosphorus; 26 mg calcium; 1 mg iron; 21 mg sodium; 205 mg potassium; 12365 IU vitamin A; 10 mg vitamin C; 0 mg cholesterol

Glycemic Index: Low

Cajun Catfish Stew

This stew is the kind of warming meal that tastes great at the end of a cold day. You can vary the heat from mild to hot based on the amount of Tabasco you add.

2 pounds (900 g) catfish

1 cup (160 g) onions, diced

¾ cup (113 g) green bell peppers, diced

8 ounces (225 g) no-salt-added tomato sauce

2 cups (360 g) no-salt-added tomatoes, diced

½ teaspoon Worcestershire sauce

2 slices low-sodium bacon, diced

1 clove garlic, minced

2 medium potatoes, diced

½ cup (65 g) carrot, diced

Tabasco sauce to taste

¼ cup (15 g) fresh parsley, chopped

Place fish in soup pot. Cover with water. Simmer until fish is just done (about 20 minutes). Strain, reserving liquid. Flake fish, removing any bones, and set aside. Lightly sauté onion and garlic with bacon until lightly browned. Add fish broth, green peppers, carrots, potatoes, tomatoes, and seasoning to taste. Simmer for at least one hour. Add fish and cook a few minutes longer. Serve in bowls; sprinkle parsley on top.

Yield: 6 servings

Each with: 376 g water; 352 calories (33% from fat, 32% from protein, 34% from carb); 29 g Protein; 13 g total fat; 3 g saturated fat; 6 g monounsaturated fat; 3 g polyunsaturated fat; 30 g carb; 5 g fiber; 7 g sugar; 439 mg phosphorous; 71 mg calcium; 3 mg iron; 137 mg sodium; 1440 mg potassium; 2384 IU vitamin A; 23 mg ATE vitamin E; 46 mg vitamin C; 74 mg cholesterol

Glycemic Index: Low

Cajun Hot Mustard

This mustard is not for the faint of heart. It packs a pretty good kick, but I like it particularly on turkey burgers, which tend to be kind of plain.

1 tablespoon (11 g) Dijon mustard

1 tablespoon (8 g) flour

1 tablespoon (9 g) dry mustard

1 teaspoon horseradish, gated

½ teaspoon white pepper

5 ounces (150 ml) water, hot

Combine all ingredients except water and mix well. Then add the water, mix well, and simmer for 2 minutes. Remove from heat and allow to cool to room temperature. Transfer to an air-tight jar and store sealed in the refrigerator. Serve with steak and hamburgers.

Yield: 12 servings

Each with: 13 g water; 5 calories (24% from fat, 17% from protein, 59% from carb); 0 g Protein; 0 g total fat; 0 g saturated fat; 0 g monounsaturated fat; 0 g polyunsaturated fat; 1 g carb; 0 g fiber; 0 g sugar; 2 mg phosphorous; 2 mg calcium; 0 mg iron; 16 mg sodium; 6 mg potassium; 2 IU vitamin A; 0 mg ATE vitamin E; 0 mg vitamin C; 0 mg cholesterol

Glycemic Index: Low

17

Low-GI Breads and Baked Goods

Breads and baked goods are by their very nature higher in GI than many foods. Most consist primarily of flour and sugar. We've reduced the GI count of the ones in this chapter by relying mostly on whole grain flours and by replacing the sugar with a sweetener like Splenda. You'll still need to be aware of how much you eat, but you don't need to give these kinds of foods up completely.

Oatmeal Bread

This bread has a wonderful, slightly sweet flavor. It's great toasted for breakfast or for sandwiches.

1 cup (80 g) quick-cooking oats

2/3 cup (160 ml) skim milk

1/3 cup (80 ml) water

1 tablespoon (14 g) unsalted butter

1/2 cup (60 g) whole wheat flour

2 cups (275 g) bread flour

3 tablespoons (3 g) brown sugar substitute, such as Splenda

1 teaspoon yeast

Spread the oats in a baking pan and toast in an oven heated to 350°F (180°C, gas mark 4) until lightly browned, about 15 minutes, stirring occasionally. Place ingredients in bread machine in order specified by manufacturer. Process on whole grain cycle.

Yield: 12 servings

Each with: 24 g water; 167 calories (13% from fat, 15% from protein, 72% from carb); 6 g protein; 2 g total fat; 1 g saturated fat; 1 g monounsaturated fat; 1 g polyunsaturated fat; 30 g carb; 3 g fiber; 1 g sugar; 127 mg phosphorus; 32 mg calcium; 2 mg iron; 10 mg sodium; 131 mg potassium; 58 IU vitamin A; 0 mg vitamin C; 3 mg cholesterol

Glycemic Index: Low

Sesame Wheat Bread

This makes a good sandwich bread that has a little crunch and the flavor of sesame seeds.

1½ cups (355 ml) water

2 tablespoons (28 g) unsalted butter

1½ cups (205 g) bread flour

1½ cups (180 g) whole wheat flour

1 cup (80 g) uncooked multigrain cereal

½ cup (72 g) sesame seeds

3 tablespoons (3 g) brown sugar substitute, such as Splenda

1½ teaspoons yeast

Place ingredients in bread machine in order specified by manufacturer. Process on wheat cycle. It makes a 1½-pound (680 g) loaf.

Yield: 12 servings

Each with: 35 g water; 162 calories (15% from fat, 13% from protein, 71% from carb); 6 g protein; 3 g total fat; 1 g saturated fat; 1 g monounsaturated fat; 0 g polyunsaturated fat; 30 g carb; 2 g fiber; 1 g sugar; 115 mg phosphorus; 14 mg calcium; 2 mg iron; 4 mg sodium; 132 mg potassium; 64 IU vitamin A; 0 mg vitamin C; 5 mg cholesterol

Glycemic Index: Low

Buttermilk Bread

The buttermilk makes this bread a little higher in sodium than most here, but it also gives it an excellent flavor.

1 cup (235 ml) buttermilk

3¼ cups (455 g) bread flour

2 tablespoons (30 ml) canola oil

3 tablespoons (60 g) honey

¼ teaspoon sodium-free baking soda

1½ teaspoons yeast

Place ingredients in bread machine in the order specified by manufacturer. Process on white bread cycle.

Yield: 12 servings

Each with: 9 g water; 173 calories (15% from fat, 11% from protein, 74% from carb); 5 g protein; 3 g total fat; 0 g saturated fat; 1 g monounsaturated fat; 2 g polyunsaturated fat; 32 g carb; 1 g fiber; 5 g sugar; 61 mg phosphorus; 30 mg calcium; 2 mg iron; 23 mg sodium; 56 mg potassium; 2 IU vitamin A; 0 mg vitamin C; 0 mg cholesterol

Glycemic Index: Medium

Italian Peasant Bread

This is a recipe we've been using for a while and our favorite for Italian bread. I use the bread machine to make my dough and then bake it in the oven to get that traditional look.

2 cups (275 g) bread flour

1 cup (120 g) whole wheat flour

2 tablespoons (30 ml) olive oil

2 teaspoons sugar substitute, such as Splenda

2 teaspoons active dry yeast

1 cup (235 ml) warm water

2 tablespoons (18 g) cornmeal, for baking sheet

1 egg white, slightly beaten

Add flour, oil, salt, sugar, yeast, and water to your bread machine according to its instructions. Set on dough setting. Remove when signal beeps and cycle is done. Preheat oven to 375°F (190°C, gas mark 5). Sprinkle cornmeal onto a baking sheet. Punch dough down and form into a long or oval loaf. Cover and let rise for 25 more minutes. It should be doubled again by this time. Uncover and slash the top with a sharp knife or razor. Brush all over with the beaten egg white. Bake 25 to 35 minutes until hollow sounding when tapped on bottom.

Yield: 12 servings

Each with: 26 g water; 146 calories (18% from fat, 13% from protein, 69% from carb); 5 g protein; 3 g total fat; 0 g saturated fat; 2 g monounsaturated fat; 0 g polyunsaturated fat; 26 g carb; 2 g fiber; 0 g sugar; 68 mg phosphorus; 8 mg calcium; 2 mg iron; 7 mg sodium; 84 mg potassium; 5 IU vitamin A; 0 mg vitamin C; 0 mg cholesterol

Glycemic Index: Low

Barley Bread

You should be able to find barley flour at a store that carries a selection of grains. Health food stores and those that specialize in organic foods are a good choice. The barley gives this bread a unique flavor and also helps to hold down the GI count.

1½ teaspoons yeast

1 cup (235 ml) water

1 tablespoon (21 g) honey

1 cup (148 g) barley flour

1 cup (120 g) whole wheat flour

1 cup (137 g) bread flour

1 tablespoon (15 ml) olive oil

Place ingredients in bread machine pan in order specified by manufacturer. Process on white bread cycle.

Yield: 12 servings

Each with: 24 g water; 134 calories (11% from fat, 12% from protein, 76% from carb); 4 g Protein; 2 g total fat; 0 g saturated fat; 1 g monounsaturated fat; 0 g polyunsaturated fat; 26 g carb; 3 g fiber; 2 g sugar; 89 mg phosphorous; 10 mg calcium; 1 mg iron; 2 mg sodium; 101 mg potassium; 1 IU vitamin A; 0 mg ATE vitamin E; 0 mg vitamin C; 0 mg cholesterol

Glycemic Index: Low

Multigrain Bread

This makes a fairly heavy loaf that's good for sandwiches or with a soup and salad meal.

1 ⅛ cups (265 ml) water

2 tablespoons (28 g) unsalted butter

1 ⅓ cups (185 g) bread flour

1 cup (120 g) whole wheat flour

¼ cup (20 g) seven-grain cereal

3 tablespoons (3 g) brown sugar substitute, such as Splenda

2 ¼ teaspoons (9 g) yeast

TIP *You could use any multigrain, long-cooking cereal in this recipe that your grocer happens to stock.*

Place ingredients in bread machine in the order specified by the manufacturer. Process on whole wheat cycle.

Yield: 12 servings

Each with: 26 g water; 118 calories (19% from fat, 13% from protein, 69% from carb); 4 g protein; 2 g total fat; 1 g saturated fat; 1 g monounsaturated fat; 0 g polyunsaturated fat; 21 g carb; 2 g fiber; 1 g sugar; 69 mg phosphorus; 9 mg calcium; 1 mg iron; 3 mg sodium; 82 mg potassium; 61 IU vitamin A; 0 mg vitamin C; 5 mg cholesterol

Glycemic Index: Low

Light Rye Bread

We made this to use for sandwiches with leftover New Year's roast beef, using my new Christmas bread maker. I prefer it without the caraway seeds, but you can suit yourself. It makes a nice, light loaf either way.

1½ tablespoons (25 ml) canola oil

1 egg

1½ teaspoons sugar substitute, such as Splenda

1 cup (128 g) rye flour

2 cups (275 g) bread flour

1 tablespoon (7 g) caraway seed

1½ teaspoons yeast

1 cup (235 ml) water

Place ingredients in the bread machine in the order specified by the manufacturer. Process on wheat or whole grain cycle.

Yield: 12 servings

Each with: 28 g water; 137 calories (16% from fat, 13% from protein, 71% from carb); 4 g protein; 2 g total fat; 0 g saturated fat; 1 g monounsaturated fat; 1 g polyunsaturated fat; 24 g carb; 2 g fiber; 0 g sugar; 55 mg phosphorus; 13 mg calcium; 1 mg iron; 11 mg sodium; 78 mg potassium; 21 IU vitamin A; 0 mg vitamin C; 0 mg cholesterol

Glycemic Index: Low

Carrot Bread

This is an unusual vegetable yeast bread. The carrot color and flavor make this great sandwich bread.

½ cup (120 ml) water, boiling

¼ cup (30 g) cracked wheat

1¾ teaspoons yeast

¼ cup (60 ml) water

2²/₃ cups (365 g) bread flour

⅓ cup (80 ml) skim milk, warm

¼ cup (55 g) unsalted butter

¼ cup (4 g) brown sugar substitute, such as Splenda

1 cup (110 g) carrot, shredded

1 egg

²/₃ cup (63 g) oat bran

In small bowl, pour boiling water over cracked wheat; let stand 15 minutes. Drain excess water. Place ingredients in bread machine pan in order specified by manufacturer. Process on white bread cycle.

Yield: 12 servings

Each with: 38 g water; 175 calories (26% from fat, 12% from protein, 62% from carb); 5 g Protein; 5 g total fat; 3 g saturated fat; 1 g monounsaturated fat; 1 g polyunsaturated fat; 27 g carb; 2 g fiber; 2 g sugar; 83 mg phosphorous; 28 mg calcium; 2 mg iron; 30 mg sodium; 121 mg potassium; 1978 IU vitamin A; 51 mg ATE vitamin E; 1 mg vitamin C; 28 mg cholesterol

Glycemic Index: Low

Apple Butter Bread

This yeast bread is flavored with apple butter. It makes great breakfast bread with cream cheese.

1 tablespoon (12 g) yeast

1 cup (240 g) whole wheat flour

2 cups (274 g) bread flour

1 tablespoon (13 g) sugar

½ cup (141 g) apple butter

2 tablespoons (30 ml) canola oil

1 cup (235 ml) water

Place ingredients in bread machine pan in order specified by manufacturer. Process on white bread cycle.

Yield: 12 servings

Each with: 30 g water; 164 calories (16% from fat, 11% from protein, 73% from carb); 5 g Protein; 3 g total fat; 0 g saturated fat; 1 g monounsaturated fat; 1 g polyunsaturated fat; 30 g carb; 2 g fiber; 5 g sugar; 70 mg phosphorous; 10 mg calcium; 2 mg iron; 4 mg sodium; 94 mg potassium; 2 IU vitamin A; 0 mg ATE vitamin E; 0 mg vitamin C; 0 mg cholesterol

Glycemic Index: Low

Sun-Dried Tomato and Basil Bread

This is the perfect bread for tomato sandwiches.

1 cup (235 ml) plus 2 tablespoons (30 ml) water

1½ cups (205 g) bread flour

1½ cups (180 g) whole wheat flour

¼ teaspoon garlic powder

2 tablespoons (3 g) sugar substitute, such as Splenda

1½ teaspoons basil

2 teaspoons yeast

⅓ cup (35 g) sun-dried tomatoes, in oil

Place all ingredients except tomatoes in bread machine in order specified by manufacturer. Process on white bread cycle. Add the tomatoes at the beep or 5 minutes before the end of the kneading cycle.

Yield: 12 servings

Each with: 65 g water; 123 calories (7% from fat, 14% from protein, 78% from carb); 5 g protein; 1 g total fat; 0 g saturated fat; 0 g monounsaturated fat; 0 g polyunsaturated fat; 25 g carb; 3 g fiber; 1 g sugar; 82 mg phosphorus; 13 mg calcium; 2 mg iron; 11 mg sodium; 143 mg potassium; 49 IU vitamin A; 3 mg vitamin C; 0 mg cholesterol

Glycemic Index: Low

Pepper and Onion Bread

This makes a great accompaniment to soup. It's also good for sandwiches. I use it for a quick and filling breakfast on the go with just a scrambled egg or some microwaved egg substitute.

1 cup (235 ml) water

¼ cup (40 g) finely chopped onion

¼ cup (38 g) finely chopped green bell pepper

2 tablespoons (28 g) unsalted butter

1¼ cups (150 g) whole wheat flour

2 cups (275 g) bread flour

⅓ cup (47 g) cornmeal

2 tablespoons (3 g) sugar substitute, such as Splenda

1¾ teaspoons yeast

Place ingredients in bread machine in order specified by manufacturer. Process on white bread cycle.

Yield: 12 servings

Each with: 31 g water; 163 calories (14% from fat, 12% from protein, 73% from carb); 5 g protein; 3 g total fat; 1 g saturated fat; 1 g monounsaturated fat; 0 g polyunsaturated fat; 30 g carb; 2 g fiber; 1 g sugar; 80 mg phosphorus; 10 mg calcium; 2 mg iron; 3 mg sodium; 103 mg potassium; 82 IU vitamin A; 3 mg vitamin C; 5 mg cholesterol

Glycemic Index: Low

Curry Bread

I know if sounds a little strange, but it really does work. The curry powder gives this bread just enough flavor to make it great as an accompaniment to a curry meal or for a sandwich with an otherwise plain filling like roast chicken.

1 tablespoon (12 g) dry yeast

1 cup (235 ml) water

2 cups (274 g) bread flour

1 cup (120 g) whole wheat flour

¼ cup (60 ml) canola oil

1 teaspoon curry powder

½ teaspoon parsley

1 teaspoon garlic powder

Place ingredients in bread machine pan in order specified by manufacturer. Process on white bread cycle.

Yield: 12 servings

Each with: 24 g water; 162 calories (29% from fat, 11% from protein, 60% from carb); 5 g Protein; 5 g total fat; 0 g saturated fat; 3 g monounsaturated fat; 2 g polyunsaturated fat; 24 g carb; 2 g fiber; 0 g sugar; 71 mg phosphorous; 9 mg calcium; 2 mg iron; 2 mg sodium; 89 mg potassium; 7 IU vitamin A; 0 mg ATE vitamin E; 0 mg vitamin C; 0 mg cholesterol

Glycemic Index: Low

Whole Wheat Flatbread

Use this to make your own flatbread for roll-ups or other filled sandwiches.

1½ teaspoons yeast

¾ cup (175 ml) water, warm (100° to 110°F or 38° to 43°C)

1½ cups (205 g) bread flour

1½ cups (180 g) whole wheat flour

2 tablespoons (28 g) unsalted butter, melted

In small bowl dissolve yeast in warm water. Let stand 5 minutes. Place flours in bowl of food processor. Turn on machine and slowly add yeast-water mixture. Keep machine running until dough just forms a ball. Place ball in greased bowl. Cover with towel and let rise 1 hour in warm place. Punch down dough and turn out on lightly floured surface. Roll dough into a log about 1½ inches (3½ cm) thick. Cut log vertically into 12 equal pieces. Roll each piece into a 6-inch (15 cm) circle. In large cast-iron or heavy skillet over high heat, cook breads one at a time, 1 to 2 minutes until they begin to form bubbles. With tongs, turn and cook other side about 1 to 2 minutes, until golden brown. Brush with melted butter. Store tightly wrapped in the refrigerator for 1 week. To reheat, cook in microwave on high 1 minute on microwave-safe dish lightly covered with plastic wrap.

Yield: 12 servings

Each with: 19 g water; 131 calories (17% from fat, 13% from protein, 70% from carb); 4 g protein; 3 g total fat; 1 g saturated fat; 1 g monounsaturated fat; 0 g polyunsaturated fat; 23 g carb; 2 g fiber; 0 g sugar; 76 mg phosphorus; 9 mg calcium; 1 mg iron; 2 mg sodium; 89 mg potassium; 61 IU vitamin A; 0 mg vitamin C; 5 mg cholesterol

Glycemic Index: Medium

Whole Wheat Pizza Dough

We used this dough to make a pizza full of fresh veggies from the garden, but you could use it with any toppings you desire.

2 teaspoons (8 g) active dry yeast

2 cups (275) bread flour

1½ cups (180 g) whole wheat flour

1 tablespoon (13 g) sugar substitute, such as Splenda

2 tablespoons (30 ml) olive oil

1½ cups (355 ml) water

Place ingredients in bread machine in order specified by manufacturer and process on dough cycle. Turn out the dough onto a floured board. At this point you may form the pizzas or refrigerate the dough for several hours, well wrapped in plastic so it won't dry out. It makes enough dough for two 12-inch (30 cm) pizzas or two 10-inch (25 cm) thick-crust pizzas. Bake at 400°F (200°C, gas mark 6) until lightly browned around the edges. Top as desired and return to oven until cheese is melted and crust browned, about 15 minutes total.

Yield: 16 servings

Each with: 26 g water; 119 calories (16% from fat, 12% from protein, 71% from carb); 4 g protein; 2 g total fat; 0 g saturated fat; 1 g monounsaturated fat; 0 g polyunsaturated fat; 22 g carb; 2 g fiber; 1 g sugar; 62 mg phosphorus; 7 mg calcium; 1 mg iron; 2 mg sodium; 73 mg potassium; 1 IU vitamin A; 0 mg vitamin C; 0 mg cholesterol

Glycemic Index: Low

Citrus Bread

Orange juice and grated citrus peel give this bread its characteristic flavor. It's a great breakfast bread, but also surprisingly good for sandwiches.

¼ cup (60 ml) water

⅔ cup (160 ml) orange juice

3 tablespoons (45 g) unsalted butter, melted

3 tablespoons sugar substitute, such as Splenda

1 tablespoon (6 g) orange rind, finely grated

1 teaspoon lemon rind, finely grated

2¼ teaspoons (9 g) yeast

2½ cups (343 g) bread flour, unsifted

Place ingredients in bread machine pan in order specified by manufacturer. Process on white bread cycle.

Yield: 12 servings

Each with: 22 g water; 150 calories (21% from fat, 10% from protein, 69% from carb); 4 g Protein; 3 g total fat; 2 g saturated fat; 1 g monounsaturated fat; 0 g polyunsaturated fat; 26 g carb; 1 g fiber; 3 g sugar; 40 mg phosphorous; 8 mg calcium; 1 mg iron; 2 mg sodium; 72 mg potassium; 102 IU vitamin A; 24 mg ATE vitamin E; 5 mg vitamin C; 8 mg cholesterol

Glycemic Index: Low

Chili Cheese Corn Bread

Unlike the corn muffin recipe, which goes with any kind of meal, this corn bread begs to be eaten with Mexican food, with its chili and cheese flavors.

1 cup (140 g) yellow cornmeal

2 teaspoons (9.2 g) baking powder

½ teaspoon baking soda

¼ cup (150 g) whole wheat flour

1¼ cups (285 ml) buttermilk

1 egg, lightly beaten

1 egg white, lightly beaten

¼ cup (30 g) cheddar, shredded

2 tablespoons (15 g) mild green chilies

Preheat oven to 450°F (230°C, or gas mark 8). Coat an 8 x 8-inch (20 x 20 cm) baking pan with nonstick cooking spray and dust with cornmeal. Sift into a large bowl the cornmeal, baking powder, baking soda, and flour. In another bowl, combine buttermilk, eggs, cheese, and chilies, then stir into the dry ingredients. Pour batter into the prepared baking pan and place in upper third of oven. Bake 10 minutes or until dough is firm in center.

Yield: 12 servings

Each with: 32 g water; 88 calories (21% from fat, 17% from protein, 63% from carb); 4 g Protein; 2 g total fat; 1 g saturated fat; 1 g monounsaturated fat; 0 g polyunsaturated fat; 14 g carb; 1 g fiber; 2 g sugar; 85 mg phosphorous; 99 mg calcium; 1 mg iron; 144 mg sodium; 83 mg potassium; 93 IU vitamin A; 16 mg ATE vitamin E; 1 mg vitamin C; 21 mg cholesterol

Glycemic Index: Low

Orange Corn Bread

Here's corn bread with a twist—orange flavor. This is great with chicken or pork.

1 cup (125 g) flour

1 cup (140 g) yellow corn meal

¾ cup (18 g) sugar substitute, such as Splenda

4 teaspoons (18.4 g) baking powder

2 eggs

½ cup (112 g) unsalted butter, melted

1 cup (235 ml) skim milk

1 teaspoon orange extract

8 ounces (225 g) mandarin oranges

Grease an 8 x 8-inch (20 x 20 cm) pan. Mix together well, stirring so that orange slices break apart. Pour mixture into pan. Bake at 425°F (220°C, or gas mark 7) for 30 minutes or until a toothpick inserted in the center comes out clean.

Yield: 12 servings

Each with: 47 g water; 194 calories (41% from fat, 9% from protein, 50% from carb); 4 g Protein; 9 g total fat; 5 g saturated fat; 2 g monounsaturated fat; 1 g polyunsaturated fat; 25 g carb; 1 g fiber; 4 g sugar; 104 mg phosphorous; 131 mg calcium; 1 mg iron; 191 mg sodium; 109 mg potassium; 513 IU vitamin A; 89 mg ATE vitamin E; 7 mg vitamin C; 60 mg cholesterol

Glycemic Index: Low

Real Corn Muffins

We like corn muffins, especially these that have real corn mixed in. They go well with everything from chicken to chili.

1 cup (140 g) cornmeal

½ cup (63 g) flour

1 tablespoon (13.8 g) baking powder

1 cup (235 ml) buttermilk

1 cup (164 g) fresh corn, or frozen thawed

1 egg, slightly beaten

¼ cup (60 ml) canola oil

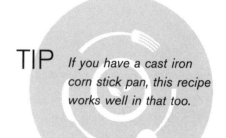

TIP *If you have a cast iron corn stick pan, this recipe works well in that too.*

Combine first 3 ingredients in medium mixing bowl. Add corn, egg, oil, and buttermilk, stirring well. Pour batter into 8 nonstick muffin cups or muffin pan with paper liners sprayed with nonstick vegetable oil spray. Bake at 475°F (240°C, or gas mark 9) for 20–25 minutes or until brown.

Yield: 8 servings

Each with: 51 g water; 204 calories (38% from fat, 9% from protein, 53% from carb); 5 g Protein; 9 g total fat; 1 g saturated fat; 5 g monounsaturated fat; 2 g polyunsaturated fat; 28 g carb; 2 g fiber; 3 g sugar; 118 mg phosphorous; 143 mg calcium; 2 mg iron; 229 mg sodium; 124 mg potassium; 93 IU vitamin A; 13 mg ATE vitamin E; 1 mg vitamin C; 28 mg cholesterol

Glycemic Index: Low

Pumpkin Pancakes

Pumpkin, rather than the usual amount of sugar, sweetens these pancakes. I like them just as is or maybe with a little cottage cheese.

1 egg

1 cup (235 ml) milk

½ cup (123 g) pumpkin, cooked or canned

¾ cup (94 g) flour

¾ cup (90 g) whole wheat flour

2 teaspoons (9.2 g) baking powder

1 tablespoon sugar substitute, such as Splenda

¼ teaspoon cinnamon

⅛ teaspoon nutmeg

⅛ teaspoon ginger

2 tablespoons (10 ml) canola oil

Combine all the ingredients in a mixing bowl and stir just until blended. Pour the batter onto a hot griddle that has been lightly oiled. Flip the pancakes over when bubbles break around the edges.

Yield: 6 servings

Each with: 64 g water; 194 calories (29% from fat, 13% from protein, 59% from carb); 6 g Protein; 6 g total fat; 1 g saturated fat; 3 g monounsaturated fat; 2 g polyunsaturated fat; 29 g carb; 3 g fiber; 5 g sugar; 167 mg phosphorous; 160 mg calcium; 2 mg iron; 197 mg sodium; 196 mg potassium; 3318 IU vitamin A; 40 mg ATE vitamin E; 1 mg vitamin C; 36 mg cholesterol

Glycemic Index: Low

Whole Wheat Biscuits

This recipe offers a small variation of the standard biscuit recipe. I added a little dill to them when we had them with the Swedish Salmon Stew. You could also add a little cheese or other herbs and spices. If you don't have a biscuit cutter, you can use a glass or just cut it into squares with a knife.

1½ cups (185 g) flour

½ cup (60 g) whole wheat pastry flour

2 teaspoons sugar substitute, such as Splenda

3 tablespoons (42 g) baking powder

¼ cup (56 g) unsalted butter

⅔ cup (160 ml) skim milk

Stir together dry ingredients. Cut in butter until mixture resembles coarse crumbs. Add milk. Stir until just mixed. Knead gently on floured surface a few times. Press to ½-inch (1 cm) thickness. Cut out circles with 2½-inch (6 cm) biscuit cutter. Transfer to ungreased baking sheet. Bake at 450°F (230°C, gas mark 8) for 10 to 12 minutes or until golden brown.

Yield: 10 servings

Each with: 19 g water; 139 calories (31% from fat, 10% from protein, 59% from carb); 3 g protein; 5 g total fat; 3 g saturated fat; 1 g monounsaturated fat; 0 g polyunsaturated fat; 21 g carb; 1 g fiber; 0 g sugar; 151 mg phosphorus; 273 mg calcium; 2 mg iron; 450 mg sodium; 76 mg potassium; 176 IU vitamin A; 0 mg vitamin C; 13 mg cholesterol

Glycemic Index: Low

Whole Grain Soda Bread

Soda bread is typically associated with Ireland. This recipe makes a loaf that has the traditional texture, raisins, etc., but it also has the nutritional advantage of mostly whole grain flour.

1 cup (125 g) flour

¾ cup (90 g) whole wheat flour

¾ cup (96 g) rye flour

¾ cup (105 g) graham flour

¾ cup (60 g) rolled oats

1 tablespoon (13.8 g) baking powder

1 teaspoon baking soda

3 tablespoons (45 ml) canola oil

¾ cup (110 g) raisins

1¾ cup (425 ml) buttermilk

TIP *If you do not have all the different kinds of flour, use what you do have to make 3¼ cups or try ¼ cup wheat germ or bran plus 3 cups flour.*

Combine dry ingredients in a bowl. Cut in oil. Stir in raisins and add buttermilk to make a soft dough. Knead lightly on a floured surface until smooth. Place on a greased baking sheet and flatten into a circle about 2½-inches (6 cm) thick. Cut large X about ¼-inch (5 mm) deep on top. Bake at 350°F (180°C, or gas mark 4) for about 1 hour or until toothpick inserted in the center comes out clean.

Yield: 16 servings

Each with: 28 g water; 156 calories (19% from fat, 11% from protein, 70% from carb); 4 g Protein; 3 g total fat; 0 g saturated fat; 2 g monounsaturated fat; 1 g polyunsaturated fat; 28 g carb; 3 g fiber; 6 g sugar; 125 mg phosphorous; 94 mg calcium; 1 mg iron; 121 mg sodium; 177 mg potassium; 8 IU vitamin A; 2 mg ATE vitamin E; 0 mg vitamin C; 1 mg cholesterol

Glycemic Index: Low

Apricot Muffins

These muffins, fruit-sweetened and with the subtle taste of cardamom, are sure to be a hit.

½ cup (65 g) apricots, finely snipped

⅓ cup (80 ml) apple juice, unsweetened

1 cup (120 g) whole wheat flour

2 teaspoons (9.2 g) baking powder

¼ teaspoon baking soda

¼ teaspoon cardamom

⅓ cup (40 g) walnuts, chopped

2 tablespoons (30 ml) canola oil

1 tablespoon (13 g) sugar substitute, such as Splenda

Soak the apricots in the apple juice for 10 minutes. Combine the flour, baking powder, baking soda, spice, and walnuts in a bowl. Beat together the oil, sugar, and egg. Add the apricots, with the juice and egg mixture to the flour. Mix just until all the ingredients are blended. Spoon into oiled muffin tins or (my choice) paper muffin cups (sprayed with nonstick spray). Fill cups ¾ full. Bake in 350°F (180°C, or gas mark 4) oven for 10 to 15 minutes or until golden brown.

Yield: 8 servings

Each with: 24 g water; 133 calories (44% from fat, 10% from protein, 46% from carb); 3 g Protein; 7 g total fat; 0 g saturated fat; 3 g monounsaturated fat; 3 g polyunsaturated fat; 16 g carb; 2 g fiber; 4 g sugar; 108 mg phosphorous; 79 mg calcium; 1 mg iron; 124 mg sodium; 127 mg potassium; 261 IU vitamin A; 0 mg ATE vitamin E; 1 mg vitamin C; 0 mg cholesterol

Glycemic Index: Low

Carrot Cake Muffins

Carrot cake is one of my favorite desserts, but I don't have it very often because it tends to be high in carbohydrates and other not so healthy stuff. These muffins are a bit better, giving a healthy dose of fruits and vegetables and a reasonable low GI.

1½ cups (180 g) whole wheat flour

1 teaspoon baking soda

1 tablespoon (13.8 g) baking powder

1 teaspoon ground cinnamon

¼ teaspoon ground nutmeg

¼ teaspoon ground ginger

1 egg

2 tablespoons (30 ml) vegetable oil

¼ cup (36 g) raisins

¼ cup (30 g) walnuts, chopped

⅓ cup (80 ml) skim milk

8 ounces (225 g) crushed pineapple

1½ cups (165 g) carrots, grated

Combine the dry ingredients in a bowl. Add the remaining ingredients and stir to blend. Spoon into oiled muffin tins or paper muffin cups. Bake at 350°F (180°C, or gas mark 4) for 20 to 25 minutes.

Yield: 12 servings

Each with: 41 g water; 125 calories (32% from fat, 11% from protein, 56% from carb); 4 g Protein; 5 g total fat; 1 g saturated fat; 1 g monounsaturated fat; 2 g polyunsaturated fat; 19 g carb; 3 g fiber; 5 g sugar; 117 mg phosphorous; 98 mg calcium; 1 mg iron; 146 mg sodium; 191 mg potassium; 2742 IU vitamin A; 12 mg ATE vitamin E; 3 mg vitamin C; 18 mg cholesterol

Glycemic Index: Low

Pumpkin Muffins

Pumpkin gives these muffins both great flavor as well as additional nutrition. They taste a little like pumpkin pie, and who can argue with pumpkin pie for breakfast.

1 cup (125 g) flour

½ cup (56 g) wheat bran

1 tablespoon (13 g) sugar

2 teaspoons (4.8 g) baking powder

½ teaspoon baking soda

½ teaspoon ground cinnamon

2 tablespoons (30 ml) vegetable oil

½ cup (123 g) pumpkin, canned or cooked

1 egg

¾ cup (175 ml) orange juice

⅓ cup (48 g) raisins

1 tablespoon (7 g) wheat germ

Combine all the ingredients except the wheat germ in a mixing bowl. Stir to blend. Spoon into lightly oiled muffin tins (or paper baking cups sprayed with nonstick spray). Sprinkle on the wheat germ. Bake in a 400°F (200°C, or gas mark 6) oven for 10 to 15 minutes or until lightly browned.

Yield: 8 servings

Each with: 42 g water; 153 calories (27% from fat, 9% from protein, 64% from carb); 4 g Protein; 5 g total fat; 1 g saturated fat; 1 g monounsaturated fat; 2 g polyunsaturated fat; 26 g carb; 3 g fiber; 6 g sugar; 116 mg phosphorous; 88 mg calcium; 2 mg iron; 136 mg sodium; 205 mg potassium; 2445 IU vitamin A; 11 mg ATE vitamin E; 9 mg vitamin C; 26 mg cholesterol

Glycemic Index: Low

Oat Bran Muffins

These are soo good that you won't guess that they are good for you.

2¼ cups (225 g) oat bran

1 tablespoon (14 g) baking powder

¼ cup (35 g) raisins

¼ cup (28 g) chopped pecans

2 eggs

2 tablespoons (30 ml) olive oil

¼ cup (85 g) honey

1¼ cups (295 ml) water

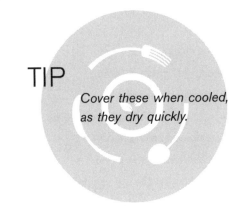

TIP

Cover these when cooled, as they dry quickly.

Preheat oven to 425°F (220°C, gas mark 7). Put dry ingredients, raisins, and nuts in mixing bowl. Beat egg whites, olive oil, honey, and water lightly. Add this mixture to dry ingredients and stir until moistened. Line muffin pans with paper liners or coat with nonstick vegetable oil spray and fill about half full. Bake for 15 to 17 minutes.

Yield: 12 servings

Each with: 34 g water; 113 calories (39% from fat, 9% from protein, 52% from carb); 3 g protein; 5 g total fat; 1 g saturated fat; 3 g monounsaturated fat; 1 g polyunsaturated fat; 16 g carb; 1 g fiber; 9 g sugar; 97 mg phosphorus; 93 mg calcium; 3 mg iron; 168 mg sodium; 89 mg potassium; 129 IU vitamin A; 1 mg vitamin C; 39 mg cholesterol

Glycemic Index: Low

Whole Wheat Banana Muffins

Here's another fresh muffin idea, this time with a way to get rid of those overripe bananas.

1 egg

¾ cup (175 ml) skim milk

⅓ cup (80 ml) canola oil

½ cup (115 g) mashed banana

1 cup (125 g) flour

½ cup (60 g) whole wheat flour

¼ cup (25 g) wheat germ

2½ teaspoons (12 g) sodium-free baking powder

¼ teaspoon cinnamon

Combine egg, milk, oil, and banana. Stir to mix. Stir together dry ingredients. Add milk mixture and stir until just mixed. Spoon into 12 lined or greased muffin cups. Bake at 375°F (190°C, gas mark 5) for 20 to 25 minutes.

Yield: 12 servings

Each with: 26 g water; 140 calories (45% from fat, 10% from protein, 46% from carb); 4 g protein; 7 g total fat; 1 g saturated fat; 2 g monounsaturated fat; 4 g polyunsaturated fat; 16 g carb; 1 g fiber; 1 g sugar; 148 mg phosphorus; 75 mg calcium; 1 mg iron; 19 mg sodium; 225 mg potassium; 66 IU vitamin A; 1 mg vitamin C; 18 mg cholesterol

Glycemic Index: Low

Oatmeal Applesauce Muffins

These tasty muffins get most of their sweetness from applesauce, helping to hold down the calorie count and GI level.

½ cup (123 g) applesauce, unsweetened

½ cup (120 ml) skim milk

¾ cup (60 g) quick cooking oats

2 tablespoons (30 ml) canola oil

¾ cup flour

2 eggs

2 teaspoons (10 ml) vanilla

2 teaspoons (4.6 g) cinnamon

1 teaspoon ginger

2 teaspoons (9.2 g) baking powder

5 teaspoons (1.7 g) brown sugar substitute, such as Splenda

Combine oatmeal, applesauce, milk, and oil. Let stand for 20 minutes. In another bowl, combine flour, cinnamon, ginger, and baking powder. Add slightly beaten eggs, vanilla, and brown sugar to oatmeal mixture. Add dry ingredients. Stir just enough to moisten. Spray muffin tins with nonstick vegetable oil spray. Fill tins ⅔ full. Bake at 350°F (180°C, or gas mark 4) for 15–20 minutes.

Yield: 12 servings

Each with: 27 g water; 99 calories (34% from fat, 13% from protein, 53% from carb); 3 g Protein; 4 g total fat; 1 g saturated fat; 2 g monounsaturated fat; 1 g polyunsaturated fat; 13 g carb; 1 g fiber; 2 g sugar; 80 mg phosphorous; 74 mg calcium; 1 mg iron; 101 mg sodium; 69 mg potassium; 69 IU vitamin A; 19 mg ATE vitamin E; 0 mg vitamin C; 40 mg cholesterol

Glycemic Index: Low

Oatmeal Blueberry Muffins

I love breads and muffins with oatmeal in them, and this recipe is no exception. Add in the flavor of fresh blueberries, and you have a real winner.

1 cup (125 g) flour

6 ounces (170 g) oats

1 tablespoon (13.8 g) baking powder

2 tablespoons (3 g) sugar substitute, such as Splenda

1 cup (235 ml) skim milk

1 egg

¼ cup (60 ml) canola oil

1 cup (145 g) fresh blueberries

1 teaspoon ground cinnamon

Combine flour, oats, baking powder, and sugar substitute in a medium bowl; make a well in center of mixture. Combine milk, egg, and oil; add to dry ingredients, stirring just until moistened. Gently fold in blueberries. Spoon batter into muffin pans coated with cooking spray, filling two-thirds full. Sprinkle cinnamon over muffins and bake at 425°F (220°C, or gas mark 7) for 20 to 25 minutes or until lightly browned.

Yield: 12 servings

Each with: 34 g water; 160 calories (36% from fat, 12% from protein, 52% from carb); 5 g Protein; 6 g total fat; 1 g saturated fat; 3 g monounsaturated fat; 2 g polyunsaturated fat; 21 g carb; 2 g fiber; 2 g sugar; 143 mg phosphorous; 111 mg calcium; 1 mg iron; 142 mg sodium; 126 mg potassium; 77 IU vitamin A; 20 mg ATE vitamin E; 1 mg vitamin C; 18 mg cholesterol

Glycemic Index: Low

Banana Pumpkin Muffins

These moist pumpkin muffins have a spiced brown sugar topping.

½ cup (113 g) pureed banana

½ cup (122 g) canned pumpkin

½ cup (12 g) sugar substitute, such as Splenda

¼ cup (60 ml) milk

¼ cup (60 ml) canola oil

1 egg

1¾ cups (210 g) whole wheat pastry flour

2 teaspoons (9.2 g) baking powder

1 teaspoon pumpkin pie spice

Topping

½ cup (115 g) packed brown sugar substitute, such as Splenda

½ cup (40 g) rolled oats

½ teaspoon pumpkin pie spice

Puree banana in blender to make ½ cup. Mix pureed banana, pumpkin, sugar substitute, milk, oil, and egg until well blended. Combine flour, baking powder, and pumpkin pie spice. Spoon into greased muffin tins. Top each with 1 tablespoon of the topping mixture. Bake in an oven preheated to 375°F (190°C, gas mark 5) for 20 minutes or until toothpick inserted into muffin comes out clean.

Yield: 12 servings

Each with: 19 g water; 169 calories (30% from fat, 9% from protein, 62% from carb); 4 g protein; 6 g total fat; 1 g saturated fat; 3 g monounsaturated fat; 2 g polyunsaturated fat; 27 g carb; 3 g fiber; 11 g sugar; 112 mg phosphorus; 73 mg calcium; 1 mg iron; 96 mg sodium; 151 mg potassium; 1,629 IU vitamin A; 0 mg vitamin C; 18 mg cholesterol

Glycemic Index: Low

Blueberry Buttermilk Muffins

Blueberries and strawberries have both been on sale around here lately, so I decided it had been too long since I'd had fresh blueberry muffins. This one makes a big batch, so the family doesn't need to argue over the last one.

2½ cups (300 g) whole wheat pastry flour

1½ teaspoons baking powder

½ teaspoon baking soda

¾ cup (18 g) sugar substitute, such as Splenda

2 eggs

1 cup (235 ml) buttermilk

4 ounces (112 g) unsalted butter

1½ cups (120 g) blueberries

Sift dry ingredients together in a large bowl. In another bowl, whisk eggs, buttermilk, and butter that has been melted and browned slightly. Make a well in dry ingredients and pour in liquid ingredients, mixing quickly. Fold in blueberries. Spoon batter into greased muffin cups and bake at 400°F (200°C, gas mark 6) for 20 to 30 minutes until golden brown.

Yield: 24 muffins

Each with: 23 g water; 97 calories (41% from fat, 11% from protein, 48% from carb); 3 g protein; 5 g total fat; 3 g saturated fat; 1 g monounsaturated fat; 0 g polyunsaturated fat; 12 g carb; 2 g fiber; 3 g sugar; 70 mg phosphorus; 37 mg calcium; 1 mg iron; 49 mg sodium; 81 mg potassium; 150 IU vitamin A; 1 mg vitamin C; 30 mg cholesterol

Glycemic Index: Low

Pizza Snack Muffins

These are good as a snack or for those who have always wanted pizza for breakfast.

2 cups (240 g) whole wheat pastry flour

2 teaspoons baking powder

1 teaspoon basil

1 teaspoon oregano

¾ cup (175 ml) skim milk

1 egg

2 tablespoons (30 ml) olive oil

½ cup (90 g) chopped tomatoes

½ cup (75 g) finely chopped pepperoni

2¼ ounces (65 g) black olives, sliced ripe

¾ cup (90 g) shredded mozzarella cheese

In a bowl, mix flour, baking powder, basil, and oregano. Add milk, egg, and oil; stir to moisten. Add tomatoes, pepperoni, olives, and half of the cheese; mix well. Divide batter equally among 10 oiled muffin cups (2 to 2½ inches or 5 to 6 cm); top with remaining cheese. Bake in oven heated to 350°F (180°C, gas mark 4) until muffins are well browned, 30 to 35 minutes. Let stand about 5 minutes and then remove from pan. Serve warm or cool.

Yield: 12 servings

Each with: 37 g water; 138 calories (35% from fat, 17% from protein, 47% from carb); 6 g protein; 6 g total fat; 2 g saturated fat; 3 g monounsaturated fat; 1 g polyunsaturated fat; 17 g carb; 3 g fiber; 1 g sugar; 158 mg phosphorus; 147 mg calcium; 1 mg iron; 189 mg sodium; 149 mg potassium; 119 IU vitamin A; 1 mg vitamin C; 25 mg cholesterol

Glycemic Index: Low

Whole Wheat Banana Bread

Whole wheat flour has more flavor and is lower in GI the white flour. And in this case, the whole wheat taste just seems to go particularly well with the natural sweetness of the bananas.

1½ cups (180 g) whole wheat flour, divided

½ cup (43 g) coconut, unsweetened shredded.

2 teaspoons (9.2 g) baking powder

½ teaspoon baking soda

¼ teaspoon salt

1 cup (225 g) banana, mashed

2 tablespoons (30 ml) vegetable oil

2 tablespoons (42 g) honey

Mix together 1¼ cup (150 g) of flour, coconut, baking powder, baking soda, and salt in a bowl. Combine banana, oil, and honey. Stir into flour mixture quickly but gently until just combined. Add remaining ¼ cup (30 g) flour if batter is thin. Batter will be lumpy. Spread batter evenly in a lightly greased 8 x 4-inch (20 x 19 cm) loaf pan. Bake at 350°F (180°C, or gas mark 4) about 45 minutes until tester inserted in center comes out clean. Cool 10 minutes in pan. Turn out of pan and cool completely on rack.

Yield: 14 servings

Each with: 15 g water; 97 calories (27% from fat, 8% from protein, 65% from carb); 2 g Protein; 3 g total fat; 1 g saturated fat; 1 g monounsaturated fat; 1 g polyunsaturated fat; 17 g carb; 2 g fiber; 5 g sugar; 65 mg phosphorous; 44 mg calcium; 1 mg iron; 71 mg sodium; 120 mg potassium; 11 IU vitamin A; 0 mg ATE vitamin E; 1 mg vitamin C; 0 mg cholesterol

Glycemic Index: Low

Cranberry Bread

This makes a nice holiday breakfast loaf, but we like it so much that we don't wait for a holiday.

1 cup (110 g) cranberries, chopped

½ cup (55 g) pecans, chopped

1 tablespoon (6 g) grated orange peel

2 cups (240 g) whole wheat pastry flour

1 cup (25 g) sugar substitute, such as Splenda

1½ teaspoons baking powder

½ teaspoon baking soda

2 tablespoons (28 g) unsalted butter

¾ cup (175 ml) orange juice

1 egg, well beaten

TIP *You can buy fresh cranberries when they are in season and freeze them right in the bag they came in so you have them for recipes like this one.*

Preheat oven to 350°F (180°C, or gas mark 4). Generously grease and lightly flour a 9 x 5-inch (23 x 13 cm) loaf pan. Prepare cranberries, nuts, and orange peel. Set aside. In a bowl, mix together flour, sugar, baking powder, and soda. Cut in butter. Stir in orange juice, egg, and orange peel mixing just to moisten. Fold in cranberries and nuts. Spoon into prepared pan. Bake 60 minutes or until wooden pick inserted into center comes out clean. Cool on a rack 15 minutes before removing from pan.

Yield: 12 servings

Each with: 28 g water; 149 calories (35% from fat, 10% from protein, 55% from carb); 4 g Protein; 6 g total fat; 2 g saturated fat; 3 g monounsaturated fat; 1 g polyunsaturated fat; 22 g carb; 3 g fiber; 4 g sugar; 106 mg phosphorous; 50 mg calcium; 1 mg iron; 70 mg sodium; 145 mg potassium; 111 IU vitamin A; 23 mg ATE vitamin E; 7 mg vitamin C; 23 mg cholesterol

Glycemic Index: Low

Strawberry Bread

This is a fairly sweet bread and probably wouldn't suffer at all from a reduction in sugar. It did make wonderful breakfasts almost all week, though.

1½ cups (190 g) flour

1 cup (25 g) sugar substitute, such as Splenda

1 teaspoon sodium-free baking soda

1½ teaspoons cinnamon

2 eggs

½ cup (120 ml) canola oil

2 cups (340 g) sliced strawberries

Mix together dry ingredients. Mix together remaining ingredients and add to dry. Stir together. Pour into greased 9-inch (23 cm) loaf pan. Bake at 350°F (180°C, gas mark 4) for about 1 hour until knife inserted in center comes out clean. Cool 10 minutes before removing from pan.

Yield: 12 servings

Each with: 34 g water; 168 calories (51% from fat, 7% from protein, 42% from carb); 3 g protein; 10 g total fat; 1 g saturated fat; 3 g monounsaturated fat; 5 g polyunsaturated fat; 18 g carb; 1 g fiber; 5 g sugar; 36 mg phosphorus; 15 mg calcium; 1 mg iron; 19 mg sodium; 92 mg potassium; 41 IU vitamin A; 15 mg vitamin C; 0 mg cholesterol

Glycemic Index: Low

18

Desserts, Drinks, and Sweets

It's easy to find high-GI desserts. But you can limit the GI content by replacing white flour with whole wheat pastry flour and by limited the quantity you eat. Along with the cookies and cakes, we also have some good fruit desserts and a couple of tasty low-GI drinks.

Peanut Butter Cookies

The use of sugar substitutes makes these cookies good for anyone who is watching their carbo-hydrates and trying to eat a lower GI diet. And the taste is every bit as good as the regular peanut butter cookies they are patterned after.

⅓ cup (42 g) flour

¼ teaspoon baking soda

¼ teaspoon baking powder

¼ cup (55 g) unsalted butter

4 tablespoons (64 g) peanut butter

1 tablespoon (1 g) brown sugar substitute, such as Splenda

½ cup (12 g) sugar substitute, such as Splenda

1 egg, well beaten

Preheat oven to 375°F (190°C, or gas mark 5). Grease cookie sheet lightly. Sift together flour, baking soda, and baking powder. Work butter and peanut butter with spoon until creamy; gradually add brown sugar replacement and continue working until light. Add granulated sugar replacement and egg; beat well. Mix in dry ingredients thoroughly. Drop by teaspoonfuls onto cookie sheet; flatten with tines of fork in a criss-cross pattern. Bake until done, 8–10 minutes.

Yield: 18 servings

Each with: 3 g water; 62 calories (67% from fat, 9% from protein, 24% from carb); 1 g Protein; 5 g total fat; 2 g saturated fat; 2 g monounsaturated fat; 1 g polyunsaturated fat; 4 g carb; 0 g fiber; 2 g sugar; 21 mg phosphorous; 8 mg calcium; 0 mg iron; 13 mg sodium; 34 mg potassium; 97 IU vitamin A; 26 mg ATE vitamin E; 0 mg vitamin C; 18 mg cholesterol

Glycemic Index: Low

Carrot Cookies

These make a quick grab-and-go breakfast option or a tasty dessert.

1 cup (110 g) grated carrot

½ cup (115 g) fat-free plain yogurt

¼ cup (4 g) brown sugar substitute, such as Splenda

2 tablespoons (30 ml) canola oil

1 teaspoon vanilla

1½ cups (267 g) dates

1½ cups (180 g) whole wheat pastry flour

¼ cup (29 g) crunchy wheat-barley cereal, such as Grape-Nuts

½ teaspoon baking soda

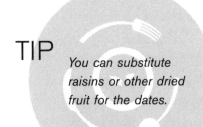

TIP

You can substitute raisins or other dried fruit for the dates.

Preheat oven to 350°F (180°C, gas mark 4). Coat baking sheets with nonstick vegetable oil spray or line with parchment paper or silicone sheets. In medium mixing bowl, stir carrot, yogurt, sugar substitute, oil, vanilla, and dates. Let stand 15 minutes. Stir in remaining dry ingredients until well blended. Drop rounded tablespoonfuls of mixture onto baking sheets, spacing 1½ inches (3½ cm) apart. Reduce to teaspoonful drops for mini-size cookies. Bake 15 minutes or until cookie top springs back when lightly touched. Cool.

Yield: 30 servings

Each with: 10 g water; 62 calories (16% from fat, 8% from protein, 76% from carb); 1 g protein; 1 g total fat; 0 g saturated fat; 1 g monounsaturated fat; 0 g polyunsaturated fat; 13 g carb; 2 g fiber; 6 g sugar; 36 mg phosphorus; 15 mg calcium; 1 mg iron; 12 mg sodium; 109 mg potassium; 733 IU vitamin A; 0 mg vitamin C; 0 mg cholesterol

Glycemic Index: Low

Orange Cookies

This is a different kind of oatmeal cookie with a nice, unexpected orange flavor.

1 cup (225 g) unsalted butter

1 cup (25 g) sugar substitute, such as Splenda

2 eggs

¼ cup (60 ml) orange juice

1 teaspoon vanilla

2 teaspoons (4 g) grated orange peel

2 cups (240 g) whole wheat pastry flour

1 teaspoon baking soda

2 cups (160 g) quick-cooking oats

1 cup (75 g) raisins

½ cup (55 g) chopped pecans

Cream butter and sugar substitute until light. Beat in eggs, juice, vanilla, and orange peel. Add dry ingredients and mix well. Stir in by hand the oats, raisins, and nuts. Drop by rounded teaspoonfuls on greased baking sheet. Bake at 375°F (190°C, gas mark 5) for 10 to 15 minutes.

Yield: 42 servings

Each with: 6 g water; 102 calories (50% from fat, 8% from protein, 42% from carb); 2 g protein; 6 g total fat; 3 g saturated fat; 2 g monounsaturated fat; 1 g polyunsaturated fat; 11 g carb; 1 g fiber; 3 g sugar; 52 mg phosphorus; 10 mg calcium; 1 mg iron; 5 mg sodium; 79 mg potassium; 151 IU vitamin A; 1 mg vitamin C; 23 mg cholesterol

Glycemic Index: Low

Fudge Brownies

Yes, you can have brownies. This quick brownie recipe gets a fiber and nutrition boost from the whole wheat flour.

1 cup (225 g) unsalted butter

½ cup (40 g) cocoa powder

2 cups (50 g) sugar substitute, such as Splenda

4 eggs

2 teaspoons (10 ml) vanilla

1 cup (120 g) whole wheat pastry flour

Heat oven to 350°F (180°C, gas mark 4). In microwave, melt butter and cocoa together, stirring once or twice. When melted, add sugar substitute, eggs, and vanilla. Stir to mix well and then add flour. Pour into greased 13 × 9-inch (33 × 23 cm) pan. Bake 25 minutes.

Yield: 18 servings

Each with: 13 g water; 155 calories (66% from fat, 7% from protein, 27% from carb); 3 g protein; 12 g total fat; 7 g saturated fat; 3 g monounsaturated fat; 1 g polyunsaturated fat; 11 g carb; 2 g fiber; 4 g sugar; 67 mg phosphorus; 15 mg calcium; 1 mg iron; 20 mg sodium; 84 mg potassium; 376 IU vitamin A; 0 mg vitamin C; 80 mg cholesterol

Glycemic Index: Low

Apple Cake

Everyone wants something sweet every once in a while. But that doesn't mean that it still can't still be good for you. Whole wheat flour and apples bump up the nutrition and fiber levels of this cake, but the taste just says "good."

2¼ cups (250 g) whole wheat pastry flour

1 cup (25 g) sugar substitute, such as Splenda

¾ cup (12 g) brown sugar substitute, such as Splenda

1 tablespoon (7 g) cinnamon

2 teaspoons baking powder

½ teaspoon baking soda

¾ cup (175 ml) canola oil

1 teaspoon vanilla

3 eggs

2 cups (250 g) finely chopped apple

1 cup (120 g) chopped walnuts

¼ cup (25 g) powdered sugar, sifted

Generously grease and flour a 10-inch (25 cm) fluted tube pan; set aside. In a large mixing bowl, combine the flour, sugar substitutes, cinnamon, baking powder, and baking soda. Add oil, vanilla, and the eggs; beat until well mixed. Stir in the chopped apple and walnuts. Spoon batter evenly into prepared pan. Bake in an oven heated to 350°F (180°C, gas mark 4) for 45 to 50 minutes or until cake tests done. Cool in pan 12 minutes; invert cake onto a wire rack. Cool thoroughly. Sprinkle with powdered sugar.

Yield: 16 servings

Each with: 23 g water; 246 calories (58% from fat, 9% from protein, 34% from carb); 6 g protein; 17 g total fat; 1 g saturated fat; 8 g monounsaturated fat; 6 g polyunsaturated fat; 22 g carb; 3 g fiber; 8 g sugar; 133 mg phosphorus; 56 mg calcium; 1 mg iron; 77 mg sodium; 139 mg potassium; 62 IU vitamin A; 1 mg vitamin C; 44 mg cholesterol

Glycemic Index: Low

Chocolate Carrot Cake

Carrots and whole wheat flour boost the nutrition levels of this tasty cake, while the use of sugar substitute helps to keep the GI value low.

1½ cups (165 g) carrot, grated

¾ cup (18 g) sugar substitute, such as Splenda

½ cup (120 ml) canola oil

1 cup (235 ml) water, boiling

1½ cups (180 g) whole wheat flour

½ cup (90 g) cocoa powder, unsweetened

1 teaspoon cinnamon

1½ teaspoons baking powder

Preheat oven to 350°F (180°C, or gas mark 4). In a large bowl, combine carrots, sugar, and oil. Pour water over the mixture. In a separate bowl, combine the rest of the ingredients. Add to the carrot mixture and mix well. Pour into a nonstick or lightly oiled 8 x 8-inch (20 x 20 cm) pan. Bake for 35 minutes.

Yield: 6 servings

Each with: 72 g water; 317 calories (53% from fat, 7% from protein, 40% from carb); 6 g Protein; 20 g total fat; 2 g saturated fat; 11 g monounsaturated fat; 6 g polyunsaturated fat; 35 g carb; 7 g fiber; 7 g sugar; 193 mg phosphorous; 103 mg calcium; 3 mg iron; 148 mg sodium; 336 mg potassium; 5383 IU vitamin A; 0 mg ATE vitamin E; 2 mg vitamin C; 0 mg cholesterol

Glycemic Index: Low

Banana Cake

A couple of past-their-prime bananas that needed to be used up and a bit of a sweet tooth resulted in this recipe.

1 teaspoon vinegar

½ cup (120 ml) skim milk

¾ cup (165 g) unsalted butter

1½ cups (37 g) sugar substitute, such as Splenda

2 eggs

1 teaspoon vanilla extract

1 cup (225 g) mashed bananas

2 cups (240 g) whole wheat pastry flour

1 teaspoon baking powder

Powdered sugar for dusting (optional)

Mix vinegar into milk and let stand 5 minutes to sour. Cream butter and sugar together. Add eggs, milk mixture, vanilla, and bananas. Mix until smooth. Stir together flour and baking powder. Add to creamed mix and mix well. Pour into a greased 9 × 13-inch (23 × 33 cm) baking pan. Bake at 350°F (180°C, gas mark 4) until done, about 35 to 40 minutes. Sprinkle with powdered sugar if desired.

Yield: 24 servings

Each with: 18 g water; 112 calories (50% from fat, 8% from protein, 43% from carb); 2 g protein; 6 g total fat; 4 g saturated fat; 2 g monounsaturated fat; 0 g polyunsaturated fat; 12 g carb; 1 g fiber; 4 g sugar; 57 mg phosphorus; 27 mg calcium; 1 mg iron; 31 mg sodium; 92 mg potassium; 217 IU vitamin A; 1 mg vitamin C; 35 mg cholesterol

Glycemic Index: Low

Lite Lemon Cheesecake

Do you think that you can't have cheesecake on your low GI diet? Think again. This cheesecake is full of flavor but not full of carbs or fat, so it works for just about anyone.

⅓ cup (40 g) graham cracker crumbs

1 small box sugar-free lemon gelatin

⅔ cup (160 ml) water, boiling

1 cup (225 g) fat-free cottage cheese

8 ounces (225 g) fat-free cream cheese

2 cups (150 g) whipped topping, like Cool Whip

Spray 8- or 9-inch (20 x 23 cm) springform pan or 9-inch (23 cm) pie plate lightly with nonstick cooking spray. Sprinkle with graham cracker crumbs. Completely dissolve gelatin in boiling water; pour into blender container. Add cottage cheese and cream cheese; cover. Blend at medium speed, scraping down sides occasionally, about 2 minutes or until mixture is completely smooth. Pour into large bowl. Gently stir in whipped topping. Pour into prepared pan; smooth top. Chill until set, about 4 hours.

Yield: 8 servings

Each with: 70 g water; 141 calories (57% from fat, 21% from protein, 22% from carb); 7 g Protein; 9 g total fat; 5 g saturated fat; 3 g monounsaturated fat; 0 g polyunsaturated fat; 8 g carb; 0 g fiber; 3 g sugar; 107 mg phosphorous; 66 mg calcium; 1 mg iron; 247 mg sodium; 99 mg potassium; 307 IU vitamin A; 82 mg ATE vitamin E; 0 mg vitamin C; 28 mg cholesterol

Glycemic Index: Low

Easy Apple Pie

The microwave preparation makes this especially quick and easy.

½ cup (60 g) crushed graham crackers

5 apples, cored and peeled

½ teaspoon cinnamon

¼ teaspoon allspice

¼ cup (35 g) raisins

⅓ cup (80 ml) apple juice

Coat a microwave-safe pie plate with nonstick vegetable oil spray. Spread the cracker crumbs in the plate. Cover with apple slices. Sprinkle with spices. Sprinkle raisins over top. Pour juice over. Cover and microwave for 15 minutes.

Yield: 6 servings

Each with: 106 g water; 108 calories (7% from fat, 3% from protein, 90% from carb); 1 g protein; 1 g total fat; 0 g saturated fat; 0 g monounsaturated fat; 0 g polyunsaturated fat; 26 g carb; 2 g fiber; 18 g sugar; 27 mg phosphorus; 14 mg calcium; 1 mg iron; 44 mg sodium; 175 mg potassium; 42 IU vitamin A; 5 mg vitamin C; 0 mg cholesterol

Glycemic Index: Low

Grilled Fruit

We never seem to eat as much fruit as we should. This recipe makes it easy to get people to eat more. It's a great choice for dessert if you already are using the grill for the main course, but it's also worth firing up the grill just for dessert.

1 apple

1 pear

1 banana

⅓ cup (75 g) unsalted butter, melted

3 tablespoons (3 g) brown sugar substitute, such as Splenda

1 teaspoon ground cinnamon

½ teaspoon ground ginger

Cut the fruit in half or wedges. Do not peel. Banana should be cut lengthwise, then in half. Remove cores. Combine butter, brown sugar, and spices. Baste fruit with mixture. Place fruit on grill with skin up. Grill on medium 8 to 10 minutes for halves, 4 to 5 minutes for smaller wedges.

Yield: 6 servings

Each with: 95 g water; 182 calories (49% from fat, 2% from protein, 49% from carb); 1 g Protein; 11 g total fat; 7 g saturated fat; 3 g monounsaturated fat; 0 g polyunsaturated fat; 24 g carb; 3 g fiber; 14 g sugar; 25 mg phosphorous; 13 mg calcium; 0 mg iron; 2 mg sodium; 319 mg potassium; 373 IU vitamin A; 85 mg ATE vitamin E; 8 mg vitamin C; 27 mg cholesterol

Glycemic Index: Low

Jellied Sangria

This makes a dessert fancy enough for any celebration or company meal, but it's easy and tasty enough that you won't want to wait for that special occasion.

1½ cups (355 g) dry white wine

2½ cups (570 ml) club soda, cold

1 tablespoon (15 ml) lime juice

1 large sugar-free lemon gelatin

1 cup (170 g) strawberries, sliced

1 cup (150 g) red grapes, sliced

1 cup (150 g) green grapes, sliced

Bring wine to a boil in small saucepan. Completely dissolve gelatin in the boiling wine; pour into medium bowl. Stir in club soda and lime juice. Place bowl in a larger bowl of ice and water; let stand about 10 minutes until slightly thickened, stirring occasionally. Stir in fruit. Pour into 6-cup (1.4 L) mold which has been sprayed with nonstick cooking spray. Chill until firm, about 4 hours. Unmold.

Yield: 12 servings

Each with: 100 g water; 40 calories (4% from fat, 5% from protein, 91% from carb); 0 g Protein; 0 g total fat; 0 g saturated fat; 0 g monounsaturated fat; 0 g polyunsaturated fat; 5 g carb; 0 g fiber; 3 g sugar; 17 mg phosphorous; 10 mg calcium; 0 mg iron; 17 mg sodium; 72 mg potassium; 17 IU vitamin A; 0 mg ATE vitamin E; 8 mg vitamin C; 0 mg cholesterol

Glycemic Index: Low

Creamy Yogurt Cups

Yogurt adds a creaminess to this low fat, low carb dessert. It's perfect for those times when you just want a little something sweet.

1 small box sugar-free gelatin, any flavor

¾ cup (175 ml) water, boiling

ice cubes

8 ounces (225 g) vanilla yogurt

½ teaspoon vanilla extract

Completely dissolve gelatin in boiling water. Combine cold water and enough ice cubes to measure 1 cup (235 ml). Add to gelatin; stir until slightly thickened. Remove any unmelted ice. Stir in yogurt and vanilla. Pour into 5 individual dishes. Chill until set, about 30 minutes. Garnish if desired.

Yield: 5 servings

Each with: 72 g water; 42 calories (12% from fat, 22% from protein, 66% from carb); 2 g Protein; 1 g total fat; 0 g saturated fat; 0 g monounsaturated fat; 0 g polyunsaturated fat; 7 g carb; 0 g fiber; 6 g sugar; 78 mg phosphorous; 79 mg calcium; 0 mg iron; 42 mg sodium; 101 mg potassium; 20 IU vitamin A; 5 mg ATE vitamin E; 0 mg vitamin C; 2 mg cholesterol

Glycemic Index: Low

Baked Apples

This simple baked apple recipe contains no added sugar, letting the flavor of the apples come through.

4 apples

¼ cup (36 g) raisins

½ cup (120 ml) apple juice, unsweetened

Preheat oven to 375°F (190°C, or gas mark 5). Wash and core apples. Pare a strip from top of each apple. Put tablespoon (9 g) of raisins in each apple. Pour apple juice over apples. Bake 40 minutes or until done. Baste apples with juice during cooking. Serve warm or chilled.

Yield: 4 servings

Each with: 139 g water; 106 calories (2% from fat, 2% from protein, 96% from carb); 1 g Protein; 0 g total fat; 0 g saturated fat; 0 g monounsaturated fat; 0 g polyunsaturated fat; 28 g carb; 2 g fiber; 22 g sugar; 27 mg phosphorous; 13 mg calcium; 0 mg iron; 3 mg sodium; 230 mg potassium; 49 IU vitamin A; 0 mg ATE vitamin E; 6 mg vitamin C; 0 mg cholesterol

Glycemic Index: Low

Frozen Cherry Dessert

This frozen dessert makes a great low GI alternative to ice cream.

8 ounces (225 g) sweet cherries, undrained, pitted

1 small box sugar-free gelatin, cherry flavor

1 cup (235 g) water, boiling

8 ounces plain fat-free yogurt

2 cups (150 g) whipped topping, like Cool Whip

Line bottom and sides of 9 x 5-inch (23 x 13 cm) loaf pan with plastic wrap; set aside. Drain cherries, reserving syrup. If necessary, add enough cold water to reserved syrup to measure ½ cup (120 ml). Cut cherries into quarters. Completely dissolve gelatin in boiling water. Add measured syrup. Stir in yogurt until well blended. Chill until mixture is thickened but not set, about 45 minutes to 1 hour, stirring occasionally. Gently stir in cherries and whipped topping. Pour into prepared pan; cover. Freeze until firm, about 6 hours or overnight. Remove pan from freezer about 15 minutes before serving. Let stand at room temperature to soften slightly. Remove plastic wrap. Cut into slices. Cover and store leftovers in freezer.

Yield: 12 servings

Each with: 58 g water; 46 calories (42% from fat, 13% from protein, 44% from carb); 2 g Protein; 2 g total fat; 1 g saturated fat; 1 g monounsaturated fat; 0 g polyunsaturated fat; 5 g carb; 0 g fiber; 4 g sugar; 48 mg phosphorous; 50 mg calcium; 0 mg iron; 33 mg sodium; 88 mg potassium; 100 IU vitamin A; 19 mg ATE vitamin E; 1 mg vitamin C; 8 mg cholesterol

Glycemic Index: Low

Pineapple Kabobs

Try these sweet grilled pineapple wedges with grilled ham or pork chops or serve as dessert.

¼ cup (85 g) honey

2 tablespoons (28 g) unsalted butter

1 teaspoon cinnamon

1 pineapple

Combine honey, butter, and cinnamon. Pare and cut fresh pineapple into long wedges. Grill over medium heat 15 minutes, basting with sauce. Turn frequently.

Yield: 4 servings

Each with: 15 g water; 123 calories (40% from fat, 1% from protein, 60% from carb); 0 g protein; 6 g total fat; 4 g saturated fat; 1 g monounsaturated fat; 0 g polyunsaturated fat; 20 g carb; 1 g fiber; 19 g sugar; 4 mg phosphorus; 12 mg calcium; 0 mg iron; 2 mg sodium; 28 mg potassium; 183 IU vitamin A; 1 mg vitamin C; 15 mg cholesterol

Glycemic Index: Low

Mocha Spread

You can use this on the muffins or as a not-too-sweet frosting for cakes.

4 ounces (115 g) cream cheese

1 tablespoon (13 g) sugar substitute, such as Splenda

½ teaspoon instant coffee granules

½ teaspoon vanilla

¼ cup (44 g) miniature chocolate chips

Combine ingredients in a food processor or blender. Cover and process until well blended.

Yield: 12 servings

Each with: 5 g water; 54 calories (69% from fat, 6% from protein, 25% from carb); 1 g protein; 4 g total fat; 3 g saturated fat; 1 g monounsaturated fat; 0 g polyunsaturated fat; 4 g carb; 0 g fiber; 3 g sugar; 15 mg phosphorus; 9 mg calcium; 0 mg iron; 28 mg sodium; 26 mg potassium; 127 IU vitamin A; 0 mg vitamin C; 10 mg cholesterol

Glycemic Index: Low

Cappuccino Mousse

This is great for those times when you want a fancy dessert that no one knows has a low-GI rating.

3 cups (705 ml) 1 percent milk

1 sugar-free chocolate pudding mix

6 teaspoons (11 g) decaffeinated instant coffee

½ teaspoon cinnamon

2 cups (150 g) fat-free whipped topping

Pour milk into 5-quart (5 L) mixer bowl. Add pudding mix, instant coffee, and cinnamon. Blend by hand with a wire whip, scraping the sides of bowl to moisten completely. Whip at medium speed with electric mixer for 3 minutes or until pudding is smooth and creamy. Fold in whipped topping. Immediately portion ½ cup into stemmed glasses or coffee mugs. Chill at least 1 hour. Keep refrigerated.

Yield: 10 servings

Each with: 74 g water; 117 calories (36% from fat, 10% from protein, 54% from carb); 3 g protein; 5 g total fat; 4 g saturated fat; 1 g monounsaturated fat; 0 g polyunsaturated fat; 16 g carb; 0 g fiber; 12 g sugar; 165 mg phosphorus; 91 mg calcium; 0 mg iron; 178 mg sodium; 156 mg potassium; 165 IU vitamin A; 0 mg vitamin C; 4 mg cholesterol

Glycemic Index: Low

Lime Fizz

If you are looking for something cool and refreshing to drink, give this a try. You can also use lemon juice to make a lemon fizz. Adjust the amount of juice and sweetener to your own taste.

2 tablespoons (30 ml) lime juice

2 teaspoons sugar substitute, such as Splenda

¼ cup (60 ml) water

1 cup (235 ml) seltzer water

Combine juice, artificial sweetener, and water in a tall glass. Stir until dissolved. Add ice. Fill glass with seltzer.

Yield: 1 serving

Each with: 324 g water; 41 calories (1% from fat, 1% from protein, 98% from carb); 0 g protein; 0 g total fat; 0 g saturated fat; 0 g monounsaturated fat; 0 g polyunsaturated fat; 11 g carb; 0 g fiber; 9 g sugar; 37 mg calcium; 0 mg iron; 4 mg sodium; 34 mg potassium; 15 IU vitamin A; 9 mg vitamin C; 0 mg cholesterol

Glycemic Index: Low

Lemonade

When the weather is hot, a tall cold glass of lemonade sure tastes good. Fresh-squeezed lemon juice is best, but you can still get good lemonade using bottled juice.

½ cup (100 g) sugar substitute, such as Splenda

1½ cups (355 ml) lemon juice

5 quarts (5 L) water

Heat sugar and lemon juice just until sugar dissolves. Add to water. Stir and serve over ice.

Yield: 20 servings

Each with: 253 g water; 24 calories (0% from fat, 1% from protein, 99% from carb); 0 g protein; 0 g total fat; 0 g saturated fat; 0 g monounsaturated fat; 0 g polyunsaturated fat; 7 g carb; 0 g fiber; 5 g sugar; 1 mg phosphorus; 8 mg calcium; 0 mg iron; 7 mg sodium; 25 mg potassium; 3 IU vitamin A; 8 mg vitamin C; 0 mg cholesterol

Glycemic Index: Low

Fruit Slush

This is sort of like sherbet but without as much preparation effort. This works either as a dessert or just a cooling snack on a hot day.

6 ounces (170 g) lemonade concentrate undiluted

6 ounces (170 g) orange juice concentrate undiluted

½ cup (12 g) sugar substitute, such as Splenda

16 ounces (475 g) lemon-lime carbonated beverage

15 ounces (425 g) crushed pineapple, drained

14 ounces (400 g) fruit cocktail

2 cups banana, sliced

Mix by hand. Freeze. Let thaw 10 minutes before serving. Stir to make slush.

Yield: 6 servings

Each with: 274 g water; 274 calories (1% from fat, 3% from protein, 96% from carb); 2 g Protein; 0 g total fat; 0 g saturated fat; 0 g monounsaturated fat; 0 g polyunsaturated fat; 70 g carb; 3 g fiber; 60 g sugar; 49 mg phosphorous; 32 mg calcium; 1 mg iron; 14 mg sodium; 617 mg potassium; 386 IU vitamin A; 0 mg ATE vitamin E; 58 mg vitamin C; 0 mg cholesterol

Glycemic Index: Low

19

Cooking Terms, Weights and Measurements, and Gadgets

Cooking Terms

Are you confused about a term I used in one of the recipes? Take a look at the list here and see if there might be an explanation. I've tried to include anything that I thought might raise a question.

Al Dente

"To the tooth," in Italian—The pasta is cooked just enough to maintain a firm, chewy texture.

Bake

To cook in the oven—Food is cooked slowly with gentle heat, concentrating the flavor.

Baste

To brush or spoon liquid, fat, or juices over meat during roasting to add flavor and to prevent it from drying out

Beat

To smoothen a mixture by briskly whipping or stirring it with a spoon, fork, wire whisk, rotary beater, or electric mixer

Blend

To mix or fold two or more ingredients together to obtain equal distribution throughout the mixture

Boil

To cook food in heated water or other liquid that is bubbling vigorously

Braise

A cooking technique that requires browning meat in oil or other fat and then cooking slowly in liquid—The effect of braising is to tenderize the meat

Bread

To coat the food with crumbs (usually with soft or dry bread crumbs), sometimes seasoned

Broil

To cook food directly under the heat source

Broth or Stock

A flavorful liquid made by gently cooking meat, seafood, or vegetables (and/or their by-products, such as bones and trimming) often with herbs and vegetables, in liquid, usually water

Brown

A quick sautéing, pan/oven broiling, or grilling done either at the beginning or end of meal preparation, often to enhance flavor, texture, or eye appeal

Brush

Using a pastry brush to coat a food such as meat or bread with melted butter, glaze, or other liquid

Chop

To cut into irregular pieces

Coat

To evenly cover food with flour, crumbs, or a batter

Core

To remove the inedible center of fruits such as pineapples

Cream

To beat butteror margarine, with or without sugar, until light and fluffy—This process traps in air bubbles, later used to create height in cookies and cakes.

Cut In

To work margarine or butter into dry ingredients

Dash

A measure approximately equal to $1/16$ teaspoon

Deep Fry

To completely submerge the food in hot oil—It's a quick way to cook some food and as a result, this method often seems to seal in the flavors of food better than any other technique.

Dice

To cut into cubes

Direct Heat

Heat waves radiate from a source and travel directly to the item being heated with no conductor between them. Examples are grilling, broiling, and toasting.

Dredge

To coat lightly and evenly with sugar or flour

Dumpling

A batter or soft dough, which is formed into small mounds that are then steamed, poached, or simmered

Dust

To sprinkle food lightly with spices, sugar, or flour for a light coating

Fold

To cut and mix lightly with a spoon to keep as much air in the mixture as possible

Fritter

Sweet or savory foods coated or mixed into batter, then deep-fried

Glaze

A liquid that gives an item a shiny surface—Examples are fruit jams that have been heated or chocolate that has been thinned.

Grease

To coat a pan or skillet with a thin layer of oil

Grill

To cook over the heat source (traditionally over wood coals) in the open air

Grind

To mechanically cut a food into small pieces

Hull

To remove the leafy parts of soft fruits such as strawberries or blackberries

Knead

To work dough with the heels of your hands in a pressing and folding motion until it becomes smooth and elastic

Marinate

To combine food with aromatic ingredients to add flavor

Mince

To chop food into tiny, irregular pieces

Mix

To beat or stir two or more foods together until they are thoroughly combined

Panfry

To cook in a hot pan with small amount of hot oil, butter, or other fat, turning the food over once or twice

Poach

To simmer in a liquid

Pot Roast

A large piece of meat, usually browned in fat, cooked in a covered pan

Puree

Food that has been mashed or sieved

Reduce

To cook liquids down so that some of the water they contain evaporates

Roast

To cook uncovered in the oven

Sauté

To cook with a small amount of hot oil, butter, or other fat, tossing the food around over high heat

Sear

To brown a food quickly on all sides using high heat to seal in the juices

Shred

To cut into fine strips

Simmer

To cook slowly in a liquid over low heat

Skim

To remove the surface layer (of impurities, scum, or fat) from liquids such as stocks and jams while cooking—This is usually done with a flat slotted spoon.

Smoke

To expose foods to wood smoke to enhance their flavor and help preserve and/or evenly cook them

Steam

To cook in steam by suspending foods over boiling water in a steamer or covered pot

Stew

To cook food in liquid for a long time until tender, usually in a covered pot

Stir

To mix ingredients with a utensil

Stir-fry

To cook quickly over high heat with a small amount of oil by constantly stirring—This technique often employs a wok.

Toss

To mix ingredients lightly by lifting and dropping them using two utensils

Whip

To beat an item to incorporate air, augment volume, and add substance

Zest

The thin, brightly colored outer part of the rind of citrus fruits—It contains volatile oils, used as a flavoring.

Weights and Measurements

First of all, here is a quick refresher on measurements.

3 teaspoons = 1 tablespoon

2 tablespoons = 1 fluid ounce

4 tablespoons = 2 fluid ounces = ¼ cup

5⅓ tablespoons = 16 teaspoons = ⅓ cup

8 tablespoons = 4 fluid ounces = ½ cup

16 tablespoons = 8 fluid ounces = 1 cup

2 cups = 1 pint

4 cups = 2 pints = 1 quart

16 cups = 8 pints = 4 quarts = 1 gallon

Metric Conversions

The information below is intended to be helpful to those readers who use the metric system of weights and measures.

Measurements of Liquid Volume
The following measures are approximate, but they're close enough for most, if not all, of the recipes in this book.

1 quart = 1 liter

1 cup = 235 milliliters

¾ cup = 175 milliliters

½ cup = 120 milliliters

⅓ cup = 80 milliliters

¼ cup = 60 milliliters

1 fluid ounce = 30 milliliters

1 tablespoon = 15 milliliters

1 teaspoon = 5 milliliters

Measurements of Weight
Much of the world measures dry ingredients by weight, rather than volume as is done in the United States. There is no easy conversion for this, as each item is different. However the following conversions may be useful.

1 ounce = 28.4 grams

1 pound = 454 grams (about half a kilo)

Oven Temperatures

Finally, we come to one that is relatively straightforward, the Fahrenheit to Celsius conversion.

100°F = 38°C
150°F = 66°C
200°F = 95°C
225°F = 110°C
250°F = 120°C
275°F = 140°C
300°F = 150°C
325°F = 165°C
350°F = 180°C
375°F = 190°C
400°F = 205°C
425°F = 220°C
450°F = 230°C
475°F = 240°C
500°F = 260°C

Gadgets I Use

The following are some of the tools that I use in cooking. Some are used very often and some very seldom, but all help make things a little easier or quicker. Why are some things here and others not? No reason except that most of these are things I considered a little less standard than a stove, oven, grill, and mixer.

Blender

Okay, so everyone has a blender. And it's a handy little tool for blending and pureeing things.

Bread Machine

A bread machine can reduce the amount of effort required to make your own bread to a manageable level. It takes at most 10 minutes to load it and turn it on. You can even set it on a timer to have your house filled with the aroma of fresh bread when you come home.

Canning Kettle

If you are planning on making batches of things like pickles and salsa in volume so you don't have to go through the process every couple of weeks, then you are going to need a way to preserve things. Most items can be frozen, of course, if that is your preference. But some things just seem to me to work better in jars. What you need is a kettle big enough to make sure the jars can be covered by water when being processed in a boiling water bath. There are also racks to sit the jars in and special tongs to make lifting them in and out of the water easier. I've had a porcelain covered kettle I use for this for a lot of years, and it also doubled as a stockpot before I got the one described below. It's better for canning than for soup because the relatively thin walls allow the water to heat faster (and the soup to burn).

Deep Fryer

Obviously, if you are watching your fat intake, this should not be one of your most often-used appliances. I don't use it nearly as often as I used to, but it still occupies a place in the appliance garage in the corner of the kitchen counter. It's a Fry Daddy, big enough to cook a batch of fries or fish for three or four people at a time.

Food Processor

I'm a real latecomer to the food processor world. It always seemed like a nice thing to have, but something I could easily do without. I use it now all the time to grind bread into crumbs or chop the peppers and onions that seem to go into at least three meals a week. It's a low-end model that doesn't have the power to grind meat and some of the heavier tasks, but I've discovered it's a real time-saver for a number of things.

Contact Grill

The George Foreman models are the most popular example of this item. I much prefer the way it does burgers or steak when it's too cold to grill them outside. And the design allows the fat to drain away, giving you a healthier, lower-fat meal.

Grinder

MANY years ago we bought an Oster Kitchen Center. It was one of those all-in-one things that included a stand mixer, blender (the one we still use), food chopper, and a grinder attachment. The grinder was never a big deal that got any use until I started experimenting with sausage recipes. Since then I've discovered that grinding your own meat can save you both money and fat.

Buying a beef or pork roast on sale, trimming it of most fat, and grinding it yourself can give you hamburger or sausage meat that is well over 90 percent lean and still less expensive than the fattier stuff you buy at the store. So now the grinder gets fairly regular use.

Pasta Maker

I bought this toy after seeing it on a Sunday morning TV infomercial. It's a genuine Ronco/Popiel "As Seen On TV" special, but try not to hold that against it. Unlike the pasta cutters that merely slice rolled dough into flat noodles, this one mixes the whole mess are then extrudes it through dies with various-shaped holes in them. The recipes say you can use any kind of flour, but I've found that buying the semolina flour that is traditionally used for pasta gives you dough that's easier to work with, as well as better texture and flavor. The characterization of it as a "toy" is pretty accurate. There aren't really any nutritional advantages over store-bought pasta. If you buy the semolina, the cost is probably about the same as some of the more expensive imported pasta. But it's fun to play with, makes a great conversation piece, and the pasta tastes good.

Salad Shooter

We seem to end up with a lot of these gadgets, don't we? This is another one that's been around for a while, but it's still my favorite implement for shredding potatoes for hash browns or cabbage for coleslaw.

Sausage Stuffer

This is really an addition to the Kitchen Center grinder. I found it at an online appliance repair site. It is really just a series of different-size tubes that fit on the end of the grinder to stuff your ground meat into casings. I do this occasionally to make link sausage, but most of the time I just make patties or bulk sausage.

Slicer

This was a closeout floor model that I bought years ago. Before going on the low-sodium diet I used to buy deli meat in bulk and slice it myself. Now it's most often used to slice a roast or smoked piece of meat for sandwiches.

Slow Cooker

I've tried to avoid calling it a Crock-Pot, which is a trademark of Rival. Anyway, whatever the brand, no kitchen should be without one.

Smoker

This was another pre-diet purchase that has been used even more since. I started with a Brinkman that originally used charcoal. Then I bought an add-on electric heat source for it that works a lot better in cold weather. Last year the family gave me a fancy MasterChef electric one that seals like an oven and has a thermostat to hold the temperature. Not only do I like the way it does ribs and other traditional smoked foods, but we also use it fairly regularly to smoke a beef or pork roast or turkey breast to use for sandwiches.

Springform Pan

This is a round, straight-sided pan. The sides are formed into a hoop that can be unclasped and detached from its base.

Steamer (Rice Cooker)

I use this primarily for cooking rice, but it's really a Black and Decker Handy Steamer Plus that does a great job steaming vegetables too. For those of you who have trouble making rice like me should consider getting one of these or one of the Japanese-style rice cookers.

Stockpot

The key here is to spend the extra money to get a heavy-gauge one (another thing I eventually learned from personal experience.). The lighter-weight ones not only will dent and not sit level on the stove, but they will burn just about everything you put in them. Mine also has a heavy glass lid that seals the moisture in well.

Turbocookers

This was another infomercial sale. It is a large dome-lidded fry pan with racks that fit inside it. You can buy them at many stores too, but mine is the "Plus" model that has two steamer racks and a timer. It really will cook a whole dinner quickly, "steam frying" the main course and steaming one or two more items. The only bad news is most of the recipes involve additions and changes every few minutes, so even if you only take a half hour to make dinner, you spend that whole time at the stove.

Wok

This is a round-bottomed pan popular in Asian cooking.

Index